Microiontophoresis and Pressure Ejection

IBRO HANDBOOK SERIES:
METHODS IN THE NEUROSCIENCES

General Editor: **A. D. Smith**
Department of Pharmacology
University of Oxford

Volume 1: **Tracing Neural Connections with Horseradish Peroxidase**
Edited by M-Marsel Mesulam
0 471 10028 5   267 pages   (cloth)   1982
0 471 10029 3   267 pages   (paper)   1982

Volume 2: **Brain Microdissection Techniques**
Edited by A. C. Cuello
0 471 10523 6   196 pages   (cloth)   1983
0 471 90019 2   196 pages   (paper)   1983

Volume 3: **Immunohistochemistry**
Edited by A. C. Cuello
0 471 10245 8   518 pages   (cloth)   1983
0 471 90052 4   518 pages   (paper)   1983

Volume 4: **Methods for Neuronal Recording in Conscious Animals**
R. Lemon
0 471 90174 1   174 pages   (cloth)   1983
0 471 90237 3   174 pages   (paper)   1983

Volume 5: **Intracellular Perfusion of Excitable Cells**
Edited by P. G. Kostyuk and O. A. Krishtal
0 471 90379 5   145 pages   (cloth)   1984
0 471 90392 2   145 pages   (paper)   1984

Volume 6: **Measurement of Neurotransmitter Release** *In Vivo*
Edited by C. A. Marsden
0 471 90444 9   244 pages   (cloth)   1984
0 471 90445 7   244 pages   (paper)   1984

Volume 7: **Molecular Biology Approach to the Neurosciences**
Edited by H. Soreq
0 471 90386 8   264 pages   (cloth)   1984
0 471 90437 6   264 pages   (paper)   1984

Volume 8: **Microiontophoresis and Pressure Ejection**
T. W. Stone

Microiontophoresis and Pressure Ejection

T. W. STONE
Reader in Neurosciences
University of London

A Wiley–Interscience Publication

JOHN WILEY & SONS
Chichester · New York · Brisbane · Toronto · Singapore

Copyright © 1985 The International Brain Research Organization

All rights reserved.

No part of this book may be reproduced by any means, nor transmitted, nor translated into a machine language without the written permission of the publisher

Library of Congress Cataloging in Publication Data:
Stone, T. W.
   Microiontophoresis and pressure ejection.
   (IBRO handbook series. Methods in the neurosciences; v.8)
   'A Wiley–Intersciences publication.'
   Bibliography: p.
   Includes index.
   1. Action potentials (Electrophysiology)   2. Iontopophoresis.
3. Microinjections.   4. Neurotransmitters.
I. Title.   II. Series.
QP363.S786   1985   599'.0188   84-17361

   ISBN 0 471 90607 7
   ISBN 0 471 90608 5 (pbk.)

British Library Cataloguing in Publication Data:
Stone, T. W.
   Microiontophoresis and pressure ejection. —
   (IBRO handbook series. Methods in the neurosciences; v.8)
   1. Brain — Research   2. Iontophoresis
   I. Title   II. Series
   599.01'88   QP376

   ISBN 0 471 90607 7
   ISBN 0 471 90608 5 Pbk

Phototypeset by Dobbie Typesetting Service, Plymouth, Devon
Printed by St Edmundsbury Press, Bury St Edmunds, Suffolk

Contents

Series Preface	vii
Preface	ix
1. Historical Introduction and Underlying Principles	1
2. Electrode Assemblies for Microiontophoresis and Pressure Ejection	6
3. Equipment	23
4. The Release of Compounds from Micropipettes and the Tissue Concentrations Achieved	39
5. Analysis of Results	76
6. Limitations and Problems of Interpretation	104
7. Practical Applications: An Introduction to the Microiontophoretic Literature	133
8. The Ejection of Dyes and Other Markers	181
References	185
Addresses of Manufacturers	210
Subject Index	211

Preface for IBRO Handbook Series

During the last 50 years there have been two changes in the way in which scientists have studied the nervous system. First of all, the traditional and largely independent major scientific disciplines of physics, chemistry, physiology, pharmacology, and pathology gave rise to the more specialized subdisciplines of neurophysiology, neurochemistry, neuropharmacology, etc., and the science of experimental psychology was born. Then, after about another generation, it became clear that a deeper understanding of the brain could not be achieved by separate and unrelated studies in each of these subdisciplines. Rather, a unified approach was needed in which the specialized methods were applied in a coordinated way to solve a particular problem. Indeed, combinations of methods could often yield results not obtainable by the application of any individual technique. Thus, scientists studying the nervous system began to call themselves neurobiologists or neuroscientists because they did not wish to be identified with any particular experimental discipline. Very soon metings took place (e.g. in 1955 the First International Meeting of Neurobiologists) and organizations (Neuroscience Research Program, MIT) were founded to give formal recognition of this new approach to the study of the brain. In 1958 the decision was taken in Moscow to establish the International Brain Research Organization (IBRO), which became incorporated as an independent organization through a Bill in the Parliament of Canada at Ottawa in 1961.

IBRO now has 2000 members, most of whom hold senior positions in research or teaching, in 52 countries of all political complexions. Through its National Corporate members, many of which are academies of sciences or national societies for neuroscience, the body of neuroscientists reflected in IBRO must be of the order of 15 000. One of the programmes of IBRO, all of which aim to serve the international community of neuroscientists, is the publication programme. IBRO publications include *IBRO News*, *Neuroscience* and the *IBRO Symposia Series*. With the present *Handbook Series*, IBRO aims to fill a major gap in the world literature. The neuroscientist needs to be able to turn to whichever specialized method that is most suited for the problem he is currently studying. The series on *Methods in the Neurosciences* will help to provide expert advice on exactly how to carry out the experiments, on what difficulties can occur and on the limitations of the method.

It is planned as a continuing series, so that new volumes can be published as and when new methods are developed, tested, and found useful. It is my hope that books in this series will have a significant impact on neuroscience throughout the world, by helping to provide the tools with which the scientist can tackle his problems.

                        A. David Smith,
                        Director of Publications, IBRO,
                        University Department of Pharmacology,
                        South Parks Road,
                        Oxford OX1 3QT, UK.

Preface

There can be few scientists using the technique of microiontophoresis who have not been dismayed at some time by inexplicably unusable electrodes, variable responses to a given compound, sudden changes of firing rate which ruin an otherwise unblemished recording. Many is the time I have promised myself, late at night, that this will be my last iontophoretic experiment.

But a few days later I may be demonstrating the method to an undergraduate student, and I share the sense of awe as a switch is flicked to eject glutamate and a lethargic neurone jumps into top gear within a second or two, to stop just as quickly when the glutamate is stopped. Or a rapidly firing cell is silenced by the ejection of GABA.

Arguably the micron-sized microiontophoretic electrode tip allows us to create the nearest thing we have to an artificial synapse. Microiontophoresis is a powerful tool, fascinating and flexible, but the more widespread its use, and thus the relevant literature, becomes, the more difficult it becomes for people wishing to use the technique anew to trace those snippets of information, buried in methods, results or even discussion sections of papers, which make the difference between success and failure, jubilation and frustration.

It is the purpose of this book to try and draw together a few of those details and to provide an introductory guide to the literature on microiontophoresis and the related micropressure methodologies.

My thanks are due to the authors and publishers who have allowed the reproduction of figures, to Miss Penny Forster for photographing those figures, and to my wife Anne for her unfailing help and encouragement.

CHAPTER 1

Historical Introduction and Underlying Principles

I BASIC PRINCIPLES	3
I.1 Pressure Ejection	4
I.2 The Microtap	5

The ancient Greeks used the term φορετικος to refer to the production or induction of movement. The modern term electrophoresis was originally used in physical chemistry to refer to the movement of charged molecules under the influence of an applied voltage, usually for the purposes of separation and analysis. The word was subsequently introduced into medical science to describe the movement of ions into a part of the body resulting from the passage of an electric current through a solution with which that tissue was in contact.

Early investigators using this technique applied histamine to the skin of the forearm in experiments to determine the relationship between histamine and Lewis's H-substance. Sir Henry Barcroft and colleagues (1943) were later to apply adrenaline by 'iontophoresis' from adrenaline-soaked bandages wrapped around the arm in an attempt to ascertain the cause of forearm blood flow changes after deep nerve blockade. This kind of 'limb iontophoresis' is still used today (Kuyihar-Csillik *et al.*, 1982).

The word iontophoresis was soon used interchangeably with electrophoresis by biologists who were almost invariably concerned with the movement of relatively small ions rather than the complex molecules and charged polypeptides studied by the physical chemists.

In investigating the phenomenon of synaptic transmission at the neuromuscular junction, in the early 1950s, a technique became very desirable for mimicking artificially the effects of transmitter release from somatic motor nerve terminals. The most critical requirement was for a means of applying the suspected transmitter, acetylcholine, to a very limited area of muscle membrane.

Several ingenious devices were in existence which allowed drug application to areas of tissue only a fraction of a square millimetre in size. Such was Kuffler's hooked wire method in which a tiny drop of solution was held in a fine wire loop by surface tension and carefully lowered until touching the tissue under study. Contact between drug and tissue could be as brief as a fraction of a second if required.

Even this method, however, does not allow the refinement necessary for a study of subsynaptic receptors. The area of tissue involved is measurable in microns and application times of only a few milliseconds would be needed to mimic transmitter release. Such methods are also inappropriate for non-superficial areas, such as structures in the brain.

A technique appropriate for the study of synaptic pharmacology was first realized by Nastuk (1953) and later developed by del Castillo and Katz (1955) and consisted essentially of the iontophoresis method, i.e. movement of charged particles produced by an electric current, restricted to a micropipette with a tip diameter of the order of 1 μm. Thus solutions of acetylcholine chloride were used and by passing a suitable current through this solution acetylcholine ions could be ejected from the 1 μm orifice onto a correspondingly localized area of subsynaptic membrane at the neuromuscular junction. Furthermore, by the use of automatic timing devices, acetylcholine ejections of a few milliseconds' duration could be effected, and the similarity between the effect of such ejections and of motor neurone stimulation was a powerful piece of evidence in favour of a transmitter function of acetylcholine at the neuromuscular juntion (del Castillo and Katz, 1955).

Independently of this line of development, Suh *et al.* (1936) had ejected acetylcholine from micropipettes by the use of an applied voltage into different regions of the hindbrain in attempts to localize areas of cardiovascular control. This work was not known to researchers in Europe and America until relatively recently.

Curtis and his colleagues soon adopted the new technique, now appropriately renamed microiontophoresis or microelectrophoresis for use in studying the mammalian central nervous system. Reports of its use in this situation first appeared in 1958 (Curtis and Eccles, 1958 a,b) in which these workers confirmed previous reports that acetylcholine probably acted as a transmitter between motor axon collaterals and inhibitory interneurones (Renshaw cells) in the spinal cord.

The experiments of Curtis and coworkers, however, involved an important modification of the original method, for this group used multi-barrel micropipettes. In the production of these, several lengths of tubing are fused together and then pulled so as to produce a single collective tip, but with each barrel having its own orifice. Multibarrel pipettes may be composed of two to nine barrels, although five or seven barrels give an adequate and conveniently sized assembly for most purposes.

Historical Introduction and Underlying Principles

PART I: BASIC PRINCIPLES

In the simplest case each barrel of a micropipette assembly to be used for drug ejection is filled with a solution of the ionized compound and the solution connected to the iontophoresis machine by a suitable lead.

As for other electrophysiological situations, the business end of the lead which is in contact with the drug solutions should be of the non-polarizing variety, i.e. platinum or silver/silver chloride. We have found platinum to be the more satisfactory. The establishment of a potential difference between the drug solution and the medium surrounding the barrel tip will then cause the movement of ions through the solution and out of the pipette tip (Figure 1a). An outward current will cause the 'ejection' of positively charged ions, an inward current the ejection of negatively charged particles. (As the direction of current flow is traditionally viewed as the movement of positive charges, the terms outward and inward relate respectively to the transport of positive charges *out* of or *into* the pipette, and of course the movement of negative charges in the opposite direction. Some authors use the terms cationic or positive current to refer to the current ejecting cations — positively charged — from the pipette and anionic or negative current to that ejecting anions.)

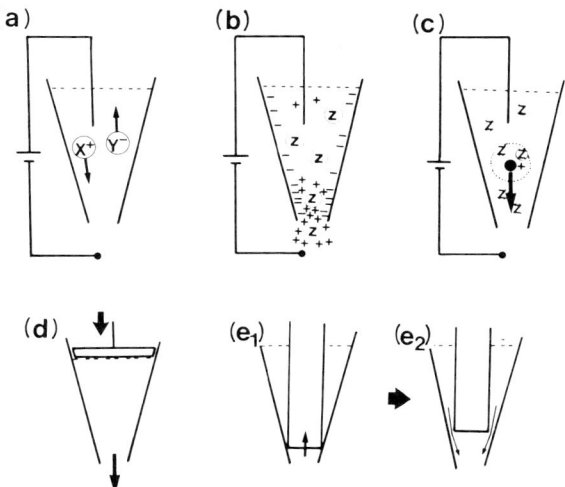

Figure 1 A summary of the main methods currently available for ejecting substances from micropipettes. (a) Microiontophoresis proper; ion movement results directly from the application of a potential difference between the inside and outside of the pipette barrel. (b) Electro-osmosis; this usually contributes to the total release resulting from an applied voltage. It is due to the existence of an electrical 'double layer' at a glass/water interface, giving the solution a net positive charge. A volume of solution, with dissolved drug molecules (Z) is, therefore, ejected by outward current. (c) Hydration effects. The ejection by microiontophoresis of an ion which carries a hydration shell will cause movement of drug molecules (Z) dissolved in the water of hydration. (d) Pressure. (e) The microtap; a central plunger is withdrawn, usually by electrical means, a few microns from the barrel tip. Solution can then escape through the opening created (e2)

As drug molecules would tend to diffuse from the solution in the pipette tip into the extracellular environment it is normal to apply a small current to reduce that efflux. This is known as a holding, backing, braking or retaining current. It is also usual practice to include a barrel containing a sodium chloride solution which can be used to control for the effects of current itself. This may be done either by periodically passing through the control barrel the same current used for drug ejection: this is a direct test for the effect of current on the cell, or by passing continuously a current adequate to cancel out the instantaneous sum of ejecting and retaining currents passing through the drug-containing barrels. This is known as current balancing.

Clearly the use of microiontophoresis as just described is suitable for any ionized molecule, but un-ionized compounds can be ejected by the closely related variant, electro-osmosis which is attributable to the presence of an electrical 'double layer' within the barrel tip. When an aqueous solution is in contact with glass, negative ions are tightly adsorbed on to the glass surface, leaving the bulk of solution carrying a net positive charge. The passage of positive (or outward) current then causes the ejection of a small volume of solution containing the compound of interest (Figure 1b). It should be noted that this mechanism has nothing whatever to do with the osmotic pressure of a solution or the establishment of any osmotic gradient. The term electro-osmosis derives simply from the fact that the driving force is the movement of the *solvent* not the solute, just as in the case of osmotic movements across a semipermeable membrane.

Un-ionized compounds may also be ejected dissolved in the water of hydration of mobile ions such as sodium, and NaCl may be added to solutions to increase the size of this phenomenon (Figure 1c). It should be noted, however, that the addition of such an electrolyte may divert the applied current from producing ejection by electro-osmosis: electro-osmosis and hydration effects involving cations are competing events.

It is often forgotten (or ignored) that some bulk fluid ejection will, therefore, occur with any outward current, even if this is being used for the conventional iontophoresis of a cation. Similarly some ejection of fluid will occur during the passage of an outward retaining current, although at the retaining currents normally used of around 5–10 nA the amount of presumably active anion ejected by this means will almost certainly be negligible in view of the opposing withdrawal of anions from the tip fluid (see Ch. 4, Pt. II).

I.1 Pressure ejection

As alternative method of applying both ionized and non-ionized compounds from micropipettes is the use of pressure. A suitable source of pressure, usually a cylinder of compressed gas, is connected to the open end of a micropipette barrel. Pressures usually up to about 20 pounds per square inch (p.s.i.) will eject fluid from a 1 μm pipette tip (Figure 1d). This method is finding increasing popularity not only because it is so readily applicable to all compounds, but also because the amount of solution (and therefore dissolved compound) can be easily and accurately determined simply by applying pressure while viewing the tip under a laboratory microscope and measuring the diameter of the extruded droplet. Pressure ejection is not without its complement of problems and artefacts, however, and is unlikely to replace microiontophoresis as a microapplication method.

I.2 The microtap

The microtap concept involves blocking the orifice of a drug-containing micropipette with a second, internal microtube (which can be a recording electrode). When the central barrel is raised hydrostatic pressure causes a flow of drug solution from the outer barrel (Figure 1e). This ingenious method has been used to apply picolitre volumes of fluid where the composition of the solution is important, as in studies of osmosensitive neurones (Leng, 1980), but the difficulties of constructing the pipette assemblies and obtaining the necessarily very small but controlled movements of the gate pipette have meant that it has not achieved great popularity. The most satisfactory method of inducing the small movements required seems to be to couple the inner barrel to a piezo-electric crystal or tube (Comis et al., 1972; Leng, 1980).

In the following pages of this volume these basic principles of drug microapplication will be expanded. In the years since Nastuk (1953) reported results with his 'electrically controlled microjet', microiontophoresis has been used to study systems ranging from single neurones and glia in culture (Hösli and Hösli, 1978) to the processes of thrombus formation in blood vessels (Begent and Born, 1970). The iontophoretic application of ATP has even been used to activate the flagella of isolated spermatozoa (Shingyoji et al., 1977). Ejected materials have ranged from the simplest ions, protons, to suspensions of synaptosomes (Krnjević and Whittaker, 1965). It remains an enormously valuable, flexible and informative technique but only if it is used wisely, its advantages and limitations are clearly understood, and the many pitfalls of interpretation are taken carefully into account.

CHAPTER 2

Electrode Assemblies for Microiontophoresis and Pressure Ejection

I Electrode Blanks	6
I.1 Intracellular Pipettes	9
II Pullers	10
II.1 The Pulling Process	11
III Breaking the Tip; 'Bumping'	12
IV Filling	12
V Cleaning	14
VI Combination Electrodes	15
VI.1 Manufacture	16
VI.2 Combined Metal and Glass Pipettes	18
VI.3 Artefact Suppression	19
VI.4 Iontophoresis in Oil	19
VII Special Considerations for Pressure Microinjection	19
VIII Drug Solutions	20
VIII.1 Preparation	20
VIII.2 Use of Sodium Chloride	20
VIII.3 Acidity	21
VIII.4 Use of Antioxidants	21
IX The Assessment of Electrodes	22

PART I ELECTRODE BLANKS

Microelectrodes and microiontophoretic assemblies can be readily manufactured from borosilicate glass tubing. For the commonly used five- or seven-barrelled multibarrel assemblies (Figures 2 and 3) several pieces of tubing are fused together before pulling. The appropriate number of tubes are fastened together at their ends by a strong (heat-resistant) adhesive, a metal collar, heat-shrink tubing, etc., and the top and bottom of this electrode 'blank' are then held by chucks in the electrode puller. The heating coil is used to melt gently the glass in the central portion of the assembly and the lower chuck is then rotated slowly by hand while exerting a small amount of pull on the glass. This rotation and slight pulling cause the lengths of tubing to fuse together. The coil is now switched off and the tubing allowed to cool, after which the position of the blank may be adjusted if necessary (it usually requires raising slightly) before pulling in the normal way.

It probably does not matter greatly which of the various types of capillary tubing available is used in the manufacture of multibarrel blanks for extracellular use; it is more important if intracellular iontophoresis or pressure ejection is to be used. For example the use of thin-walled capillaries (Corning, Haer) will produce pipettes with longer shanks and smaller external tip size for a given resistance than the more usual capillary tubing and these would clearly be preferable for intracellular penetration. Pipette assemblies made with thin-walled tubing, however, must be made with great care and tested very thoroughly to ensure that there is no significant electrical coupling between barrels resulting from the thinness of the glass wall near the tip or breaks in the wall produced during manufacture.

Some thought must also be given to the method of filling to be used. This will determine whether plain or fibre-filled (omega-dot, Haer) tubing is used, and will depend in part on the properties of the compound to be applied (e.g. its stability in solution).

While the above method for fabricating multibarrels from single tubing is undoubtedly the cheapest, several varieties of multibarrel blank are available commercially. The simplest and cheapest of these consist of fused straight lengths of tubing available in three- to seven- barrel configurations from Clark Electromedical Instruments, UK or WPI Ltd, USA. As each capillary tube has an external diameter of 1.2 mm, even the seven-barrelled assemblies can be pulled with no difficulty on a fairly small and lightweight puller. As two micro-iontophoretic assemblies result from pulling one of these blanks, they are quite economical to use.

Because these commercial blanks are simply cut from the very long lengths produced during their manufacture, the ends of the barrels are flush. This means that some care is required when filling. An advantage of the home-made variety of blank is that the tubes can be fixed together in a staggered conformation (Figure 2c) or the ends of the tubes even bent outwards from each other at some stage of the pulling process (Figure 2d) so as to reduce subsequent cross-contamination when filling.

The blanks from Wesley Coe Ltd, UK, consist of five barrels each having an external diameter of 4 mm. The bulk of these blanks means that only the larger pullers, such as the Narashige vertical puller, can cope adequately with them even though they are presented in a partially pulled format (Figure 2a) with or without a length of tubing fused to the narrow end to facilitate fixing in the lower chuck of the puller. The open ends of the tubes are also splayed to facilitate access.

Between these two extremes lie the assemblies introduced by Medical Systems Corp. (USA) to complement their Neurophore and pressure ejection system (see Ch. 3, Pt. III.2). The overall splayed, partially pulled design is similar to that of the Wesley Coe electrodes, but each barrel has an external diameter of

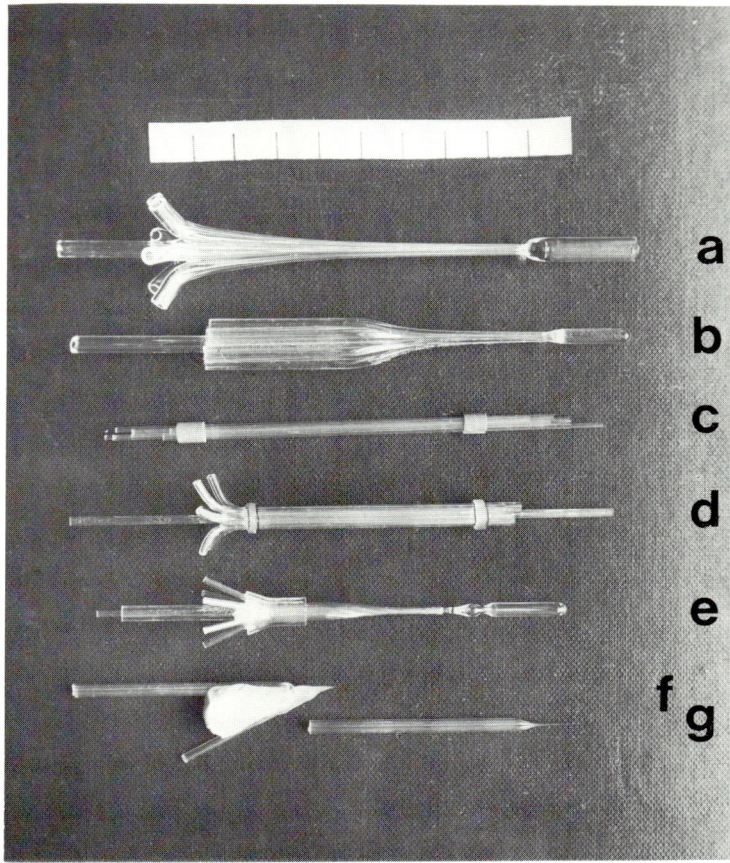

Figure 2 Some commonly used varieties of multibarrel pipettes and 'blanks'. A scale marked in centimetres is shown at the top. (a) A six-barrelled splayed blank from Wesley Coe. (b) A custom-made non-splayed version. (c) Here seven lengths of single 1 mm fibre-containing capillaries have been fastened together in a staggered arrangement using rubber tubing. When twisted and pulled this will yield two multibarrels in which the ends are sufficiently separated to permit access to several of them, for example for pressure ejection. (d) An alternative home-made blank using 1.5 mm tubing and bending the ends before pulling, for subsequent access. (e) A multibarrel blank from Medical Systems Corp. (f) Parallel electrode assembly as used routinely in the author's laboratory, and made by gluing together a single recording electrode with an angled tip, and a multibarrelled assembly. (g) Pulled from seven-barrelled lengths of tubing (Clark Electromedical)

only 1.5 mm (Figure 2e). While these blanks can of course be used with any iontophoresis system, their special value lies in their compatibility with Medical Systems equipment. An additional attractive feature for busy labs with money, or labs using iontophoresis so occasionally that major investment in pulling equipment is a waste, is that these electrodes can be supplied already pulled.

Both the Wesley Coe and Medical Systems blanks result in multibarrel assemblies costing at least ten times more than those produced from the unassuming straight blanks which in turn cost about three times more than the home-made variety. The larger, splayed blanks can be produced by a competent glass-blower, but their construction is time consuming and a requirement for a continuous supply may represent a significant drain on his work schedule. The larger assemblies of course are easier to handle and to fill than the smaller, while the latter may be essential if a number of items are to be manoeuvred within a confined working space. The ease of filling of home-made electrodes can be greatly improved, as noted above, by fusing the barrels in a staggered arrangement (Figure 2c,d). This would also be necessary if pressure ejection were to be anticipated since access to each barrel must be independent.

The smaller assemblies also drink much smaller volumes of solution: if some of the more exotic or expensive compounds are to be used this may be an important consideration.

Finally, various modifications of the more widely used blanks described above have been suggested at different times for specific purposes. For example Curtis (1964) suggested that the coupling between iontophoretic barrels themselves, caused by electrical leakage through the barrel walls or actual breakdown of the wall near the tip, might be a problem leading to serious interbarrel artefacts. The suggested remedy was to space the iontophoretic barrels apart using fibreglass rods when making the pipette blanks. This does not seem to have been put into practice to any significant extent, but it still seems a good idea.

I.1 Intracellular pipettes

If intracellular iontophoresis of compounds or current injection or voltage clamping is planned then it is unlikely that any of the above commercial multibarrels will be suitable, partly because they are all constructed from relatively thick-walled tubing which makes it very difficult to obtain a fine enough tip for cell penetration ($<0.5~\mu$m) without causing closing of the barrel tip, a situation clearly incompatible with iontophoresis. Even the home-made blanks using thin-walled tubing suffer from the disadvantage that, since they are composed of several separate tubes fused alongside each other the pulled tips also have a non-circular cross-section which may increase the risk of dimpling of cell membranes and thus mitigate against clean penetration.

For intracellular work it is, therefore, advisable to use single capillary tubing with internal partitions. The simplest variety contains a single partition, giving two channels, and is known as theta, θ, tubing because of its cross-sectional appearance (Figure 3c). Three-channelled and four-channelled tubing (Figures 3b,d) is also available from Clark Electromedical and WPI. Electrodes made from blanks such as these may yield relatively noisy recordings due to the thinness of the partitions, and there is no doubt that if large cells are being studied in which it is feasible to insert separate iontophoretic and recording electrodes (e.g. invertebrate neurones or muscle cells) then this would

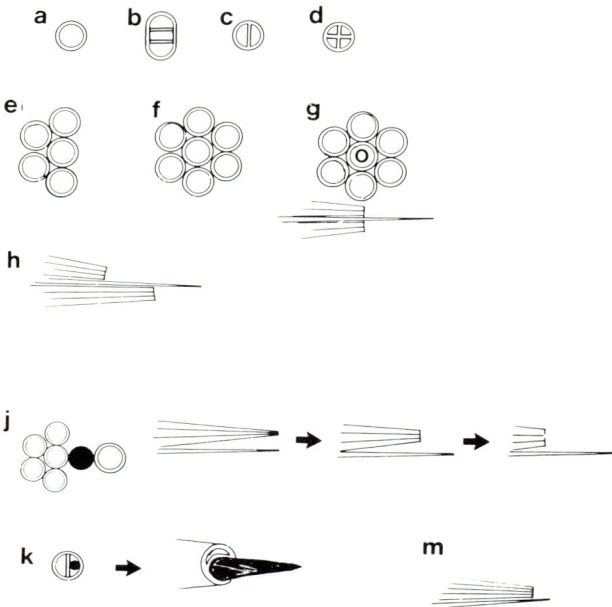

Figure 3 Examples of pipette configurations used in microiontophoresis. (a) Single fibre-containing capillary. (b) Three-channelled single tubing. (c) Theta capillary. (d) Four-channel tubing. (e) Five-barrel assembly. (f) Seven-barrel assembly. (g) A cross-section and longitudinal section through a combined multibarrel/single barrel assembly in which the single electrode is inserted through the centre barrel. (h) A combination of two multibarrels and recording electrode as used by Zieglgänsberger and Champagnat (1979) and Cherubini et al. (1982). (j) Begins with a cross-section of the blank assemblies advocated by Carette (1978). Subsequent illustrations show the tip profile after pulling and on two successive stages of tip enlargement. Note that the single to multibarrel tip distance is necessarily related to the multibarrel tip size. (k) Cross-section and pulled profile of a metal-in-glass combination (see Ch. 2, Pt. VI.2). The iontophoretic barrel tip is crescent shaped in this case (Kasser and Cheney, 1983). (m) As used in the author's laboratory (see Figure 2f)

be preferable. On the other hand these tubes can be pulled readily even on the more lightweight pullers or those designed to produce long fine tips needed for intracellular penetration.

WP Instruments has recently introduced theta tubing with a greatly thickened central partition to reduce the problems of electrical coupling.

PART II PULLERS

Many types of electrode puller are available which are suitable for pulling multibarrel assemblies. Some pull vertically, some horizontally; the pulling force may be manual, gravitational or electromagnetic. The choice between these possibilities is largely a matter of personal preference, though only the larger pullers, such as the vertical puller from Narashige (who also makes an excellent horizontal puller) will cope adequately with the larger species of electrode blanks. Other suppliers of pullers include Kopf Instruments, USA (vertical); Harvard Bioscience, UK (vertical), Clark Electromedical, UK (horizontal). As different sized heating coils from those routinely supplied may be required for multibarrels make sure that the supplier knows exactly what you intend to pull.

A home-made equivalent to the large vertical Narashige may be constructed by following the design of Winsbury (1956).

While any of these pullers is adequate to produce multibarrels for extracellular use, the vertical varieties are not usually ideal for producing the long fine pipettes needed for intracellular work. A horizontal puller, such as the Narashige, or those sold by Clark and WP Instruments which is based on the design of Livingston and Duggar (1934) (the Livingston puller), is virtually essential. The main difference between the vertical and horizontal pullers is that in the former the lower chuck is exerting pull on the tube, as it begins to soften, due to gravity. In most horizontal pullers this initial phase of pull can be more readily controlled electromagnetically. In the Livingston puller no tension is exerted on the tube until the glass has been heated to the experimenter's required fluidity. The full extent of a preset force is then applied to a single pull. The amount of heat applied and the delay to pull can be varied. Other methods for producing long-shanked electrodes have been described (e.g. Erhardt and Junier, 1982). Some of the major factors affecting micropipette size and profile in the Livingston puller have been discussed by Flaming and Brown (1982), and a Flaming–Brown puller, in which virtually every aspect of micropipette profile can be controlled by the experimenter, is now available commercially from Sutter Instrument Company.

II.1 The pulling process

There is a great deal to the art of pulling electrodes and especially multibarrel blanks which cannot be conveyed on paper, nor can it be easily learned in the laboratory. This is simply because the size of a multibarrel blank is such that the slightest difference between two heater coils, for example in their diameter, or in the spacing between the rings, can have a major effect on heat distribution to the glass. Adjustment of current supplies to the heating coil and the degree and timing of non-gravitational pull must, therefore, be made anew on each puller used and for each coil. The combination of heat and pull may be varied to produce pipettes with tips of different lengths and diameters, though we have found that other properties, such as the ease of breaking back the tip and even the current-passing characteristics of barrels can also change. There is much to be said for having a 'dedicated' puller which, once set, remains unadjusted. In my own laboratory a vertical Narashige puller is dedicated to multibarrel use for extracellular microiontophoresis and a Kopf to single microelectrodes for extracellular recording, while intracellular single electrodes are pulled on a horizontal Livingston.

We have, however, found it necessary to reset the pullers when a new batch of capillaries or blanks is obtained, reflecting differences in the properties of glass produced from year to year. For most consistent results it may be advisable to stock up as much as possible from a single batch of glass blanks.

For multibarrels the usual procedure is to pull so as to produce an overall tip size of about 1 μm and then to break back the extreme tip to an overall size of about 5 μm, each barrel then having an opening of about 1 μm. This size of tip represents a compromise between the need to reduce spontaneous drug diffusion from larger openings, and the poor current-passing characteristics of smaller tips.

PART III BREAKING THE TIP; 'BUMPING'

In most laboratories the breaking or bumping process is performed by aligning the micropipette, held in a micromanipulator, in the same plane as a smooth surface (a glass sphere, or the heat-fused end of a glass tube are ideal, also held in a micromanipulator) under the low power of a laboratory microscope. The pipette is then moved slowly until the tip has just touched the sphere. This usually causes a clean breakage of the tip, although on occasions the operation may need to be repeated two or three times until a completely satisfactory tip is obtained.

If it is intended to insert a two- or three-barrelled pipette or a multichannel single pipette intracellularly, it may be necessary to bevel the tip. Bevelling produces an elliptical opening with a lower electrode resistance, for a given tip diameter, than the unbevelled circular orifice. The finer points of bevelling have been discussed by Brown and Flaming (1975, 1979), Baldwin (1980), and Ogden et al. (1978). Commercial bevelling units are also available (WP Instruments, USA).

For many purposes the resistance of a barrel is of more practical relevance than its size, and it has, therefore, become quite a common practice to fill a freshly pulled electrode and then to monitor its resistance during the breaking or bevelling process. The latter is particularly important as it is often difficult or impossible to see what is happening at the electrode tip during bevelling.

PART IV FILLING

The method chosen for filling the micropipette barrels will depend mainly on the type of micropipette. The simplest to fill are those in which a glass filament has been fused along the inside wall of each barrel of the blank, the so-called omega-dot (Haer) tubing (Figure 3a). The junction between the filament and tubing wall causes the movement of any liquid, placed anywhere in the tube, to be transported along the length of the tube by capillarity. Because of the fineness of the barrel tip, and its taper, fluid is carried most rapidly into the tip. As more fluid coats the internal surface of the tip, the surface tension of the water causes the solution to occupy the whole cross-section of tube at the extreme tip. This then draws more fluid down the tube along the glass filament, due to surface tension, and the pipette fills. The whole process is very rapid, and the end few millimetres of a barrel will be filled within a second or two. The filling process can, however, be observed under a microscope.

The barrels of the Clark, WPI and Medical Systems multibarrel blanks are of the omega-dot variety and thus can all be filled simply by placing solution into the barrel immediately before use. This is a major advantage if unstable compounds are being used.

While a hypodermic syringe and needle with a fine flexible length of tubing attached is adequate for placing solution into the larger pipettes, some difficulty may be experienced with the smaller Clark and WPI barrels. We have found the best answer to be custom-made stainless steel 30 gauge Luer fitting syringe needles, 3 inches in length (exploring needles) from Shrimpton and Fletcher. These are not expensive.

If blanks are being used which are not constructed from omega-dot tubing but rapid filling is important, glass fibres can be made by hand simply by drawing out finer and finer pieces of tubing in a Bunsen flame, and a filament dropped into each barrel before pulling (Tasaki *et al.*, 1968). Although not entirely satisfactory a high rate of successful fusions of filament and tube wall within the terminal region of the pipette can be obtained (with practice and luck!)

More reproducible methods of filling non-omega-dot blanks are by centrifugation or vacuum. In the former case solution is placed as far down as possible in the pulled and broken pipette barrel, the pipette is held in a suitable clamp (a rubber bung with an appropriately sized central hole is suitable) and centrifuged at 10 000 g for 10 minutes. This is usually sufficient to force the solutions into the barrel tips (Curtis, 1964).

If drug stability is not a problem these electrodes can also be filled by holding them in a closed container with the terminal few centimetres below the surface of distilled water or methanol, and then evacuating the vessel by a vacuum pump. After about 30 minutes the liquid should have occupied the tips of the barrels. Methanol is more reliable in this by virtue of its lower surface tension and boiling point. Using a syringe and fine tube or needle the barrels can now be filled with different drug solutions, and the electrodes allowed to stand for 24 hours for the drug molecules to diffuse down to the barrel orifice (Curtis, 1964). By sucking out solutions at the end of an experiment and replacing with water for several days it is possible, if economically essential, to re-use the larger pipettes. It is said that centrifugation after such filling by replacement speeds up the access of drug into the barrel tip.

Very few attempts have been made to compare the efficiency of filling by different methods, but Kirsten and Sharma (1976a) found that the transport number of acetylcholine after filling by replacement followed by centrifugation was 0.386 ± 0.02 (mean of eight) but after filling by the glass fibre method the value was 0.473 ± 0.03 (mean of six).

It is at the filling stage that the main advantage of the splayed type of electrode blank is realized. Here there is little chance of contamination between barrels during filling, but with the non-splayed variety it is all too easy to obtain contamination. The exposed surface of the pipette must be absolutely dry, or fluid inserted into one barrel may pass back up the barrel along the glass fibre and across the cut surface into another barrel. It must be remembered that *any* fluid, no matter how microscopic a drop, in contact with the end of a barrel will be conducted down to the business end of the pipette along the glass fibre. Not only is the contaminated barrel then out of commission but also, if a potent compound is involved so is the whole multibarrel unless you complete the filling process and apply a retaining current. Even worse, of course, you may not be aware of the contamination until well into the experiment. Apart from drying thoroughly the non-pulled end of a multibarrel immediately before filling it may also be very advisable to coat the cut surface of the blank (*before* pulling) with a siliconizing medium such as Surfasil® or Aquasil® (Pierce) to minimize further the possibility of interbarrel tracking.

During the filling process, air bubbles may be introduced into the solution near the pipette tip. The incidence of this occurrence may be reduced by injecting the solution steadily into the barrel, care being taken that the solution does not spill over onto the outside surface of the pipette. Air bubbles may also be removed by inserting a fine wire into the troublesome area and manipulating it gently so as to dislodge the offending air pocket. This method of manipulating a fine wire (alternative insertion and withdrawal) has in fact been used successfully to introduce freshly made solution into the tips of micropipette barrels (Nastuk, 1953; Ito *et al.*, 1962).

Air bubbles may also be dislodged by sharp taps or flicks of the barrel with the fingers, care being taken not to aim in the direction of a friendly colleague lest the securing grip be inadequate for the power of the flick.

PART V CLEANING

Some practitioners of microiontophoresis go to considerable lengths to ensure absolutely clean micropipettes. The blanks may go through several stages, including chromic acid, nitric acid, or strong detergent, water and ether before being dried ready for pulling. This again is probably a matter of personal preference. We have found that such 'cleaning' results in a higher proportion of poor electrodes (i.e. with poor current-passing properties) than if the assemblies are used as they come. Whether this is due to dislodging minute particles which become lodged further down in the tip, or to a change in the chemical composition of the glass surface or a change in its ionic properties (the electrical double layer, Ch. 1, Pt. I) is unclear. Some of these problems are circumvented by sonication of the pipettes, but the possibility of dislodging minute particles remains. Most blanks manufacturers, however, will testify that their glass is thoroughly cleaned before fusion into the multibarrel blanks, and we have routinely used several varieties of electrodes without further cleaning with excellent results.

PART VI COMBINATION ELECTRODES

In some circumstances it is possible to use one barrel, usually the central one as it tends to have a lower resistance than the peripheral barrels, for recording unit activity. Such a barrel would be filled in the usual way with a suitable electrolyte solution such as potassium chloride, sodium chloride or potassium acetate. A metal wire contact (Ag/AgCl or platinum) can then be placed in the solution and the barrel treated as a conventional microelectrode. Many authors find this system satisfactory, and it is certainly adequate for investigating the responses of large cells, such as motoneurones and pyramidal tract cells in the mammalian central nervous system.

However, the size of the extracellularly recorded action potential is a function of the current flow in the extracellular space around the neurone, so that while 1 mV spikes may be recorded from the larger cells, potentials from the smaller interneurones, for example in superficial regions of the cerebral cortex, or cells in the striatum, may be only tens of microvolts in size. For the study of such small cells, therefore, it is probably best to combine a multibarrel micropipette with a conventional single recording electrode (Figure 3h–m) (Stone, 1973a; Crossman et al., 1974). We have found that this combination improves the signal-to-noise ratio for extracellular recording *in vivo* by at least an order of magnitude. This not only means that the sampling bias inherent in microiontophoretic work is reduced and cells will be detected which would have been missed by conventional multibarrel recording, but also that for a given signal-to-noise ratio in studies of a particular cell type, the experimenter can afford to remain slightly further away from the cell and thus reduce the risk of physical damage, effects of drug leakage or ejecting current artefacts, etc.

Various other configurations of electrodes have been used for specific purposes. For intracellular recording combined with extracellular iontophoresis, for example, it is necessary to arrange the recording electrode so that it protrudes beyond the multibarrel tip (Figure 3g). Curtis (1964) has stated that intertip distances of 40 to 60 μm are optimal for this kind of work. A suitable separation of recording and iontophoretic tips is also useful for applying compounds to different parts of the dendritic tree, for example, while recording from the neuronal soma or for studying the extent of spread of drug effects in an area (Herz et al., 1969, 1970). In these cases the intertip distance will depend on the experiment and may range from 10 μm up to 300 μm (Herz et al., 1969).

The concept of separating the iontophoretic and recording tips has been most elegantly realized in studies by Zieglgänsberger and Champagnat (1979), who combined a single pipette for intracellular recording with two multibarrel assemblies located at different distances from the recording tip in order to compare the efficacy of substances applied close to the soma with their efficacy when applied to the more distal dendritic regions (Figure 3h). Cherubini et al. (1982) have also used combinations of two multibarrel assemblies with tip separations of around 200 μm in order to compare the effects of drugs at the somatic level and in the synaptic receiving area of the dendrites on hippocampal pyramidal cells *in vivo*.

VI.1 Manufacture

Combination electrodes may be made in several ways. One of the first methods was to make a coaxial assembly using a recording electrode with a very long fine tip which could be inserted, using a micromanipulator under microscopic control, along the length of the centre barrel of a pulled multibarrel (Figure 3g). When the recording tip protrudes sufficiently a drop of strong adhesive is introduced to prevent movement of the position. This method is only feasible with the larger types of multibarrel and requires very careful preparation of the recording electrode to ensure the correct profile, as well as very precise manipulation inside the multibarrel.

It is also possible to construct a manipulator which will hold the two coaxial components separately but in a fixed position relative to each other not only for the construction process but also during the course of an experiment (Curtis, 1964).

The construction of these coaxial assemblies clearly necessitates a recording electrode which has a long fine shank for insertion along the multibarrel and methods have been described which may facilitate their production (Erhardt and Junier, 1982).

One of the biggest disadvantages of coaxial systems is that of electrical coupling of one form or another, for example noise pickup from an adjacent iontophoresis barrel. The problem is perhaps greatest where interest is focused on the shape and time-course of rapid potential changes (such as spikes or current-measuring pulses) recorded intracellularly. The capacitance between the recording and iontophoretic barrels may cause serious attenuation of such changes. One solution to the problem was described by Sonnhof (1973) and involves coating the recording electrode with gold and then driving this screen, or shield, at unit gain from the input amplifier.

The expense of this method has prompted Engberg *et al.* (1975) to devise a cheaper method in which recording electrodes are coated to within 1 mm of the tip by spraying with graphite from an aerosol can (the terminal millimetre is protected by holding it under ethanol: the electrode is filled with electrolyte first). The coated electrode is then inserted down the centre barrel of a multibarrel pipette, electrolyte solution is added to occupy part of the surrounding space down to the tip and the graphite screen or the electrolyte is then connected to a unity gain amplifier.

More recently Biscoe *et al.* (1978) attempted to facilitate the production of coaxial recording and multibarrel pipettes for use in mouse brain, since parallel assemblies caused too much damage. They, therefore, manufactured blanks in which the place of the centre barrel was taken by glass tubing which was not continuous along the blank, that is, a gap of several centimetres was left between the two pieces of tubing. The relatively large size of this tube, even after the pulling process greatly aided the manipulation of the single recording electrode along it, to protrude beyond the multibarrel opening by 15–25 μm. This idea would seem to deserve wider application where coaxial assemblies are needed or tissue damage is problematic, than it seems to have received.

An alternative arrangement which also reduces the noise and coupling problem is to fix the recording electrode alongside the multibarrel. A variety of more or less sophisticated and more or less expensive contraptions have been used for this purpose (Curtis, 1968; Oliver, 1971) though all that is required is a pair of micromanipulators which can be arranged so that the tips of electrodes held by each can be approximated under a microscope. A rapid setting adhesive (such as Rapid Araldite®, from Ciba) can then be applied to the shanks and tips of the electrodes, care being taken to use a glue which allows final adjustments of position to be made before it sets hard. It is also essential, of course, that the adhesive does not contract on hardening as this may produce an undesirable movement of the tip positions.

Carette (1978) has described a method in which a single relatively large capillary, destined to be the recording barrel, and several smaller capillaries to be used for iontophoresis are lightly fused to opposite sides of a central glass rod (Figure 3j). On pulling this assembly in two or three stages the difference in size of the capillaries, together with the lightness of fusion results in a separation of the tips such that they can be broken back independently if desired. While this method has the great advantage that the problems of combining pulled single and multibarrel electrodes are eliminated, it carries the disadvantage that the size of multibarrel tip will vary with degree of bumping, that is, with the single to multibarrel tip distance (Figure 3j) (Poulain and Carette, 1981).

In my own laboratory these 'parallel' or 'piggy-back' combinations are produced routinely without even needing a micromanipulator (Figure 2f). For the best electrodes the angle between single and multibarrel pipette should be as acute as possible to minimize tissue damage, and is essential if studies are to be made of neurones situated deep within the brain *in vivo*. Our first stage is to bend the shank of the pulled single pipette by arranging the coil of the electrode puller around the shoulder or shank of the pipette, applying heat and then nudging the tip with a seeker. An angle of 10–15° is sufficient. Next a piece of Plasticine® is pushed on to the side of the multibarrel, and the single pipette pushed into this so that the single and multibarrel tips are reasonably close, as judged by eye. The assembly is now placed in a small perspex holder on the stage of a microscope and, under ×100 magnification, while steadying the perspex holder with one hand, the position of the single pipette is adjusted to produce the desired proximity of intertip distance. Rapid Araldite® is now stroked on to the shanks and shoulder of the assembly, from as near the tip as possible. Final adjustment of position must be made immediately under the microscope as the positions cannot be changed after about 3 minutes. With a little practice the finished combination can be produced within 10 minutes of mounting the single and multibarrel blanks in their respective pullers. They can be used almost immediately, although 20 to 30 minutes is normally allowed for complete hardening before use.

A different approach entirely is to use a micromanipulator system to manoeuvre the two components of a system (e.g. intracellular recording and extracellular iontophoresis) completely independently. A manipulator system which can accomplish this although it was originally designed to facilitate the insertion of two pipettes into a single neurone has been described by Engberg *et al.* (1972). Units are also available from Narashige which are designed to permit the alignment of electrode tips to a common point. These units incorporate screw mechanisms which allow the movement of the two electrodes independently in each of three planes.

A method was also described much earlier by Tomita and Torihama (1956) for the independent manipulation of the components of coaxial assemblies.

Most of the above methods are equally suitable for combining multibarrel pipettes with the relatively coarse single electrodes adequate for extracellular spike or field potential recording, or with the superfine electrodes needed for intracellular work. In the latter case the use of multichannel tubing such as theta glass would greatly facilitate voltage clamp work by providing one clamping channel and one recording channel.

VI.2   Combined metal and glass pipettes

Metal recording electrodes may be preferable to glass if a low resistance electrode is required, say, for multi-unit recordings, if the electrode has to negotiate a thick or tough layer of tissue (such as the dura) or in circumstances where the fragility of glass may be problematic, as in chronic recordings of neuronal activity in conscious animals. However, it is not easy to combine metal electrodes with glass pipettes for iontophoresis. Theoretically it would be possible to fix a metal-insulated electrode alongside a conventional multibarrel, but it is doubtful whether this would significantly reduce the possibility of breakage. Methods have, therefore, been described in which a sharpened metal electrode is inserted into one side of a length of theta glass, the combination is mounted in an electrode puller which can be manipulated manually, and the glass is pulled over the metal (Fries and Zieglgänsberger, 1974; Kasser and Cheney, 1983).

In the method of Kasser and Cheney (1983) for example, a tungsten rod was etched to a suitable tip size (about 5 μm) and then back-fed into one side of a theta capillary. The assembly was positioned in the coil of a horizontally mounted puller and heat applied to the pipette, which was then pulled manually in the direction of the metal electrode tip. This pulling was performed in three or four stages, with the electrodes being repositioned in the coil each time. The effect of the pulling process is to cause the glass pipette to collapse down on to the metal electrode, insulating it. According to the authors, correct positioning of the pipette assembly for the final pulling stage (together presumably with a choice of optimal heating parameters and impeccable timing) will cause the glass barrels to break off a few microns from the tip of the metal electrode, leaving 5 to 25 μm exposed. This yields a tip profile similar to that in Figure 3k, with a narrow crescent-shaped opening to the barrel available for iontophoresis.

VI.3 Artefact suppression

It has been suggested by Wang and Aghajanian (1977) that the combination of a single recording electrode with a multibarrel iontophoretic pipette may be used to reduce the size of stimulus artefacts resulting from electrical stimulation at distances of several millimetres from the recording site. The idea is that one of the pipette barrels is used as the indifferent pole for the stimulation so that the separate single recording electrode picks up less of the shock artefact. However, for this to work satisfactorily there would probably need to be a greater separation between the multibarrel and recording pipettes than is useful for most iontophoretic studies. This may explain why the method does not seem to have become widely used.

VI.4 Iontophoresis in oil

The completion of an electrical circuit is a *sine qua non* of microiontophoresis. In order to obtain the release of acetylcholine by iontophoresis from a single micropipette in an oil medium, Kuffler and Yoshikami (1975a) applied a hydrophilic layer of egg albumen or saliva to the outside of the tip of their pipette, extending from the orifice to a layer of colloidal silver coated on the shank of the pipette. Electrical contact could then be made between the pipette contents and the silver layer, providing a return path for the iontophoretic current.

PART VII SPECIAL CONSIDERATIONS FOR PRESSURE MICROINJECTION

Generally speaking any micropipette barrel which is suitable for microiontophoresis is also suitable for ejection by pressure, assuming that the unpulled end of the barrel stands proud of adjacent hindrances so that the pressure application tube can be attached tightly to produce an airtight seal. A further limitation on micropipettes for pressure application is that the tip opening must be greater than 0.5 μm across unless the experimenter has access to a means of applying astronomical pressures. At this lower limit of tip size ejection by pressure also becomes extremely variable and a proportion of pipettes will fail to eject at all (Palmer *et al.*, 1980; Poulain and Carette, 1981).

Enlarging a micropipette tip by simply touching it against a smooth surface has been mentioned above, but if a single pipette is broken to about 10 μm or more, or a seven barrel assembly to about 15 μm or more, this method frequently results in irregular breakage seen either as an irregular outline to a single pipette opening or as the breakage of some barrels more than others of a multibarrel.

If relatively large tips are required, therefore, for example to pressure eject nanolitre volumes over a period of several minutes, a different method of bumping such as that described by Briano (1983) is to be preferred. This method involves inserting the pipette to be broken along the inside of a larger pipette, and then applying a force perpendicular to the long axis using something like a razor blade so as to cause fracture of the inner pipette where it protrudes from the outer one. Although the method was described for single pipettes it should be applicable, with care, to multibarrel assemblies.

One difficulty associated with pressure ejection, which can be observed under the microscope, is the tendency for an ejected droplet to run back along the outside of the tip to form a globule several tens of microns away from the orifice. Sakai *et al.* (1979) state that heating a freshly pulled micropipette for 5 minutes at 200 °C greatly reduces this tendency. A coating of (hydrophobic) wax on the outside of the pipette was used for the same purpose by Kuffler and Yoshikami (1975a). Although this droplet formation may not be a problem when the tip is inserted into tissue, it could markedly affect the reliability and accuracy of calibration.

PART VIII DRUG SOLUTIONS

VIII.1 Preparation

Since a micropipette may, if it is working well, find itself in use for many hours, there is ample time for particles of glass, dust or undissolved drug to float gently tipwards and create havoc. The tip may become blocked so that its current-passing properties are severely compromised, or no compound at all may be ejected. It is always a sensible precaution, therefore, to remove at least the larger particles from solutions by centrifugation or filtration. Both methods are applicable very easily to large volumes of solution using the traditional tubes and funnels, but they can also now be applied even to quite small volumes of a few hundred microlitres using multicompartment microcentrifuge tubes and Luer-fitting filters. These are available from most suppliers of liquid chromatography equipment (Waters, Anachem).

All solutions should be made in at least double distilled and preferably deionized water: the presence of small highly mobile ions may result in their carrying a significant fraction of the iontophoretic current, especially if the compound of interest is of high molecular weight or is poorly ionized.

VIII.2 Use of sodium chloride

The term 'osmotic artefact' is used to refer to the bulk flow of solution, carrying the active ion, which could result if the solution in the pipette were present at a substantially lower osmotic concentration than the biological fluids with which the tip is in contact. To minimize this it is usual, wherever possible, to use ionized compounds at a concentration of 150–200 mM for microiontophoresis. This is because a solution which is iso-osmolar with body fluids is approximately 165 mM (if it dissociates into two ions).

Some substances, of course, are not sufficiently soluble to be used at this concentration. Such substances may be dissolved in a solution of sodium chloride so that the total solute concentration is 165 mM. This procedure, however, may introduce complications more serious than that introduced by the use of a hypotonic solution. Firstly, if the ion of interest is negatively charged, it would be appropriate to apply an outward retaining current but this would cause the ejection of sodium ions and thus of the dissolved compound by hydration effects as well as electro-osmosis (see Ch. 1, Pt. I). Secondly, if the ion of interest has a relatively high molecular weight, then it may carry only a small fraction of any iontophoretic current in comparison with sodium (of chloride) ions. Very little of the active compound may, therefore, be ejected.

This diluting effect can, of course, be used to advantage. If a compound of very high potency is being used (for example quisqualic acid) it may be desirable to dilute the solution with NaCl in order to use sensible iontophoretic currents (bearing in mind the accuracy of ± 1 nA of some equipment) but to eject very small amounts of the active material. This should be preferable to merely diluting a solution with water since, on theoretical grounds, the amount of ion ejected for a given current should be independent of concentration (Ch. 4).

VIII.3 Acidity

The pH of drug solutions is often adjusted either to increase solubility or to optimize the degree of ionization of weak acids and bases. Lowering the pH also increases the chemical stability of compounds such as acetylcholine and catecholamines, and since in experiments on mammalian preparations the solution within the electrode tip and shank may be at 37 °C for several hours this could be important.

Against the need for stability and optimal ionization the possibility should be considered that the ejection of H^+, particularly from solutions below about pH 2.5, can cause excitation of neurones or may modify neuronal responses to other agents. This will be discussed in more detail in Chapter 6.

VIII.4 Use of antioxidants

In order to improve the stability of catecholamines in particular some workers include ascorbic acid in their solutions (see Hughes and Smith, 1978). However, there are reports that ascorbate will reduce the binding of dopamine to neuronal membranes (Heikkila et al., 1983) so that some effect on neuronal responses should be borne in mind. Controls for the ejection of ascorbate along with the ion of interest or by the retaining current will also need to be performed.

The pharmacological effects of ascorbate may be circumvented by the use of sodium metabisulphite, 1%, with corresponding controls.

PART IX THE ASSESSMENT OF ELECTRODES

Although the careful microscopic examination of an electrode tip may satisfy the observer as to the general condition, size and profile of the tip, it is unfortunately an unreliable guide as to its performance. An improvement on visual inspection is to measure the electrical resistance of the filled barrels. It does not particularly matter whether resistance to alternating (AC) or direct (DC) current is determined as long as the two are not compared between different laboratories, or with existing literature: AC resistance is the more conventional measurement and may be an order of magnitude lower than DC resistance. On the other hand, since iontophoretic current is DC, the DC measurement may provide a more appropriate guide to pipette performance. A simple multimeter and a beaker of saline or a battery, series resistor and oscilloscope are quite adequate for determining DC resistance, although a number of more or less sophisticated bridge circuits are available commercially to measure AC or DC resistance and capacitance (e.g. WP Instruments).

The values for resistance to be expected will obviously depend on the use to which the barrel will be put—resistances of the fine microelectrodes and multibarrels for intracellular use, for example, will need to be at least an order of magnitude higher than normally needed for extracellular iontophoresis. In our own electrodes the parallel single recording barrel has a tip diameter of about 2–3 μm and an AC (1 kHz) resistance of about 5 MΩ. Iontophoretic barrels containing electrolyte solutions have resistances of 10–15 MΩ, barrels filled with amino acid solutions (100 mM) are about 20–40 MΩ while amine- or alkaloid-containing barrels are usually in the range 50–100 MΩ. In general we find resistance to outward currents to be greater than that to inward currents, though whether this is related merely to the well-known rectifying properties of glass micropipettes (Purves, 1981) or to the presence of drug ions is not clear.

One of the advantages of the Medical Systems Neurophore equipment is that a readout of barrel resistance can be obtained at any time during the course of an experiment and the LED display will flash, whether set to display iontophoretic current or barrel resistance, if resistance increases to an extent which prevents passage of the desired current.

CHAPTER 3

Equipment

I MICROIONTOPHORETIC CURRENT SOURCES	23
I.1 Shielding	26
I.2 Monitoring Current Flow	27
II CURRENT BALANCING	27
II.1 Passive Method	27
II.2 'Active' Method	27
III COMMERCIALLY AVAILABLE EQUIPMENT	29
III.1 WP Instruments	29
III.2 Medical Systems Corporation	31
III.2.a Balancing	33
III.2.b Current Control	34
III.2.c External Programming	34
III.3 Dagan	34
III.3.a Current Balancing	36
IV CURRENT INJECTION	36
V PRESSURE EJECTION	36
V.1 Medical Systems	37
V.2 WP Instruments	37
V.3 The Picospritzer	38
VI RECORDING	38

PART I   MICROIONTOPHORETIC CURRENT SOURCES

In theory at least it is possible to eject compounds from a micropipette simply by connecting the iontophoretic lead to the appropriate pole of a battery and completing the circuit through a switch, to the animal or bath (Figure 4A). The current passed through the electrode can be calculated from Ohm's Law—a 1 V battery into a 10 MΩ electrode should produce 100 nA of current.

Modification of this most basic of circuits then depends on the experimenter's expertise. The use of a second battery in parallel to the first, connected with the reverse polarity and with a means of switching between the two, provides both a retaining and ejecting voltage. In order to vary the current it will be necessary to include a voltage divider of some kind (Figure 4b).

Most micropipette barrels have resistances of between 1 and 100 MΩ when filled with drug solution and during an experiment the resistance may fluctuate for a variety of reasons, mostly biological. For example particles of tissue or membrane may partially block a barrel orifice, proteins may be pulled towards or into the tip solution, or a particle of dust, glass or precipitate might settle into the electrode tip. Clearly a change of barrel resistance will have a dramatic effect on current passage through the electrode and it is usual, in the simpler circuits, to include a resistor in series with the micropipette (on the supply line) which will swamp any such variation. Resistances of around 10^8 or 10^9 ohms are common (Figure 4b). This in turn, of course, requires a high voltage supply in order to provide appropriate currents. As iontophoretic currents rarely exceed 100 nA, a 100 V supply should be adequate.

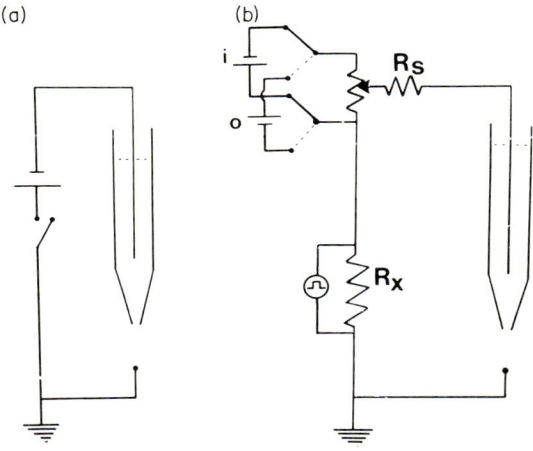

Figure 4 (a) A sketch of the simplest possible iontophoretic circuit, consisting of a battery and a switch. (b) A more advanced circuit would include a crossover facility to permit retaining as well as ejecting current, a series resistor R_s to minimize the effect of fluctuations of electrode resistance and a current monitoring device such as a pen recorder or oscilloscope placed across a small series resistor R_x

A difficulty with high voltage high resistance circuits of this kind, however, is that interference, by electrical pickup either from nearby extrinsic voltage sources, or internally generated when voltages are switched to and from a pipette barrel ('switching artefacts'), is enhanced and conducted into the micropipette. This can present major problems for the recording system. The problem can be almost entirely eliminated by separating the recording and iontophoretic electrodes (see Ch. 2, Pt. VI).

An alternative and more satisfactory solution to the problem of variable barrel resistance is to use a current pump, which should maintain a constant current flow through the barrel, independently of the tip resistance (up to the limit set by its own supply voltage). Various authors have designed current pump circuits

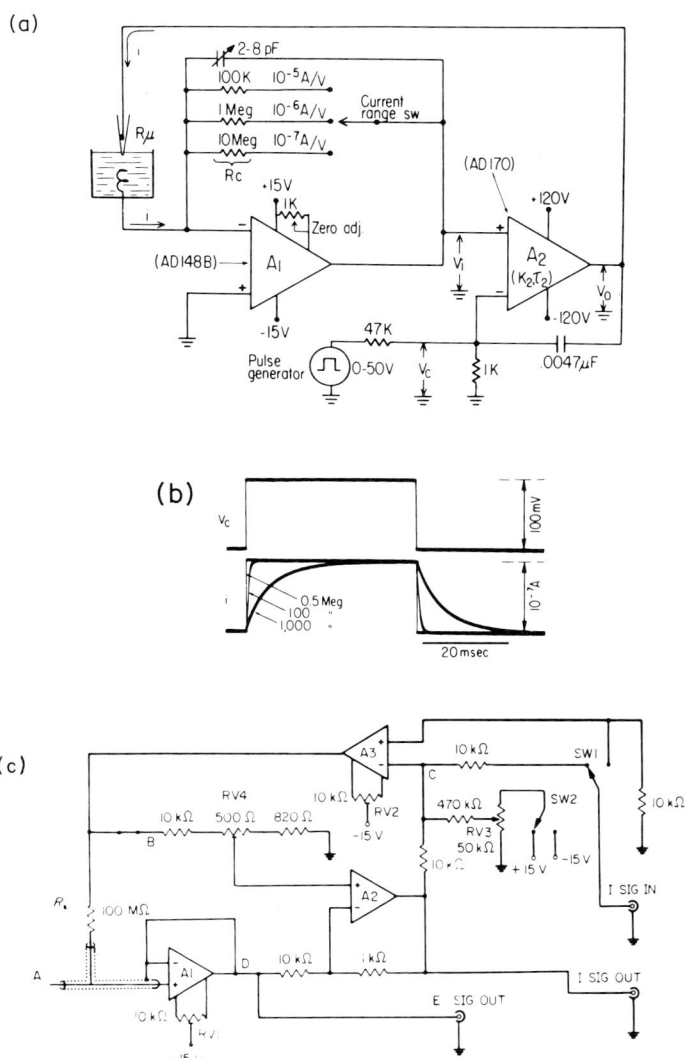

Figure 5 (a) Constant current feedback circuit. The current monitoring voltage V_i is compared to the control voltage V_c and the error is amplified by the amplifier A_2 to generate the controlled current through the microelectrode. (b) Current response to a pulse of control voltage. Upper trace: control voltage. Lower trace: current with microelectrode resistances of 0.5, 100 and 1000 MΩ. The longer time constant is associated with the larger microelectrode resistance. (c) Circuit diagram of simple current pump. All operational amplifiers are types CA3140. Switches SW1 (ejection polarity) and SW2 (bias polarity) are single pole, double-throw with centre off. RV3 is a front panel control which varies the steady bias current. (a and b reproduced with permission of Raven Press, NY. From *Microelectrophoresis* (Katz and Steinberg, 1976). c reproduced with permission from *Microelectrode Methods for Intracellular Recording and Iontophoresis* (Purves, 1981). Copyright: Academic Press Ltd.)

suitable for microiontophoresis (Spencer, 1971; Geller and Woodward, 1972; Dreyer and Peper, 1974; Katz and Steinberg, 1976; Purves, 1981). Pumps described by Katz and Steinberg (1976) and Purves (1981) are illustrated in Figures 5a and c respectively. The principle of operation is as follows: in Figure 5a the driving voltage V_c (pulse generator) is applied through the microelectrode and preparation. The current passed is monitored by the current monitoring amplifier A_1, the scale of which is determined by the current range switch, and the output voltage of A_1 ($= V_i$) is compared directly with V_c at amplifier A_2. Any imbalance between V_i and V_c will result in a voltage output from A_2 such that the 'error' is compensated. Two points may be emphasized in this type of circuit. Firstly, the total circuit gain K_c is determined by the circuit resistance R_c, microelectrode resistance R_μ and A_2 gain K_2 by

$$K_c = K_2 R_c / R_\mu$$

Thus the higher is $R\mu$ the lower the gain.

Furthermore the time constant of error correction τ_c is dependent on both the time constant of the A_2 circuit and K_c as:

$$\tau_c = \tau_2 / 1 + K_c$$

with the important result that as K_c diminishes with increasing microelectrode resistance, so τ_c increases. This is illustrated in Figure 5b. With this kind of circuit changes of τ_c could clearly be an important factor limiting the reliability of short current pulses.

The pump of Figure 5c is similar in principle. The driving voltage passes to the microelectrode via the 100 MΩ resistor. A_1 is a unity gain amplifier providing an indication of the applied voltage at E SIG OUT, and of current at I SIG OUT. Any discrepancy between the drive voltage and actual voltage levels as detected at C then appears as an appropriately correcting signal at A_3.

The pump described by Dreyer and Peper (1974) included capacity compensation features intended to facilitate release of compounds from high resistance micropipettes using very brief and intense stimuli. However, Dionne (1976) could subsequently find no effect of capacitance neutralization on release from pipettes of 20 to 60 MΩ resistance.

I.1 Shielding

As noted in Chapter 2 the close spacing of the barrels in many multibarrel assemblies results in resistive and capacitative coupling which can severely compromise the behaviour of the recording barrel. It may, therefore, be necessary, especially for intracellular work, to use a unity gain amplifier with capacitance compensation to drive a shield surrounding the recording electrode (see Ch. 2, Pt. VI.2).

I.2 Monitoring current flow

Particularly for extracellular work in the CNS, compounds may be applied for many seconds or minutes, and current flow through the micropipette can be monitored quite adequately using an ammeter in the iontophoretic circuit. However, one of the limitations of metering systems is their slow rise time, which clearly restricts their usefulness where ejection pulses of a few milliseconds are required (as at neuromuscular junctions, neurones in culture, invertebrate systems, etc.). In these cases it is preferable to monitor the voltage drop across a series resistor on an oscilloscope, pen recorder or similar device having a differential input. It should, of course, be noted that the recording device must not draw current from the circuit. If this possibility cannot be eliminated by other means, it will be necessary to interpose unity gain voltage followers on each of the input arms to the recorder. It is usual to select a value of the series resistor such that a 1 nA current will produce a 1 mV drop of potential. This voltage will give reasonable deflections in most recording systems at the sort of ejection currents (10–50 nA) used most frequently.

A current monitor with some advantages over analogue meters was described by Courtice (1976).

PART II CURRENT BALANCING

If a microiontophoretic electrode is located extracellularly very close to a neuronal membrane, the passage of current from a barrel to ground may be sufficient to cause a change of neuronal excitability. This problem, of course, will be particularly severe in the case of intracellular studies, but can be a serious source of difficulty, even in normal extracellular work, in areas where the neurones are unusually sensitive to current effects (see Ch. 6, Pt. III). The concept of current balancing (Salmoiraghi and Weight, 1967) was an attempt to minimize these problems by confining current flow as far as possible to the microelectrode assembly.

II.1 Passive method

In principle current balancing can be achieved in one of two ways. Firstly, the circuit passing current through a drug barrel can be completed through a 'neutral' or 'balance' barrel containing a suitably inert solution such as sodium chloride (Figure 6a). By connecting the return pole of each of the current pumps to the balance barrel, the flow of current during iontophoresis is confined, theoretically, to the immediate vicinity of the barrel tip.

II.2 'Active' method

The alternative method is to apply actively to the balance barrel a current which is equal in magnitude to the algebraic sum of all currents being passed

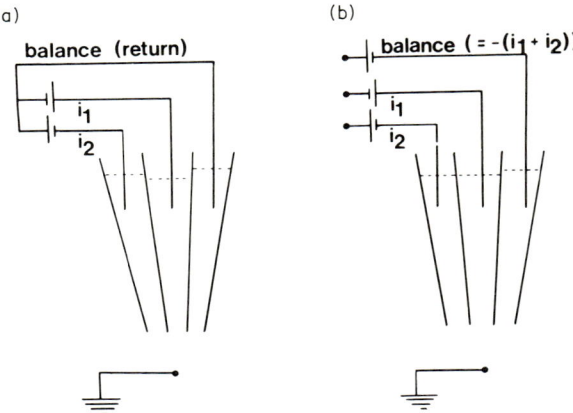

Figure 6 The two methods of 'current balancing'. (a) 'Passive' method, in which the balance barrel is merely a return channel for the iontophoretic current. (b) 'Active' method, in which a current equal in magnitude but opposite in sign to the sum of iontophoretic currents is applied via the balance barrel. The object of current balancing is to minimize current leakage through cells to ground

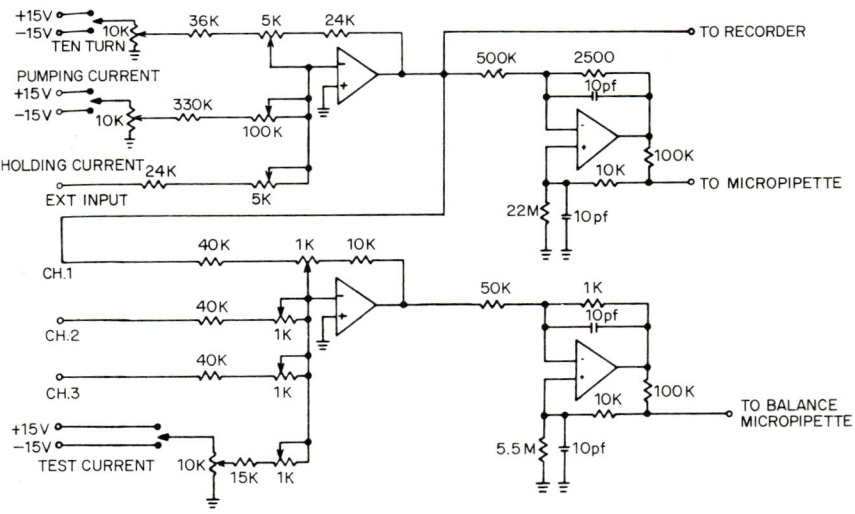

Figure 7 Schematic circuit for one of three identical drug channels. The input operational amplifier (top) sums three possible control voltage signals, pumping and holding currents and external inputs; the outputs of this operational amplifier go to the input of the pumping circuit, to a chart recorder, and to one input of the balance channel (bottom). Control voltages at CH.1, CH.2, CH.3 from the three drug injection channels are summed and the resulting voltage controls the balance current source. (Reproduced from Geller and Woodward, 1972, by permission of Elsevier Biomedical Press B.V.)

through the drug-containing barrels, but of opposite sign (Figure 6b). This may be achieved in principle by connecting the current pump output lines to a current–voltage converter, which then acts as the command input to the balance barrel current pump. The circuit published by Geller and Woodward (1972) is reproduced in Figure 7 to illustrate this concept.

PART III COMMERCIALLY AVAILABLE EQUIPMENT

III.1 WP Instruments

The first current module specifically designed for microiontophoresis was the Model 160 made by WPI. This consisted of battery operated stand alone units. Although now officially described by WPI as obsolete these useful units were widely distributed and may still be encountered frequently. The batteries provided up to 100 V output (compliance) which was adequate for most purposes. With the unit in the 'Preset' mode the pump was isolated from the preparation and both eject and retain currents could be set using the front panel meter. In the 'Operate' mode the current passing to the pipette was determined either by manually switching between Eject and Retain using the centrally located master switch, or by an external pulse (+ 5 V) applied to the Auto-Input socket. This last facility permitted regular cycles of ejection to be programmed from an external clock. The only practicable means of current balancing with this system was by the passive current return method described earlier. Although simple in operation the Model 160 did have the outstanding advantage for many workers that one need only buy one channel at a time (for some applications such as electrode marking or intracellular staining one channel may be all that is required) and each channel was portable and relatively inexpensive. It has been replaced by the Model 260 (Figure 8a), again battery powered but now by standard 9 V batteries which are far cheaper and more easily obtainable than those needed for the 160. The 260 though is still capable of generating of a 100 V output and, therefore, stands comparison with all the mains driven units to be described. Indeed the use of battery power is said to reduce greatly the equipment noise level to less than 20 μV. As for the 160 this unit may be controlled manually or from an external clock, and balancing is by the 'passive' method.

Besides these simpler and cheaper units, WP Instruments has introduced a more elaborate unit, the series 7000 modular system (Figure 8b). The 7000 series consists of a mains operated mainframe (S-7100) which includes a power source and LCD digital meter, into which can be inserted up to four iontophoresis (ionophoresis) modules (S-7061). The mainframe can be used to operate up to six such modules.

The compliance is again ± 100 V and each module can be used either in a Hold–Eject mode (i.e. for retention or ejection) or as a balance channel (Σ I mode). Each module possesses its own output socket and cable.

There is no continuous numerical indication of the current flowing in each channel, but a 'monitor' output is available for the continuous recording of current, for example on a pen recorder.

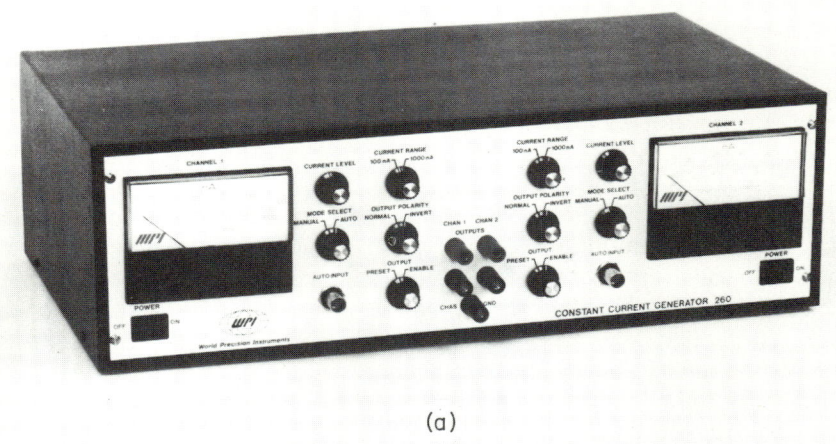

(a)

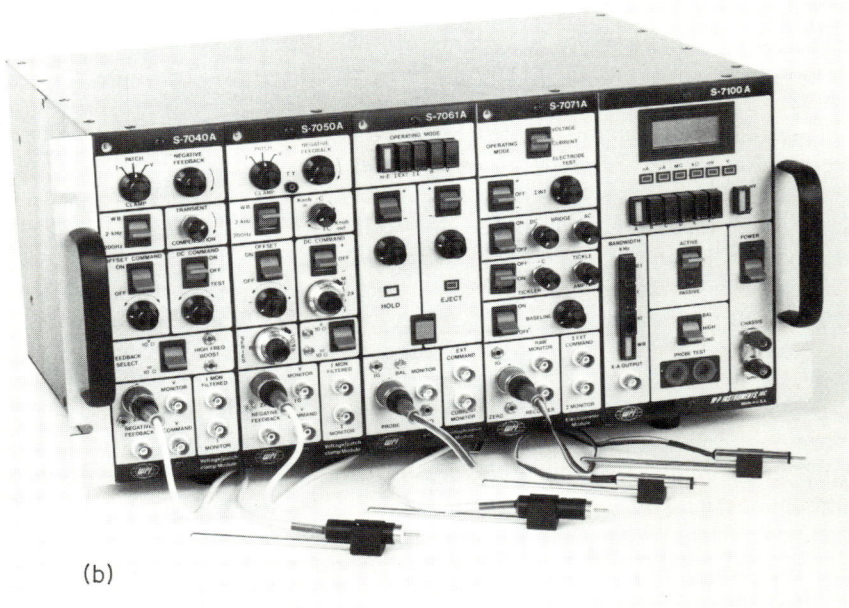

(b)

Figure 8 A photograph of (a) the Model 260 and (b) the S-7000 systems from WP Instruments. The 7000 system is a flexible modular system for electrophysiology; the 7061 module is the iontophoresis module, and up to six can be run from a single mainframe. (Reproduced by permission of World Precision Instruments, Inc.)

Equipment

If the electrode blocks and the compliance of the equipment is exceeded an 'audible alarm' will be sounded. The means available for checking the functional status of the system are: (a) by push-button selection of the channel in question (on the S-7100 control module) a readout is obtained on the 7100 LCD of the command voltage applied to the current pump. This would be of value for assessing the intactness of the command to pump connection and would be of some importance if an external command voltage were being used to drive the current pump (0.1 nA output per millivolt command); (b) by push-button selection of the R (resistance) mode on the 7061 channel in question together with push-button selection of that channel on the 7100 control module, the LCD registers the electrode resistance.

One drawback of the 7000 system is that it does not incorporate any timing facility. This is very unfortunate in view of the fact that the timing of ejection and retention is of critical importance in microiontophoretic studies (Chs. 4 and 6). The duration of ejection can be controlled by a +10 V command pulse, but this obviously requires an external (multichannel) timing device. On the other hand these external command sockets also allow the magnitude of ejecting current to be determined by an external source (1 nA/5 mV). While this would seem superfluous for the vast majority of iontophoretic experiments it does permit the programming of the ejection pulse profile. Thus a rising ramp of current, or sine wave profile may be desired for studies of receptor kinetics or desensitization. It should not, of course, be forgotten, that many factors other than current profile will have a major influence on the actual ejection of ions (see Ch. 4) and these would also need to be considered.

Finally the S-7000 claims to provide a current output accurate to within ±1% of the value displayed. This is a most valuable feature if low currents are to be used routinely.

III.2 Medical Systems Corporation

Although the WPI Model 160 was the first commercially available iontophoretic current source, the Medical Systems Neurophore holds a unique place historically because of the total control and processing system, specifically designed for microiontophoresis, of which it is a part.

The Neurophore is a mains-operated modular system based on a mainframe which includes a balance module, and a power supply. The mainframe will accommodate up to five iontophoresis (IP2) modules (Figure 9) or a mixture of these and pressure ejection modules (see below). The compliance is ±105 V. Each module boasts its own LED display, so that retention and ejection currents can be dialled up directly on each module and modified continually during the setting up of an experimental run, without the need of switching to a common meter, as in the Dagan system or monitoring an analogue output (WPI). The provision of two ranges of ejection current (0–50 nA and 0–500 nA) may be useful if very potent compounds, active in the nanoampere range, are being used interchangeably with less active compounds. During the initial setting of

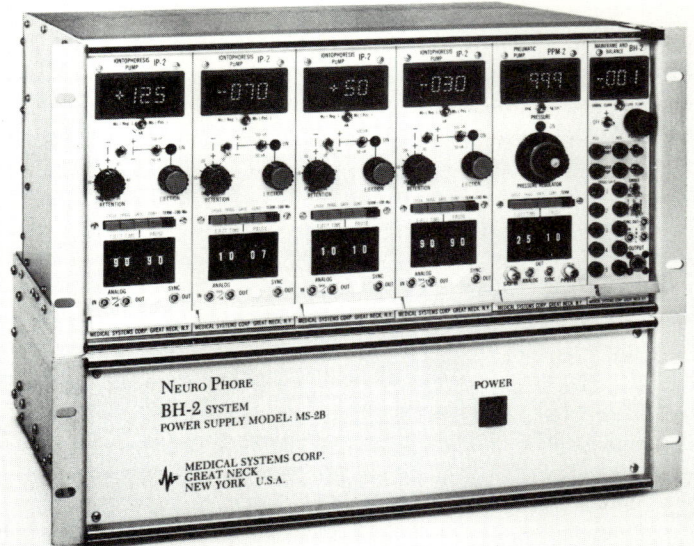

Figure 9 A photograph of the Neurophore microiontophoresis system from Medical Systems Corp. The mainframe illustrated houses four iontophoresis modules and one pressure ejection module, but any combination of iontophoresis and pressure modules can be used in the five positions. (Reproduced by permission of Medical Systems Corp.)

these currents, the output current lines may be 'terminated' into an internal load of 100 MΩ by selecting the TERM push-button. Selection of any of the other push-buttons switches the output line into the external load, usually the micropipette, seated on the end of the output lead which emerges from the balance channel module. It should be noted that the output lines from the six channels emerge through a common connector and cable from this output socket.

When the CYCLE, TRIGG or GATE functions are selected by the front panel push-buttons, a channel will rest in the Retention state. Changeover to Ejection status can then be organized as follows:

1. In CYCLE mode the duration of ejection, and retention *following* that ejection are determined by front-panel thumbwheel two-decade timing indicators. The time ranges available can be selected as 1 to 99 seconds or 10 to 990 milliseconds by a toggle switch located on the balance module, a facility which makes this apparatus useful for neuromuscular and invertebrate work as well as mammalian *in vivo* experiments.

    In addition, CYCLE mode means that after the retention period of one channel, ejection of the next channel in CYCLE mode follows automatically. Thus regular cycles of ejection and retention of up to five channels can be programmed, either in a single cycle, initiated by a push-button (CYCLE START) on the balance module, or by an input pulse delivered to

Equipment

4 mm sockets. In RECYCLE mode, selected on the balance module, the cycle of ejection/retention passes through channels 1 to 5 (those modules on CYCLE only) and the entire sequence is then repeated until the CYCLE STOP button is pressed.
2. In TRIGG mode, the timing of ejection and retention periods is determined by the thumbwheel counters on each module, but the eject phase of each module must now be initiated by an external trigger pulse delivered to the appropriate channel input sockets on the balance module.
3. In GATE mode the ejection/retention period timing is independent of the front panel controls, and is determined entirely by the duration of an external pulse applied to the appropriate sockets on the BH-2 module (Figure 9).

The duration of ejection may also be controlled manually by simply selecting the CONT button. Ejection will continue until the module is restored to the resting (retention) state by selecting CYCLE, TRIGG or GATE. Note that if none of these control switches is depressed, the channel *will* eject as if in the CONT mode!

Besides the very convenient continuous display of retaining or ejecting current passing through the micropipette, two other outputs are available from the Neurophore, an analogue output proportional to the iontophoretic current (5 mV/nA) and a SYNC output (TTL pulse) coincident with the start of the ejection and retention phases and useful for triggering oscilloscopes, signal averagers, computers, cameras, etc.

The front panel LED display has two other functions besides providing a current readout. A toggle switch immediately below the display can be displaced from its normal control central position to provide a direct indication of barrel tip resistance on the LED. Either outward or inward-going current can be selected, but it should be realized that the measurement of resistance is performed by passing a current of 50 nA through the barrel. Resistance should not, therefore, be tested during a critical experimental sequence as this imposed retention/ejection current will itself have a marked effect on ion movements.

The second use of the LED is a warning that the compliance of the apparatus is inadequate to obey the programmed command, that is, the machine cannot deliver the current level required. This usually results from a barrel becoming blocked during the course of the experiment. In this situation the LED display flashes. The numbers displayed during flashing are meaningless.

An analogue input socket is provided on each module, to allow the profiling of output current (ramp, sine wave, etc.). Comment on this feature was made in Pt. III.1 of this chapter.

III.2.a Balancing

The current output from each module is routed to the LED display panel and to a summating amplifier Σ_1 which drives the balance barrel current pump to provide a current equal to this summated value but of opposite polarity. The balance current is not displayed directly but is summed with the various channel outputs at Σ_2 before display. The balance module should, therefore, always read zero when balancing.

III.2.b Current control

The balance barrel can also be disconnected from amplifiers Σ and Σ_2 by means of a toggle switch below the display, placing the module in Current pump mode. It can now be used as a normal current pump to test the effects of current alone (as carried usually by Na^+ or Cl^- ions) on the test preparation. It can alternatively be used as a sixth iontophoretic pump module to eject drug molecules, though it would not cycle automatically, and the retention/ejection currents would need to be reset manually for each pulse. Nevertheless this is a feasible use of the BH-2 module for testing the effect of an antagonist which may require many minutes of ejection, against up to five different agonists (or doses of one agonist).

III.2.c External programming

Mention should be made here of the PDC-2 iontophoresis programmer (PDC = programmable dose/response controller). Although this can be used simply as an external timing clock to gate individual channels of the Neurophore System, its main use is as a feedback controller of drug ejection in quantitative or drug interaction studies. For example the PDC-2 will control the ejection current from a Neurophore barrel in order to achieve a preset percentage change of cell firing. This function would be most valuable for obtaining plateau responses to compounds in an attempt to obtain an estimate of relative potency (Ch. 5). The PDC-2 can also adjust continuously the ejecting current so as to maintain a constant firing rate (rate clamp mode).

III.3 Dagan

The Dagan system 6400 is illustrated in Figure 10, and consists of a mains operated mainframe capable of accommodating up to six iontophoresis channels. Unlike the WPI and Medical Systems machines, the 6400 has a compliance of only ± 50 V, providing up to 200 nA through a 200 MΩ electrode. A readout of channel current is available on an LED meter which is common to all six channels; a push-button selector is pressed to obtain a readout of current passing through a channel. The current monitor employs a FET differential amplifier to produce a floating input which makes for an accurate assessment of current while not changing the current passed.

As for the WPI equipment there is a 'block monitor': if the resistance of a barrel rises to the extent that the ± 40 V compliance is exceeded a warning light is activated both on the centre panel and on the offending channel.

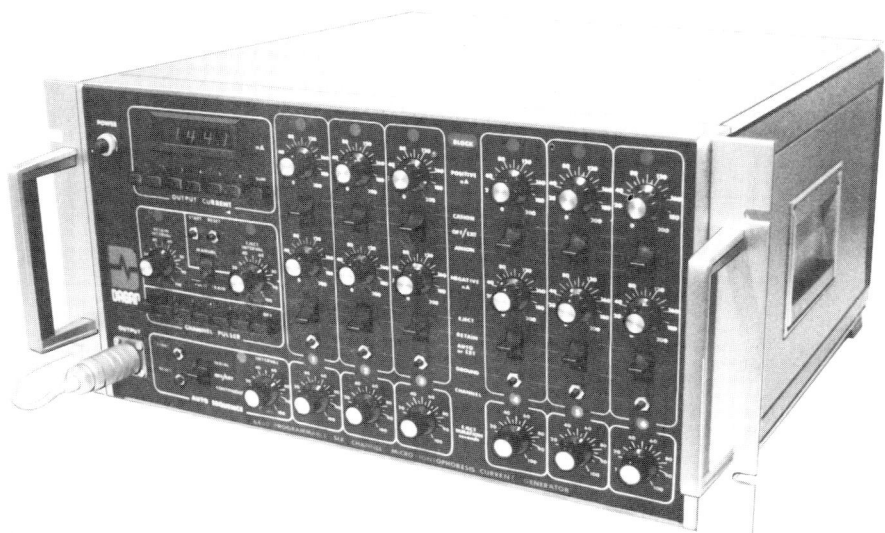

Figure 10 A photograph of the Dagan 6400 microiontophoresis system. (Reproduced by permission of Dagan Corp.)

Unlike the S-7000, however, Dagan incorporates facilities for timing the activity of the channels. A series of Channel Pulser buttons, for example, allows repeated ejections through any one selected channel, the duration of ejection and retention being determined by dials on the Channel Pulser panel. A sequence of ejections through two or more channels may be programmed by selecting the Auto Sequence mode. The duration of ejection from each channel is then determined by the Eject Duration dial at the foot of each channel panel, while the interval between ejections is determined by the Interval dial. There are two problems with this system. The first is that the interval between successive channels is necessarily constant, as it is determined by a single control. There are many examples where this is undesirable: to take one widely used example, of a sequence of excitatory amino acids and related compounds, glutamate causes a rapid but short-lasting response and neurones usually appear to recover within 10–15 seconds. A 20–30 second interval is not, therefore, unreasonable. If kainate, whose responses decline much more slowly, is used in the same sequence, however, a period of 1–2 minutes at least may be required before the next test compound. Similar timing frustrations would arise if comparing the pharmacology of rapidly acting depressants such as GABA with the more slowly acting compounds such as amines or some opiates. Of course each channel can be operated manually, or can be triggered by externally applied current into rear panel sockets. As with the WPI system, though, not all new purchasers of iontophoresis equipment will also be in a position to obtain multichannel external timing devices.

The second drawback with the Dagan timing system is the use of continuous dials. In many applications of iontophoresis it is important to know the ejection time in order quantitatively to compare drug responses, and it is important to be able to reproduce particular time intervals at random, for example when attempting to construct charge/response relationships. This is much more difficult with rotary dials than, say, thumbwheel counters.

An optional component fitted to the Dagan 6400 will permit the determination of barrel resistance, though not by merely flicking a switch as in the Medical Systems equipment. The channel of interest is first selected on the output current monitor. That channel is then set to provide a continuous ejecting current of +10 nA, while the other channels are switched off, and a push-button situated next to the LED display is depressed. The LED reading gives barrel resistance in megohms.

III.3.a Current balancing

Another option available on the Dagan machine is the Balancing Current option. This component is located inside the mainframe and provides an automatic, continuous balance current, equal in amplitude to the sum of the output currents provided at channels 1 to 6 but opposite in sign (the 'active' method). The current output from the balance channel can be monitored on the LED by depressing the SUM button It should be noted that the balance current feature cannot be switched in and out of the system at will (see Ch. 6, Pt. III).

PART IV   CURRENT INJECTION

Apart from these various units built specifically for microiontophoresis, several manufacturers produce amplifiers, usually intended for intracellular use, which incorporate or permit current injection and can, therefore, be used to iontophorese ions or dye, etc., from a recording pipette. The WP Instruments Model M-707 Microprobe, for example, delivers currents up to 5 μA on receipt of an input signal at the appropriate socket. A breakaway feature cuts out the input side of the amplifier so as to prevent damage by currents of this size.

Similarly the DC amplifier NL-102 from Neurolog incoporates a facility for the injection of up to 100 nA of current.

PART V   PRESSURE EJECTION

The pressure ejection equivalent of the Stone Age iontophoresis circuit which opened this chapter, is a cylinder of compressed gas, a length of tubing and a clip. Connecting the pressurized outflow to a micropipette and using the clip as a key will give acceptable pressure ejection. The rise time of the pressure pulse may be increased by using an electrically operated valve on the outflow line (e.g. from General Valve Corporation) and this also permits the use of an external clock to generate regular and reproducible cycles of pressure ejection.

McCaman *et al.* (1977) refer to a valve available from General Valve Corporation which exhibits a mechanical opening rise time of only 2 ms. However, it is important to note that while the rapidity of rise time of the valve may give intellectually satisfying square wave pressure pulses at the calibration stage, and may be useful if an *in vitro* system is being studied in which the micropipette tip is distanced from the target membrane by a layer of fluid, it is of little import for studies *in vivo*. Indeed as will be pointed out later (Ch. 6) some kind of flexible tubing has to be inserted into most microwave systems in order to dampen the mechanical disturbance which results from too acute a pulse rise time.

If a more sophisticated system is required, there seem to be three varieties of pressure ejection equipment available commercially.

V.1 Medical Systems

One of the outstanding advantages of the Neurophore system described above (Pt. III.2, this chapter) is that iontophoretic modules can be replaced at will by PPM-2 Pneumatic Pressure ejection modules, and any combination of pressure and iontophoresis units used as desired. The pressure ejection modules can also be used in a separate mainframe (PPS-2) which accommodates up to four pressure modules but not the iontophoresis modules. In either mainframe the timing of the pressure pulse can be controlled by CYCLE, TRIGG, GATE or CONT push-button selectors exactly analogous to those described above (Pt. III.2) for the IP-2 iontophoresis modules, in conjunction with two-decade thumbwheel timer selectors (Figure 9). A TERM selector provides for passing the pressure pulse into a dummy load for initial setting up. Available pressures range up to 100 p.s.i. (7.8 kg/cm^2). For monitoring the output an analogue voltage is available which is proportional to the output pressure (10 mV/p.s.i.) as well as a SYNC TTL pulse coincident with the start and finish of the pressure pulse.

V.2 WP Instruments

A model 1400EC nanolitre pump is a self-contained hydraulic pump available from WP Instruments. This is designed primarily for the ejection through micropipettes of volumes in the nanolitre range. (**NB** 1 nanolitre is a 100 μm sided cube and, therefore, somewhat larger than normally employed for pressure ejection studies of single cells.) Nevertheless the rate of pumping can be as low as 2 nl/min and can be accurately gated by a +5 V external timing command. It may be feasible to use this machine for ejecting volumes of tens of picolitres, though the rise time of the pumping pulse may be a limiting factor. It would be essential to ensure, under microscopic control, that the amount and time-course of an ejection pulse was adequate for the intended experiment. Fluid delivery can be achieved from micropipettes of tip size 2 to 10 μm.

V.3 The Picospritzer

The Picospritzer is a dedicated pressure microejection system from General Valve corporation (USA) which incorporates a valve system of rise time about 2 ms as well as timing facilities.

PART VI RECORDING

Electrophysiological recording, whether of EEG, evoked potentials or single units, extracellularly or intracellularly, is now so widely used a technique that a detailed discussion in a volume devoted to microiontophoresis would be wholly inappropriate; there will be very few readers of this book, contemplating microiontophoresis, who do not have some experience of single cell electrophysiology. For those people with limited experience the texts by Bureš *et al.* (1967), Thompson and Patterson (1973) and Purves (1981) should be consulted for practical advice. Nevertheless, many of the comments in Chapter 2 of this book apply equally to the preparation of recording electrodes, and Chapter 5 deals in some detail with the processing and analysis of recorded data in microiontophoretic experiments. The ready availability of a vast range (in terms of technical specifications and cost) of recording equipment from commercial sources has all but eliminated the need for home-made apparatus other than as a practical exercise.

CHAPTER 4

The Release of Compounds from Micropipettes and the Tissue Concentrations Achieved

I Spontaneous Efflux	39
II Retention	41
III Ejection by Microiontophoresis	45
III.1 Transport Numbers	45
III.1.a Measurement	45
III.1.b Values of t	48
III.2 The Quantities Released	49
III.3 Time-Course of Ejection	52
III.4 Other Considerations Affecting Iontophoretic Ejection	56
III.4.a Electrodes	56
III.4.b Receiving Medium	57
III.4.c Acidity	58
III.4.d Filling Method	59
III.4.e Ageing	59
III.4.f Effect of Drug Concentration	60
IV Electro-Osmosis	62
IV.1 Effect of Drug Concentration	63
V Ejection by Pressure	64
VI Ionic Movements and Tissue Concentrations after Iontophoresis	68

PART I SPONTANEOUS EFFLUX

At the tip orifice of a micropipette a number of factors will tend to cause some spontaneous efflux of active compound into the surrounding medium. The most obvious of these is diffusion, and since the more readily available compounds are sometimes used at concentrations of 0.1 to 1 M, it may often also be a quantitatively important factor.

Purves (1977) has shown that the amount of diffusional release, of q_D mol s^{-1} may be expressed in terms of the radius of the tip orifice, r, the angle θ between the barrel walls (the included angle) and the concentration C of compound in the pipette by the expression:

$$q_D = \pi D C \tan \theta \, r \qquad (\text{I.1})$$

D being the diffusion coefficient. The same author emphasized subsequently (Purves, 1981) that this equation implies that for a 3 M solution of compound whose diffusion coefficient is $1\,\mu m^2\,ms^{-1}$, diffusional efflux from a tip of internal diameter $0.4\,\mu m$ and included angle of 8° would approach 130 fmol s^{-1}.

A second factor causing unwanted drug leakage is the bulk flow of fluid caused by the hydrostatic pressure of several centimetres of water. Curtis (1964) has calculated that a 5 cm high column of saline would produce an efflux of around 500 fl s^{-1} from a barrel with a $5\,\mu m$ internal tip diameter. A similar estimate was derived by Purves (1981) for a barrel having an internal tip diameter of $0.4\,\mu m$ and an included angle of 8°. For a column height of 2 cm of a 3 M solution of compound the hydrostatic efflux was calculated as 390 fmol s^{-1} which corresponds to a fluid volume of 130 fl s^{-1}. When it is considered that this hydrostatic efflux is equivalent to a cube of side $10\,\mu m$ every 10 seconds, and that the drug efflux is equivalent to that produced by an iontophoretic current of 75 nA (Purves, 1981) it becomes clear that this is not a negligible factor. Of course the hydrostatic efflux will be opposed to a large extent by the forces of capillarity and, since fluid flow through a pipette tip is a function of the third power of the radius, decreasing tip size will have a particularly marked effect in reducing this efflux.

The simplest way of reducing the amount of spontaneously released substance is to use the most dilute solutions compatible with generating iontophoretic responses. In many experiments, particularly those involving isolated tissues, it may be possible to eliminate entirely the interference due to hydrostatic forces by the simple expedient of plugging the open end of the barrel and mounting the assembly horizontally. This possibility should never be overlooked, as the resting efflux of solution for an extended period of time may be quite sufficient to produce marked distortion of a tissue independently of its dissolved drug.

Actual values obtained for spontaneous leakage from pipettes vary enormously for different compounds and in different laboratories but in general they lie in the range 1 fmol s^{-1} to 1 pmol s^{-1}, for solutions in the 0.1 to 1 M concentration range, in reasonable accord with the theoretical values mentioned above. Most authors do not distinguish between that component of spontaneous efflux attributable to diffusion and that due to hydrostatic pressure, though Krnjević et al. (1963a) did suggest that the latter factor would be appreciably more significant than the former in the case of the relatively large-tipped pipettes used for iontophoresis (over $0.4\,\mu m$).

Armstrong-James et al. (1981) obtained values for the spontaneous leakage of dopamine from 0.1 M solutions in the range 15-87 fmols s^{-1}, though the size of pipette tip is not clear.

Blatt and Slayman (1983) have recently studied in some detail the leakage of ions from intracellular micropipettes of tip diameter 0.2-$0.3\,\mu m$ (50-57 MΩ) filled with 1 M KCl. The leakage was around 4-5 fmol s^{-1} in excellent agreement with a theoretical value of 1.8 fmol s^{-1} from a $0.1\,\mu m$ tip (Purves,

1981). The authors point out that intracellular K^+ concentrations with these pipettes could rise at the rate of 70 mM min^{-1} as a result of this leakage.

PART II RETENTION

In order to minimize such spontaneous drug efflux it is customary to apply a small current, variously referred to as holding, retaining, braking or backing current, of such polarity that it will tend to retain the active ion within the micropipette. Considerable argument has arisen over the most appropriate value for retaining currents. Curtis (1964) referred to optimal retaining currents being 'just adequate' to prevent the spontaneous efflux described above but qualified this by later noting that 'it is probable that absolute control of the diffusional and hydrostatic efflux is rarely obtained by the retaining potentials which are used'.

In spite of the caution implicit in this last statement most authors seem to obtain a substantial reduction of spontaneous release, below readily detectable levels, by using retaining currents of 5–25 nA. Obata et al. (1970), however, reported that in cases where the spontaneous release (of GABA) was around 1 to 300 fmol s^{-1}, retaining currents as high as 5000 nA produced no diminution. Retaining currents of the usual order were effective in controlling release from pipettes with somewhat coarser tips which exhibited spontaneous release of several picomoles per second.

Related observations were made by Bradshaw et al. (1973) who found that low retaining currents would greatly reduce the spontaneous efflux of noradrenaline from pipettes (Figure 11). However, even much higher retaining currents were unable to abolish that release entirely.

Bradshaw and Szabadi (1974) have attempted to provide a conceptual framework for the appreciation of the effects of retaining current within a microelectrode tip. Starting from the position in which a barrel is filled with solution and the tip is immersed in an external medium the authors point out that diffusion from the barrel orifice into that medium will establish a concentration gradient within the tip. The region occupied by that gradient is referred to as the interphase layer. The application of a retaining current will initiate a movement of ions throughout the barrel (Figure 12) which will have an immediate effect in preventing the diffusional efflux of a proportion of ions at the extreme barrel tip, hence there will be an immediate sharp drop in diffusional release at t_o (Figure 12). The continued withdrawal of ions by retaining current will progressively increase the thickness of the interphase layer (by withdrawing ions from the adjacent bulk solution) and correspondingly decrease the concentration of ions at the barrel tip. Bradshaw and Szabadi (1974) thus conclude that any retaining current, no matter how small, would eventually produce a drug-free region region at the barrel tip. On this basis the authors postulate a 'minimum retention time', T_{min}, defined as the minimum time for which a given retaining current must be applied in order to reduce the ionic concentration at the barrel orifice to zero, that is, to stop diffusional efflux.

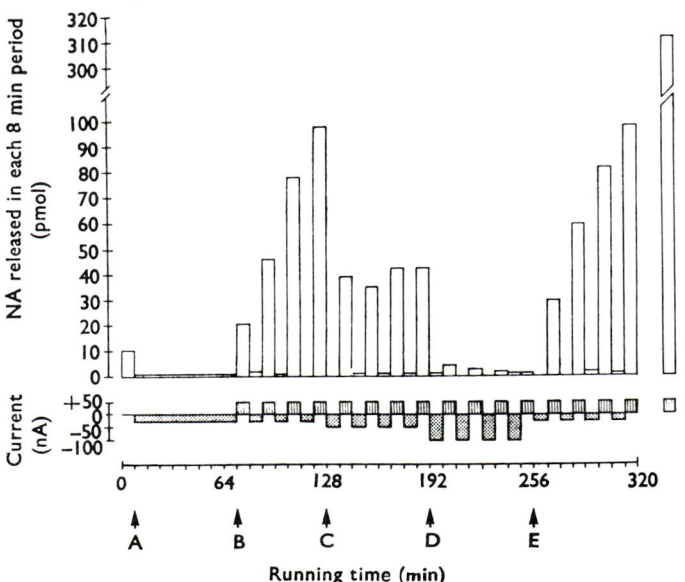

Figure 11 The effect of various retaining currents upon the electrophoretic release of noradrenaline (NA) from four barrels of micropipette No.8. Lower graph: electrophoretic current applied to each of the four NA-containing barrels. (▨), retaining current; (▥), ejecting current. Upper graph: release of NA during each 8 min period of sample collection. Ejecting and retaining currents were applied alternately: the parameters (intensity and duration) of the ejecting pulse were kept constant throughout the study. Changes in the parameters of the applied currents are indicated by capital letters under the time base. After a prolonged application of a retaining current (A–B), successive ejecting pulses (B–C) evoked progressively greater outputs. Increases in the intensity of the retaining current reduced the amount of NA released by the ejecting pulse (C–D), (D–E). Restoration of the original retaining pulse (E) was followed by progressively increasing outputs. Control (output during an ejecting pulse not preceded by a retaining pulse) is shown at the right of the figure. (Reproduced from Bradshaw *et al.*, 1973, by permission of the British Pharmacological Society.)

An expression was also derived which related the hypothetical $T_{\min}$ to the diffusion coefficient D, ionic concentration c, valency z, retaining current i, transport number t and tip radius r, by the expression

$$T_{\min} = \frac{Dc^2z^2F^2\pi^2r^4}{i^2t^2} \qquad (\text{II}.1)$$

For a given substance, therefore, retention will be more rapidly effective the lower the concentration. Reducing tip diameter would also have a particularly marked effect on retention characteristics.

The postulate that any retaining current will eventually stop diffusional loss may not be strictly true, particularly when concentrated solutions are being used,

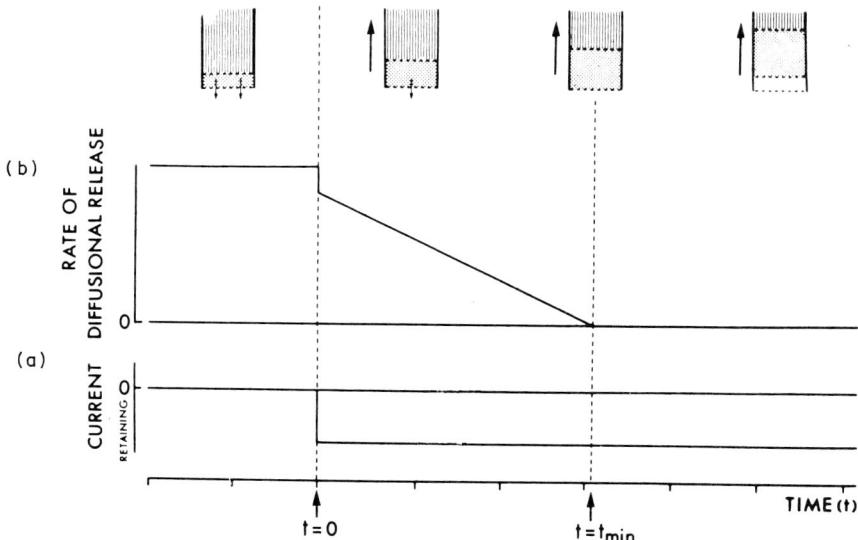

Figure 12 Hypothetical decrease in the rate of diffusional release from a micropipette in the presence of a retaining current. (a) Electrophoretic current; (b) rate of diffusional release. The positions of the concentration layers within the micropipette are shown at the top of the figure. In the presence of the retaining current the rate of diffusional release decreases in time; for the sake of simplicity this is shown as a linear function. (Reproduced from Bradshaw and Szabadi, 1974, by permission of Pergamon Press Ltd.)

since there will always be a value of retaining current at which the electrical gradient is in equilibrium with the oppositely directed concentration (diffusion) gradient. There would then be a limit on the level to which the upper edge of the interphase layer could rise and consequently on the extent of depletion attainable at the barrel tip. With this modification the T_{min} value derived by Bradshaw and Szabadi (1974) would still retain much of its practical significance, except that it would not now necessarily refer to the minimum time to achieve zero diffusional efflux but the minimum time to achieve a minimal diffusional efflux at that particular retaining current. The same mathematical description (equation II.1) would still apply. This modification of the Bradshaw and Szabadi (1974) model is more in accord with the conclusion of Purves (1977) that finite retaining currents can never suppress entirely the spontaneous leakage from micropipettes. The theoretical curves constructed by Purves (1981) and illustrated in Figure 13 indicated that retaining currents should nevertheless substantially curtail diffusional leakage, especially (relatively) for solutions more concentrated than $w = 0.1$ (i.e. about 20 mM; w is the ratio of the concentration of drug solution in the pipette to the overall molar concentration of the external medium).

It should not be forgotten when considering retention that other factors may contribute significantly to ionic movements within a barrel tip. For example

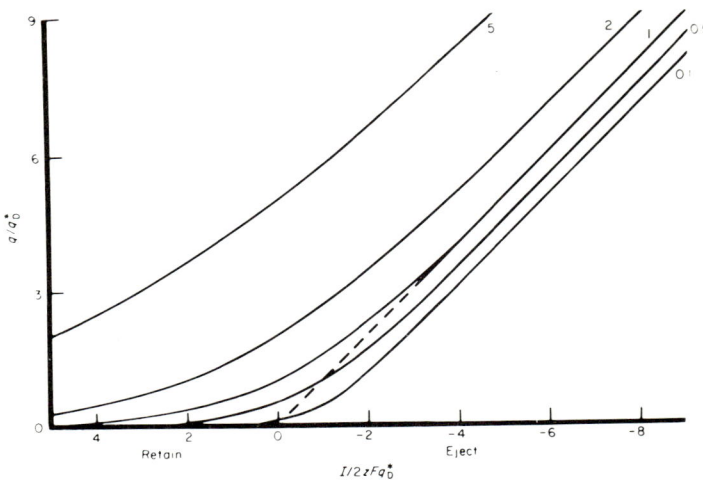

Figure 13 Theoretical relation between current flow and drug release from ionophoretic pipettes, calculated from equation (III.3). Numbers against curves are values of W. The interrupted line is the ideal relation $q = -I/2zF$. (Reproduced with permission from *Microelectrode Methods for Intracellular Recording and Ionophoresis* (Purves, 1981). Copyright: Academic Press Ltd.)

an outward (positive) retaining current will tend to restrain the diffusional loss of an anion by the mechanisms described above, but will also cause some ejection of bulk solution by electro-osmosis (see Pt. IV this chapter). It might be predicted that an extremely complex system of equilibria will be established; Obata *et al.* (1970) observed that a net ejection of (anionic) glutamate was often achieved during the application of outward (positive) supposedly retaining current. It is clearly especially important when studying substances to be retained by positive currents to use the most dilute solutions possible, in order to minimize electro-osmotic ejection.

Using the carbon fibre method of analysis (see Pt. III.1.a, this chapter), Armstrong-James *et al.* (1981) made the interesting observation that spontaneous leakage from the micropipettes could be controlled by applying a suitable retaining current, though the 'adequate' current ranged from less than 10 nA to more than 100 nA in different cases.

It should also be noted that the foregoing considerations neglect the contribution of hydrostatic efflux which, as discussed above, may be a dominant factor in determining resting leakage for barrels with tip diameters greater than about 0.5 μm.

In practical terms the size of retaining current needed to control spontaneous leakage may be determined by increasing the current in a series of steps, allowing a reasonable period of perhaps 15 minutes for equilibrium to be re-established within the pipette tip, until a level is reached at which no change of firing rate, or membrane potential is observed. This may not, of course, mean that all spontaneous leakage has ceased, merely that any residual loss is insufficient to produce an observable biological response. Factors such as desensitization, accommodation, or the fact that the concentrations achieved are subthreshold may all contribute to this situation. The importance of this point is that, even with the use of an apparently effective retaining current, enough compound may still be released to cause changes in the responses to other compounds by desensitization, antagonism, potentiation, etc.

PART III EJECTION BY MICROIONTOPHORESIS

III.1 Transport numbers

The total flux of ions in a solution, produced by 1 farad of charge (96 500 coulombs) is M/Z where M is the molecular weight and Z the valency. The molar flux Q, produced by current I is

$$Q = \frac{It}{FZ} \qquad (\text{III}.1)$$

where t is the transport number, the fraction of applied current carried by the particular ion. Ideally this simple relationship would describe the ejection of ions from micropipettes by an applied iontophoretic current, but unfortunately a number of factors conspire to reduce the practical reliability of the equation including the contribution to drug ejection made by electro-osmosis (see Pt. IV, this chapter) and the experimentally demonstrated variability of the transport number.

If any attempt at quantification of iontophoretic data is to be performed, for example in attempting to assess the relative potency of two compounds, it is necessary to eliminate as much of this variability as possible or at least minimize its contribution to the overall pattern of results. A major step towards this is to use as large a number of electrodes as possible in order to average out the effects of random variations of ejection characteristics.

An equally important step would be to determine directly the transport number for the ion of interest. Concluding that two compounds are equipotent on the basis of current or charge comparisons using 20 electrodes on 100 cells means nothing if one compound consistently has a transport number only one-tenth of the second substance.

III.1.a Measurement

The barrels to be tested are filled with a solution containing the compound of interest. Some of the first attempts to determine transport numbers employed bioassay, photometric or fluorimetric detection for acetylcholine, amines and amino acids (Krnjević *et al.*, 1963a,b; Curtis, 1964). The most satisfactory means of determining transport numbers is to use the radioactively labelled compound provided this can be obtained in a sufficiently pure form, as this provides the most sensitive means of detection. Relatively low iontophoretic currents and ejection times can, therefore, be used, more akin to those used under experimental conditions. Alternatively it may be useful to use a simple inorganic cation such as $^{24}Na^+$ to assess the characteristics of all electrodes before filling with drugs, particularly expensive ones, in order to eliminate barrels with poor ejection characteristics. Similarly, it may be desirable to check electrode properties when a new batch of glass blanks is obtained.

The micropipette is then usually arranged such that the tip is immersed in a small volume of solution, typically 0.5 ml of 200 mM NaCl. In some cases blocks of agar, or of brain have been used as the ejection medium. The protocol adopted in most studies is to leave the pipette with no applied current for periods ranging from a few minutes to a few hours, after which the ejection medium is analysed for the compound of interest. The pipette is transferred to fresh medium and iontophoretic current passed for an appropriate period of time. The combination of ejecting current and time needed to produce a measurable release of compound will depend on the ejection characteristics of the pipettes, the nature of the ejection medium, the concentration and, if radiolabelled, the specific activity of solution in the pipette. It is usually wise to perform a pilot experiment using four or five currents up to 250 nA for 60 minutes, in order to determine the adequacy of the system and to define a workable range of iontophoretic charge.

As recently pointed out by Bradshaw *et al.* (1981) it is also possible to use relatively low iontophoretic currents to determine the relative transport numbers of compounds which are not themselves radioactive, by calculating the effect which their presence has on the apparent transport number of a reference labelled compound or isotope. Thus the 'apparent' transport number of labelled noradrenaline was reduced from 0.333 to 0.119 in the presence of methoxamine and to 0.125 in the presence of equimolar phenylephrine. It was concluded that the contributions made by the unlabelled compounds to current flow, i.e. their transport numbers were similar. The method is clearly applicable to any combination of labelled and unlabelled compounds.

Armstrong-James *et al.* (1981) and Kruk *et al.* (1980) have adapted the principles of electrochemical detection, now frequently used in the biochemical analysis of amine concentrations, to the iontophoretic case. Electrical contact is made to a carbon fibre contained within a micropipette barrel. During the application of a positive going voltage pulse to this fibre, catecholamines in the vicinity are oxidized and the lost electrons set up a flow of current in the fibre. Figure 14 illustrates the voltage waveform used and the increase in peak current obtained when the electrode tip is placed in solution containing 10 μM dopamine. Non-linear current–concentration curves could be constructed for dopamine (Millar *et al.*, 1981), noradrenaline (Armstrong-James *et al.*, 1981) and 5-hydroxytryptamine (Kruk *et al.*, 1980).

These electrode assemblies were then used to examine the efflux of catecholamine from micropipettes by applying maintained currents and measuring the steady state concentration of catecholamine achieved in a large

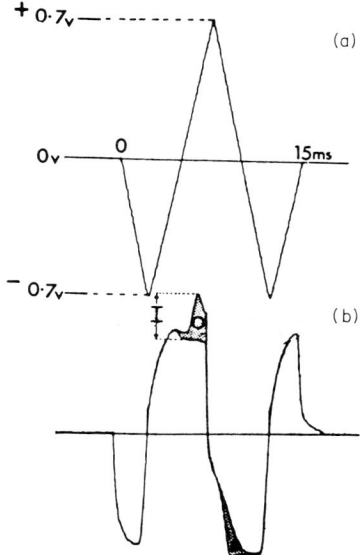

Figure 14 Carbon fibre electrode voltage and current waveform. (a) The time-course and amplitude of the standard driving voltage waveform used. (b) The resultant current waveform through the carbon fibre working electrode. (a) and (b) are on the same timescale. The smaller trace in (b) shows the current observed in saline. The larger trace shows the current observed in 1×10^{-5} M dopamine in saline. The areas between the two curves are stippled for clarity. I = the peak oxidizing current increment. The slight irregularities in (a) are due to the limitations of the digital oscilloscope. The current signals in this and subsequent figures were measured in arbitrary units. (The peak-to-peak saline control current signal is approximately 2μA in most cases.) (Reproduced from Armstrong-James et al., 1981, by permission of Elsevier Biomedical Press B.V.)

volume of saline. This concentration would clearly be dependent both on the rate of iontophoretic ejection and on the extent of diffusion of the released amine. Nevertheless a form of calibration curve could be constructed relating the ejecting current to the final external amine concentration, as illustrated in Figure 15. In common with many other groups it was found that the amount of amine released by any given current could vary between pipettes by at least an order of magnitude.

By ejecting dopamine from 100 mM solutions into small and accurately known volumes of saline (5–15μl) and measuring the concentration achieved, the total amount of amine ejected by a given electrical charge could also be determined. From these figures the transport number (apparent) was calculated to range from 0.117 to 0.355. The ejection of dopamine from 0.1 M solution was found to yield a concentration of approximately 10 μM around the micropipette tip (Millar et al., 1981).

The application of these electrochemical detection electrodes to the correlation of noradrenaline concentration with responses is discussed in Chapter 7, Part VIII.

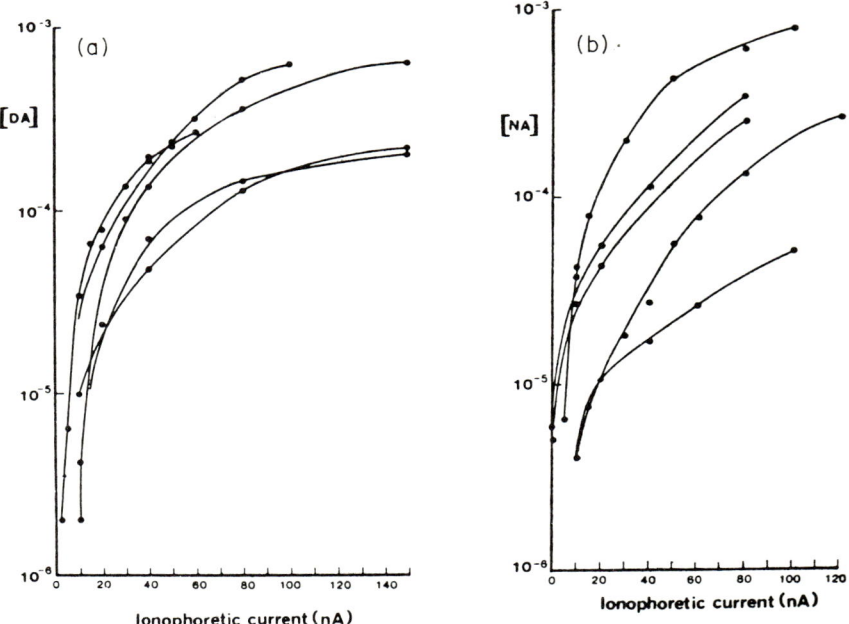

Figure 15 Ionophoresis calibration curves. From data shown elsewhere in this paper, calibration curves relating dopamine concentration at the electrode tip *in vitro* to ionophoretic current could be constructed. (a) Five curves for five carbon fibre microelectrodes with dopamine in the ionophoretic barrel. (b) A similar set of curves for five noradrenaline-containing electrodes. (Reproduced from Armstrong-James *et al.*, 1981, by permission of Elsevier Biomedical Press B.V.)

III.1.b Values of t

Among the first published estimates of transport numbers were those for acetylcholine ejected from 3 M solutions from single or multibarrelled pipettes (t = 0.42) Krnjević *et al.*, 1963a) and for a series of amines (Krnjević *et al.*, 1963b). Subsequently many authors have determined the transport numbers of ions, using a wide range of detection techniques from bioassay to the use of radioactively labelled molecules, and some of the values obtained are given in Table 1. A common finding in all these studies has been the immense variability between micropipettes and even between different barrels of any one multibarrelled pipette, emphasizing again the crucial importance of using a number of electrodes before drawing any conclusions about a compound's activity or inactivity.

Hoffer *et al.* (1971a) reported that while the transport number for noradrenaline was independent of the ejection parameters when the collecting medium was saline, it progressively increased in size when ejecting into brain.

These authors quote in support results from a pipette for which the noradrenaline transport number was 0.015 after 1 minute of ejection by 125 nA, but which rose to 0.052 after 2 minutes and 0.058 after 3 minutes. The reason for this variation was not clear, though it was presumably not attributable to the 40 nA retaining current which should have similarly affected ejection into saline.

III.2 The quantities released

Purves (1981) has derived an expression for the drug efflux q, produced by an iontophoretic current I which may be written as follows:

$$q = \frac{-It}{zF(1 - \exp[It/zFq_D])} \qquad (III.2)$$

where z is valency, t the transport number and q_D the diffusional efflux (equation I.1). This equation can be plotted graphically, as in Figure 13 for $W = 1$. The term W was introduced by Purves in an attempt to take account of differences between the molar concentration of solution in the pipette barrel and that of the external medium. Equation III.2 represents the case when these are equal, i.e. $W = 1$. For situations where the concentrations are not equal,

$$q = \frac{-It/zF + K}{1 - \exp[-(1 + It/zFK)\ln W]} \qquad (III.3)$$

giving rise to the family of curves shown in Figure 13 where W is the ratio of the concentration of solution in the pipette to the concentration of the external medium. The term K is $q_D^*(1 - W)$, q_D^* being the diffusional efflux when $W = 1$.

It is apparent in Figure 13 that at low ejecting currents (plotted as $I/2zF\, q_D^*$, assuming $t = 0.5$) the relationship between applied current and efflux is not linear. Purves (1981) calculates that the linear portion of the curves should be reached by ejecting voltages of 200 mV or greater, i.e. 2 nA through a 100 MΩ barrel. At these levels, therefore, release is directly proportional to applied current, and has the same relationship independent of W.

The non-linearities in these various predictions are due to the dilution of solution in the extreme barrel tip as a result of diffusional efflux of active material as well as diffusional influx of other substances from the external medium.

Most experimental studies of the iontophoretic release of compounds have shown an apparently linear relationship between current and efflux, but these studies have usually employed relatively large currents applied for several minutes, and it may well be impossible to detect the non-linearities under these conditions. Another factor in this apparent discrepancy is that the above theoretical discussion ignores any contribution by electro-osmosis which may account for a significant fraction of drug release by outward (positive) current.

Nevertheless, Purves (1981) has made the highly pertinent comment that the current efflux non-linearities apparent in Figure 13 could lead to serious errors

Table 1 Sample values of t, the transport number, on iontophoretic ejection

Compound	Concn	pH	t	Polarity	Reference
Acetylcholine	3 M		0.42	+	Krnjević et al. (1963a)
	1 M		0.3–0.5	+	Curtis (1964)
Noradrenaline	1%		0.09	+	Bradley and Candy (1970)
	10%		0.15	+	Bradley and Candy (1970)
	0.5 M		0.229 (radiochemical)	+	Sasa et al. (1978)
			0.153 (fluorimetric)		
	0.2 M	3.5	0.155		Barasi and Roberts (1977)
	1.7 M	3–4	0.35	+	Krnjević et al. (1963b)
	0.5 M		0.05–3	+	Hoffer et al. (1971a)
	50 mM	3.3	0.333		Bradshaw et al. (1981)
Dopamine	0.2 M	3.5	0.392	+	Barasi and Roberts (1977)
	0.1 M	3	0.117–0.355	+	Amstrong-James et al. (1981)
5-Hydroxytryptamine	0.13 M	3–4	0.10–0.18 (4)	+	Krnjević et al. (1963b)
	1%		0.18-(small tip)	+	Bradley and Candy (1970)
			0.33 (large tip)		
LSD	50 mM	4	0.219	+	Haigler and Aghajanian (1974)
	1 mM in NaCl		0.0023	+	Haigler and Aghajanian (1974)
L-Glutamate	0.1 M		0.02	–	Bradley and Candy (1970)
	2 M	8	0.22	–	Hall et al. (1979)
	0.1–1 M	8–5.9	0.3–0.6	–	Curtis (1964)
DL-glutamate	1 M	7	0.2–0.5	–	Zieglgänsberger et al. (1969)
Aspartate	0.1 M		0.126	–	Obata et al. (1970)
Kainate	0.1 M (in water, or 20 and 50 mM in NaCl)		0.28	–	Hall et al. (1979)
GABA	1 M	2.5	0.24	–	Hall et al. (1979)
		7.0	0.223	+	
		12.0	30.0	+	
			0.039	–	Obata et al. (1970)

Compound	Concentration	pH	Value	±	Reference
Glycine	0.5 M	1.4	0.135	+	
		5.9	0.695	+	
		12.7	0.024	−	
	0.5 M	2.3	0.281	+	Zieglgänsberger et al. (1974)
		6.9	0.152	+	
		9.6	0.074	−	
	0.5 M in phosphate buffer	2.2	0.283	+	Zieglgänsberger et al. (1974)
		6.7	0.531	−	
		9.5	0.132	−	
Strychnine	Saturated		0.5	+	Zieglgänsberger et al. (1974)
Substance P	7 mM	5–7	0.16	+	Curtis (1964)
	2.7 mM alone; in 170 mM Na⁺	5	0.016	+	Krnjević and Morris (1974)
			0.0008	+	Guyenet et al. (1979)
	0.8 mM in NaCl	5	0.0003	+	Belcher and Ryall (1977)
Prostaglandin E_1	20 mM	7	0.027		
	530 mM		0.069	+	Coceani and Viti (1972)
Cyclic AMP	0.5 M	4–7.3	0.482	−	Shoemaker et al. (1975)
ADP	10 mM		0.007	+	Begent and Born (1970)
17β-oestradiol	1%		0.281	+	Kelley et al. (1977)
Morphine	50 mM	4.2	0.051	+	Bradley and Dray (1974)
			0.140 (5 barrels)	−	Hosford et al. (1981)
			0.107 (7 barrels)	+	
Levallorphan	11 mM	4.4	0.074	+	Zieglgänsberger et al. (1974)
Met-enkephalin	10 mM	4.2	0.076 (5 barrels)	+	Hosford et al. (1981)
			0.031 (7 barrels)		
Chlorpromazine	20 mM	4.2	0.086	+	Zieglgänsberger et al. (1974)
Atropine	10 mM	3.7	0.131	+	Zieglgänsberger et al. (1974)
Imipramine	2 mM	4.5	0.046	+	Zieglgänsberger et al. (1974)
Haloperidol	6.7 mM	4.2	0.068	+	Zieglgänsberger et al. (1974)
Na 24	165 mM		0.27–0.37	+	Clarke et al. (1973)
Sucrose	0.32 M		70.4	+	Krnjević and Whittaker (1965)

III.3 Time-course of ejection

It has been noted above that the application of a retaining current will not merely prevent ions passing out of the pipette tip into the surrounding medium, but will also tend to deplete the tip solution of ions. While the use of a retaining current is thus essential in order to reduce the cellular responses, subliminal or otherwise, and desensitization, which may result from the uncontrolled spontaneous efflux of a potent compound or one used at high concentration, retaining currents can produce considerable complications when interpreting the time-course of drug effects in response to iontophoretic ejection.

Clarke et al. (1973) were among the first authors to examine directly the effect of retaining current on the efflux produced by a subsequent ejecting current. For this they chose to use $^{24}Na^+$ which was available at much higher specific activity than compounds such as glutamate or GABA.

The main findings of Clarke et al. (1973) are illustrated in Figure 16. Using a constant retaining current of 25 nA, there is clearly a substantial delay before a measurable release of $^{24}Na^+$ occurs during the subsequent passage of ejecting current (Figure 16). Although 25 nA is on the upper edge of the range of retaining currents often used in practice it should be noted that many of the neuroactive excitatory and inhibitory amino acids (glutamate, aspartate, N-methyl-aspartate, homocysteate, GABA, glycine) and related compounds (quisqualate, muscimol) produce marked changes of neuronal activity within a few seconds at ejecting currents of the order of those used by Clarke et al. (1973), and many other compounds (amines, peptides) act over periods of the order of 10-100 seconds. For all these compounds then, it becomes extremely hazardous to construct extensive dose-response curves on the basis of response size for a given charge passed if relatively high retaining currents are in use. This would apply particularly to the study of antagonist selectivity, since the shift of the dose-response curve will not be proportional simply to the degree of antagonism, but will depend in part on the value of retention current. As will be discussed later (Ch. 5) the problem is reduced by studying plateau responses and is also reflected in the use of time-response curves in the time-course analysis by Hill and Simmonds (1973).

A detailed experimental analysis of this same problem, but for noradrenaline, was conducted by Bradshaw et al. (1973) and is illustrated by the example of Figure 11. This group showed that the amount of noradrenaline released by repeated use of the same ejection current was highly dependent on the pre-existing retention current. Thus in Figure 11 the noradrenaline released by a 50 nA ejecting current was reduced from approximately 320 pmol per 8 minutes in the absence of retaining current to around 1 pmol per 8 minutes with a retaining current of 100 nA. A 50 nA retaining current reduced the amount of noradrenaline ejected subsequently to 10% of that obtained without retention.

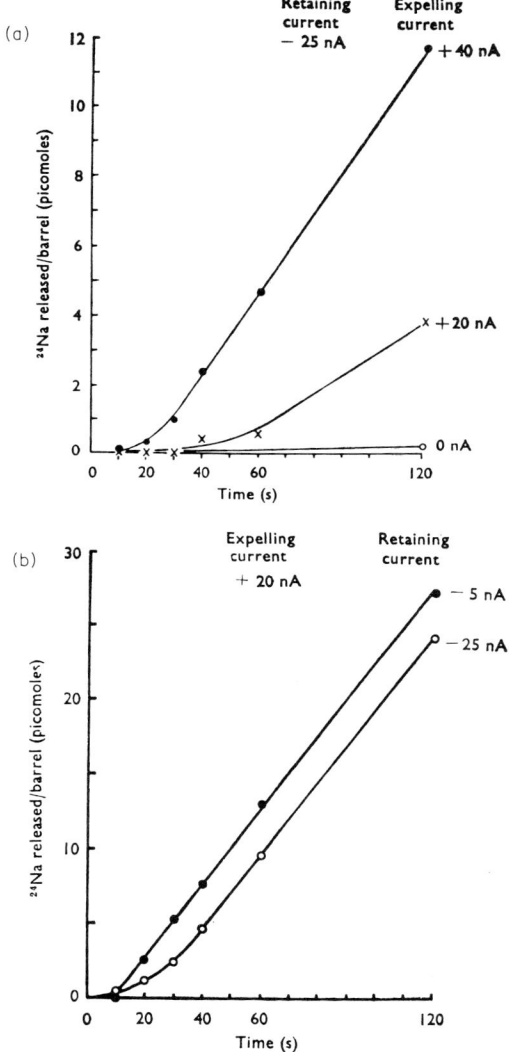

Figure 16 (a) Microiontophoretic release of $^{24}Na^+$ into rat cerebral cortex *in vitro*. Each point is the mean release/barrel from five barrels of a glass micropipette due to the passage of +40 nA (●), +20 nA (×) or 0 nA (○) through each barrel for the time shown. Before each period of release, a retaining current of −25 nA was passed through each barrel for 60 seconds. There was no detectable release of $^{24}Na^+$ during the passage of retaining current. (b) Microiontophoretic release of $^{24}Na^+$ into 0.9% NaCl solution. Each point is the mean release/barrel from five barrels of a glass micropipette due to the passage of +20 nA through each barrel for the time shown. Before each period of release, a retaining current of −25 nA (○) or −5 nA (●) was passed through each barrel for 60 seconds. With this pipette, measurable amounts of $^{24}Na^+$ diffused from the tip during the retaining period at both currents. (Reproduced from Clarke *et al.*, 1973, by permission of the British Pharmacological Society.)

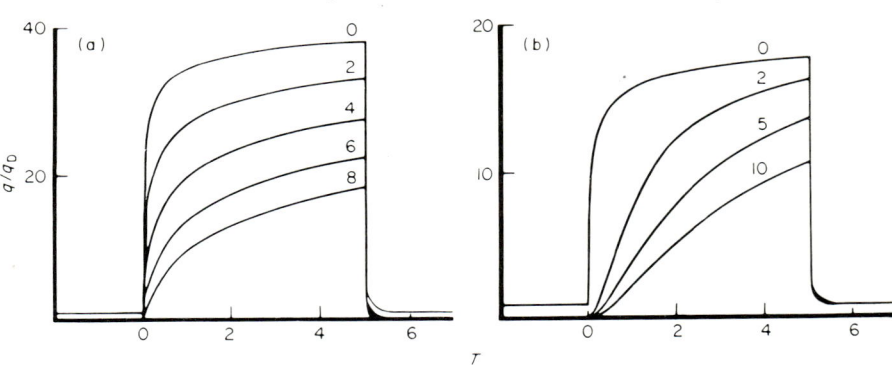

Figure 17 Computed time-course of ejection of drug from an iontophoretic pipette. The time-scale is given by the dimensionless variable $T = Dt\theta^2/r^2$, and thus depends strongly on the geometry of the pipette's tip. The ejecting pulses were applied from $T = 0$ to $T = 5$. (a) Effect of various retaining currents on ejection during a pulse of fixed strength $I/2zFq_D = -40$. Numbers against curves are values of steady retaining current applied before and after the pulse. (b) Effect of retaining current applied at various times before an ejection pulse of fixed strength $I/2zFq_D = -20$. The retaining current of fixed strength $+20$ preceded the pulse by the times shown. Note that if the ejecting pulse were continued indefinitely, all the efflux curves in (a) would tend to the same value $q/q_D = 40.0$. Similarly in (b) all curves would tend to the value 20.0. The adverse effects of retaining current on the time course of ejection are clearly evident. (Reproduced from Purves, 1979, by permission of Elsevier Biomedical Press B.V.)

These differences were undoubtedly accounted for by the retardation of iontophoretic release caused by the retaining current and indeed the authors demonstrated a slowing of the release of noradrenaline by increasing either the size or the duration of the preceding retaining current.

A theoretical analysis of the time-course of iontophoretic release has been developed by Purves (1979), and is summarized in Figure 17. An attempt has been made in that analysis to take into account the fact that the time-course of release will depend on the geometry of the micropipette tip. The time-scale is, therefore, expressed as $T = Dt\,\theta^2/r^2$ (see equation I.1 for definitions) and not in absolute units of time. Hydrostatic and electro-osmotic contributions to release are ignored in this treatment and the concentration of solution in the micropipette is assumed to be the same as that in the surrounding medium. Nevertheless, it is clear that retaining currents of up to 8 nA, comparable with those used in practice, cause a marked slowing of the time-course of iontophoretic release (Figure 17a). Indeed, even in the absence of retaining current there is a much slower onset of ejection than offset due to the relative depletion of solution in the pipette tip which results from diffusional loss of the dissolved compound.

Perhaps even more cause for concern arises out of Figure 17b in which the distortion of the release profile produced by a 20 nA ejecting pulse is illustrated when a retaining current of 20 nA is applied for up to 10 seconds before ejection. As retaining currents would normally be in use for several tens of seconds, sometimes minutes, the greatest caution must be used in describing, comparing and interpreting differences in the time-course of responses to iontophoresed substances. Armstrong-James et al. (1981) found this slowing of release to be such a problem that they applied retaining current for only 1 minute before ejection of catecholamines.

Dionne (1976) has examined the release of acetylcholine and related substances from micropipettes by using ion-sensitive electrodes to follow the time-course of efflux at a resolution of tens of milliseconds. The effect of retaining current on release was confirmed to be very marked, with release profiles remarkably similar to the curves in Figure 17.

At the end of the theoretical ejection pulses of Figure 17 there is a short period of time before the pre-ejection equilibrium efflux is re-established. This is an indication of the phenomenon of 'after-diffusion' described first by del Castillo and Katz (1957). The magnitude of retaining current and the size and duration of ejecting current will be determined empirically in each experiment, to produce the maximum control of spontaneous efflux, with responses of an appropriate size and time-course. However, at the end of the ejection period the solution in the pipette tip will be relatively more concentrated than at the end of the preceding retention period and there will be a period of relatively high spontaneous efflux, until the retention current and spontaneous leakage again bring this to a minimum. It should be evident that no constant value of retaining current can overcome this problem. The only effective method of reducing it would be to use a retaining current which was very high immediately after the ejection period in order to stem diffusional leakage and which was then decreased in size to an appropriate steady value so as not to cause excessive dilution of the tip solution for the next pulse. With the present flood of low cost microprocessors, facilities for programming retaining currents in this way may be a valuable feature of future iontophoretic equipment. At present, the use of appropriately profiled voltages into the analogue inputs of commercially available equipment (Ch. 3) does allow an approach to the manipulation of retention current profiles which would be essential where studies of the kinetics of drug–receptor interactions were being performed.

While the above treatment refers almost exclusively to retaining currents in order to convey qualitatively some feeling for ionic distribution in a micropipette tip, it should be realized that exactly analogous considerations apply to the effects of ejecting current which will cause a build-up of solute in the barrel tip and thus progressively increase the amount ejected until an equilibrium is reached. This will occur independently of the use of any retaining current, and is probably the basis of the 'warm-up' phenomenon described by Freedman et al. (1975).

The essential message from this discussion is one of the most vital for anyone practising microiontophoresis. After a change in the size or duration of the retaining or ejecting currents several cycles of ejection may be required in order for a new equilibrium to be achieved between retention and ejection phases. The experimenter must obtain at least two and preferably three or more complete cycles of similarly sized agonist responses, when any change is made in the size *or duration* of a retaining or ejecting current. This will be most essential when changes of response size are being specifically examined, whether in tests of agonist sensitivity or the effects of potentiating or antagonistic compounds.

III.4 Other considerations affecting iontophoretic ejection

One of the major factors which determines the amount of compound released by iontophoretic current is the preceding history of the micropipette in terms of retaining and ejecting currents as described above. In the following paragraphs various other facets of iontophoretic ejection and factors affecting it will be considered.

III.4.a Electrodes

Most studies of iontophoretic ejection have revealed that for any one barrel of a micropipette a roughly linear relationship exists between the amount of material ejected and the iontophoretic charge, whether expressed as total charge, constant current applied for different periods of time, or different currents applied for the same time (Krnjević *et al.*, 1963a,b; Clarke *et al.*, 1973; Candy *et al.*, 1974; Zieglgänsberger *et al.*, 1974; Shoemaker *et al.*, 1975; Kirsten and Sharma, 1976a; Sasa *et al.*, 1978). This is illustrated for the release of glycine in Figure 18 which also indicates the variability which occurs between different electrodes or barrels, as noted above. Several groups have reported that this variability extends to the extreme case in which no material at all can be ejected from a barrel. In some cases this failure is accompanied by large fluctuations in the amount of iontophoretic current passing through the electrode, together with large amounts of electrical noise (Zieglgänsberger *et al.*, 1969; Hoffer *et al.*, 1971a). In many cases, however, the absence of release follows the apparently unhindered passage of current. This phenomenon has been observed for example in the case of noradrenaline (Krnjević *et al.*, 1963b; Hoffer *et al.*, 1971a; Candy *et al.*, 1974), glutamate (Zieglgänsberger *et al.*, 1969), prostaglandins (Coceani and Viti, 1972) and a variety of drugs (Zieglgänsberger *et al.*, 1974). Krnjević *et al.* (1963b) and Zieglgänsberger *et al.* (1969) proposed as an explanation of this that the barrel tip had become blocked, perhaps by a crystalline deposit of the test material, but that this barrier was able to act as a kind of semipermeable membrane, allowing the passage of H^+ and Cl^{-1} ions for example but not the dissolved drug.

One of the most amazing findings of model release studies has been that the amount of material ejected for a given amount of charge bears no obvious relationship to the size or electrical resistance of the barrel tip (Hoffer *et al.*, 1971a; Dionne, 1976; Zieglgänsberger *et al.*, 1969, 1974). The latter group, for example, noted that multibarrelled assemblies with an overall tip size of only 1–2 μm could still yield a transport number of up to 0.3 for glutamate. This factor has been exploited in particular by Mandelbrod *et al.* (1983) who used very small tipped pipettes to reduce spontaneous leakage and therefore approach

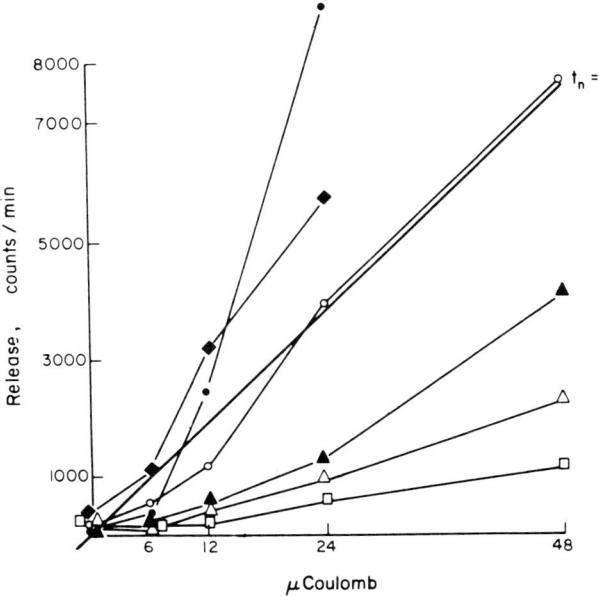

Figure 18 Release of glycine from buffered solution. Cationic currents of increasing intensities were applied. The release from six different electrodes was tested. pH of the phosphate buffer (0.2 M) was 6.7. (Reproduced from Zieglgänsberger et al., 1974, by permission of Pergamon Press Ltd.)

cells very closely, and still be sure of successful iontophoretic ejection. This approach might well be more frequently adopted.

In the case of cyclic AMP an enlargement of tip size was seen to increase the transport number. This observation may be applicable to other compounds with very low transport numbers (Shoemaker et al., 1975).

III.4.b Receiving medium

Very few groups have attempted to examine the effects of the receiving medium on iontophoretic ejection. Most workers have used a simple saline medium, but Hoffer et al. (1971a) compared the ejection of noradrenaline into saline and pieces of fresh brain. The transport numbers into brain were 'considerably less' than when the ejection was made into saline (Figure 19). These results could not be confirmed by Candy et al. (1974) who failed to detect any differences between the ejection of noradrenaline into saline and brain, and Clarke et al. (1973) subsequently found no differences between the ejection of ^{24}Na into these media.

On the other hand Roberts (1981) observed an *increased* release of histamine derivatives into brain tissue compared with saline media. Clearly the experimenter should be aware that differences such as these may exist: it may

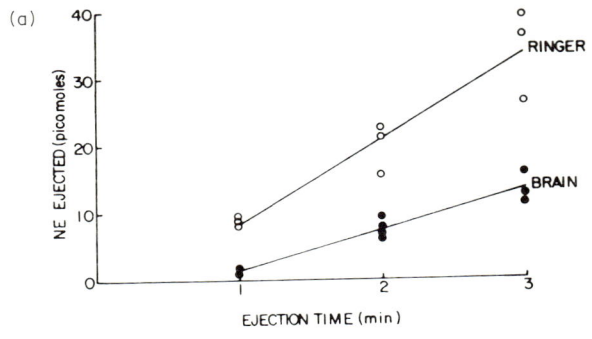

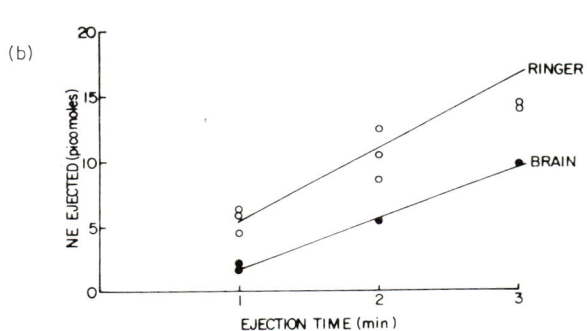

Figure 19 Quantities of norepinephrine ejected from the same pipette in brain as compared with Ringer's solution. (a) and (b) represent two different pipettes. Ejection current 125 nA for both. Each point represents a single sample. Lines were calculated for least squares fit. (Reproduced from Hoffer *et al.*, 1971, by permission of Pergamon Press Ltd.)

certainly be unwise to base comparisons of efficacy in brain tissue solely on measurements of transport number made into a saline medium (Hosford *et al.*, 1981).

III.4.c Acidity

As the pH of a drug solution may alter the degree of ionization of the dissolved compound it might be predicted that it would also change the transport number for that substance. This point assumed considerable importance in the wake of the assertion that alterations of the pH of noradrenaline solutions could affect the direction (excitatory or inhibitory) of neuronal responses (see Ch. 6, Pt. VI). The final shot of several exchanges of short communications came from Bevan *et al.* (1973a) who reported that the transport number of noradrenaline in solution at pH 5 was in the range of 0.02–0.18 while at pH 3.5 the range was 0.18–0.43. Ejections were performed using currents of 12.5–200 nA which lay within the usual iontophoretic range. The suggested explanation for this difference of transport number was that something approaching 100 mM NaOH had to be added to a simple solution of noradrenaline bitartrate in order to raise its pH from 3.5 to 5.0. These sodium ions would undoubtedly carry a significant fraction of any iontophoretic current.

Shoemaker et al. (1975) observed no differences in the (anionic) ejection of cyclic AMP from solutions of pH 4.0 to 7.3.

In the examples of noradrenaline and cyclic AMP just described there is little change in the ionization of the molecule over the pH ranges tested so that any change of transport number must be due directly to the interfering effects of H^+, Na^+, Cl^- or OH^- ions. However, for zwitterionic substances such as GABA the pH should have a major impact on the nature of ions present in a solution and this in turn would be expected to have a major influence on the amount of material ejected by iontophoretic (cationic or anionic) or electro-osmotic (cationic) currents. It is standard practice for example to adjust the pH of dicarboxylic acid solutions to around pH 8 in order to ensure a high proportion of fully ionized compound. Obata et al. (1970), however, noted that outward currents normally used for retention would still eject glutamate, presumably by electro-osmosis.

Similarly Obata et al. (1970) and subsequently Zieglgänsberger et al. (1974) found that when released from nearly neutral solutions of pH 7.0 and 5.9 respectively GABA was ejected far more readily than from more acidic or alkaline solution (Table 1). Glycine behaved more as expected, showing a higher transport number at pH 2.3 than 6.9 (Zieglgänsberger et al., 1974). If glycine was dissolved in phosphate buffer, however, the transport number at pH 6.7 was almost twice that at pH 2.2, all ejections being made using outward (positive) currents. These various observations raise the strong suspicion that the contribution of electro-osmotic bulk flow (see this chapter, Pt. IV) to drug ejection from micropipettes may be seriously underestimated.

III.4.d Filling method

Kirsten and Sharma (1976a) found a higher transport number for acetylcholine (0.473) after filling micropipettes by the glass fibre method than if they were filled initially with water under reduced pressure and the water was then replaced by drug solution (t, 0.386). It is not clear whether this indicates some limitation of drug diffusion into the extreme tip of the barrel.

III.4.e Ageing

Ageing of micropipettes has received little attention since Zieglgänsberger et al. (1974) described the phenomenon. If a freshly pulled micropipette assembly was filled with drug solutions without breaking back the pipette tip, then release remained unchanged when tested at intervals over periods of several days. If the pipette tip was broken back, however, drug release declined when tested

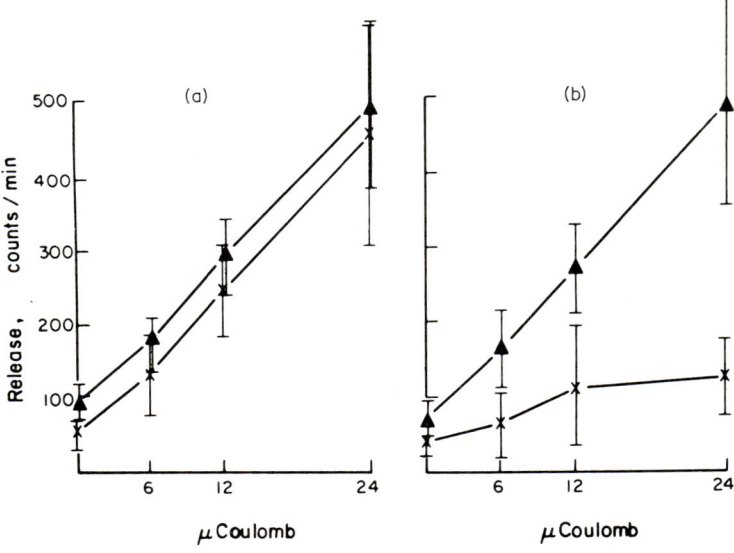

Figure 20 The effect of storing upon the release of chlorpromazine. (a) Electrodes were stored with their tips unbroken (<0.5 μm). Two different collecting media were used. Sodium chloride (0.9%) = crosses; sodium chloride (0.9%)/methanol (1 : 3) = triangles. (b) Electrodes were stored with tips broken (3.4 μm) before storing for 7 days, with their tips immersed in distilled water. Addition of methanol (triangles) to the collecting medium could restore the reduced release (crosses). Mean values and standard deviation obtained from six different electrodes. (Reproduced with permission from Zieglglänsberger *et al.*, 1974.)

over several days, though it could be restored to its original level by adding methanol to the collecting saline medium (in the proportions 3 : 1) (Figure 20). Presumably, therefore, this ageing was due to the accumulation of organic or crystalline deposits at the tip which diminished the iontophoretic release but which were soluble in methanol.

III.4.f Effect of drug concentration

The theoretical curves of Figure 13 are constructed for different values of W, where W is the ratio of the concentration of solution within the micropipette to the concentration of solute without. For ejecting currents above a certain level all these curves adopt nearly the same slope. Above that level the size of ejecting current becomes a reasonably linear reflection of the amount of material ejected, and differences in the values of q/q_D^* for the curves become an ever-diminishing proportion of the total efflux. This certainly applies over the range of values of W indicated in Figure 13, from $W = 0.1$ (pipette concentration about 20 mM) to $W = 5$ (pipette concentration about 1 molar). Purves (1981) calculates that the critical level above which the non-linearity of Figure 13 disappears (approximately $It/zFq_D^* = 3$) will be at an applied voltage of around 200–300 mV, corresponding to current of about 2 nA passing through a 100 MΩ barrel. Thus in those iontophoretic studies involving currents considerably above this level the amount of drug release for a given current should not differ appreciably from solutions within the range of concentrations 20 mM to 1 M and the amount ejected will be linearly related to the current used.

Similarly from the definition of transport number (equation III.1) a change of drug concentration in the micropipette barrel should not affect the amount of compound ejected by iontophoretic current, as there is no term involving solution concentration in equation (III.1). This is because the assumption is often made that all the charge passing through the micropipette tip is carried by the drug ion.

In practice there may be a number of factors responsible for deviations from this ideal. For example it is usual in iontophoretic experiments to increase the solubility and/or the degree of ionization of compounds by appropriate adjustment of pH. This would result in the presence of small ions (Na^+, Cl^{-1}) which could carry some of the ejecting and/or retaining current. It should also be remembered that the same problem will apply to compounds whose unadjusted solution has a high or low pH, a high pH implying the existence of hydroxyl ions arising from the non-equilibrium dissociation of water and low pH implying the existence of hydrogen ions. This effect, of course, is not dependent on the type of salt used: some free bases, such as 4-aminopyridine, can produce a substantial elevation of pH due to the protonation of amino groups.

Another factor responsible for the influence of drug concentration on iontophoretic ejection is the possible interaction between dissolved compound and the barrel wall. Many compounds are known to be adsorbed on to glass surfaces as a result of electrostatic attraction between the molecules and ionic charges in the superficial layers of glass. Since the glass surface is usually negatively charged, the problems are greatest for larger polyvalent cations and can be a particular nuisance in the case of some peptides. Substance P is an outstanding example which was shown to interact with glass surfaces by Cleugh and Gaddum, (1963). At pH 5, substance P carries three positive charges and yet, even at a concentration of 3 mM in the presence of only 17 mM Na^+, the peptide's transport number was a mere 0.016. This fell to 0.0008 in a solution of 170 mM Na^+ (Guyenet et al., 1979). Part of the reason for these low values is almost certainly the relatively low ionic mobility of the peptide but it would seem very likely that other factors such as adsorption to the glass surface make some contribution. In cases such as these, since adsorption is an exponential process, increasing the drug concentration should cause a disproportionate elevation of the transport number.

Finally those processes which involve a bulk loss of drug solution, namely hydrostatic efflux and electro-osmosis will clearly contribute to the net loss of solute in direct proportion to its concentration.

PART IV ELECTRO-OSMOSIS

An electrical double layer exists at the interface between glass and aqueous solutions such that the fluid carries a net positive charge. The passage of current through a micropipette will cause movement of this fluid volume and it is this phenomenon which is known as electro-osmosis (Figure 1b). It is in essence the opposite of iontophoresis: in the latter case an applied voltage causes the movement of charged particles relative to the bulk of solution, whereas in electro-osmosis the bulk of fluid moves relative to the surrounding layer of fixed charge.

For an ion existing primarily as a cation, the contribution of electro-osmotic movement will obviously facilitate ejection from a micropipette. However, Hill-Smith and Purves (1978) have calculated that zeta potentials comparable to those observed experimentally at glass/water interfaces would result in the movement of fluid by electro-osmosis under the influence of an applied *inward* (negative) potential sufficient to counteract the iontophoretic efflux of anions. These authors consequently argue that it is the fine balance beteen the iontophoretic and electro-osmotic efflux which causes some of the unpredictability and variability of micropipette ejections.

Several authors have derived expressions for the volume flow of solution attributable to electro-osmosis (Curtis, 1964; Hill-Smith and Purves, 1978). According to Hill-Smith and Purves, 1978, the volume flow V is given by:

$$V = \epsilon \xi I / \eta \sigma \qquad \text{(IV.1)}$$

where ϵ is the permittivity of the solution, I the applied current, η the solution viscosity and σ the conductivity. ξ is the electrokinetic or zeta potential which is the potential difference existing between the bulk of uncharged fluid and the boundary which separates freely mobile ions from the layer(s) of immobile counterions trapped electrostatically by a fixed charge (as at a glass/aqueous interface).

As first pointed out by Curtis (1964) all experimental studies of the electrically induced release of ionized substances from micropipettes must involve both iontophoresis and electro-osmosis. Strictly speaking, therefore, all reference to experimentally observed transport numbers in such studies should refer to *apparent* transport numbers. The true transport number, referring only to that fraction of *iontophoretic* current carried by an ion, can only be estimated by calculation after taking into account the electro-osmotic contribution to the observed efflux.

On the basis of calculation Krnjević *et al.* (1963a) estimated the contribution of electro-osmosis to the ejection of acetylcholine from a 3 M solution as 11% of total efflux, and Krnjević and Whittaker (1965) subsequently used radiolabelled sucrose to quantify electro-osmotic release more carefully. Although these authors noted that a maximum rate of release was achieved using currents of about 60 nA, that maximum was several nanolitres per microcoulomb. This is orders of magnitude greater than the volume flow predicted to occur with iontophoresis although the micropipettes used by Krnjević and Whittaker (1965) were substantially larger in tip diameter (12–20 μm) than those used for iontophoresis. However, it has already been noted that Obata *et al.* (1970) achieved a greater ejection of zwitterionic GABA than of the primarily cationic or anionic forms from micropipettes of a more usual size. Most of the zwitterionic ejection was presumably produced by electro-osmosis, the volume ejected on this assumption being approximately 0.3 nl μC^{-1}.

Bevan *et al.* (1979) subsequently attempted to determine the relative importance of iontophoretic and electro-osmotic ejection by performing ejections of [^{14}C]-glucose in the presence of noradrenaline bitartrate to estimate the volume of fluid released by electro-osmosis and then using that value of electro-osmotic release to calculate the proportion of efflux due to electro-osmosis and (by subtraction) iontophoresis from solutions containing [^{14}C] noradrenaline bitartrate and unlabelled glucose. The authors found that the unadjusted transport number of noradrenaline was 0.286, but that 23% of this, twice the estimate of Krnjević *et al.* (1963a) for acetylcholine could be accounted for by electro-osmosis. The 'real' transport number of the amine was estimated as 0.220.

If the movement of ions by electro-osmosis and iontophoresis is viewed as involving the passage of current through two parallel resistors, then with weak solutions (higher resistance), the electro-osmotic efflux will represent a greater proportion of total efflux than in the case of more concentrated solutions. Electro-osmosis is clearly of great practical value for the ejection of un-ionized compounds, as the bulk flow of solution achieved by an outward current will obviously carry with it the dissolved material. The amount ejected, of course, will be related to the concentration of the solution. The practice often adopted of dissolving poorly soluble substances in solutions of sodium chloride would seem to have little to recommend it since a lower proportion of any applied current will presumably be available both to the active material for direct iontophoresis and to the bulk solution for electro-osmosis. Presumably the greater part of any ejected compound is associated with the water of hydration which accompanies the ejected sodium ions (Figure 1c). (**Note** This latter phenomenon is frequently but *mistakenly* referred to as electro-osmosis, and the addition of sodium is said to increase electro-osmotic ejection. In fact, as noted above, these additions merely provide more cations which can carry current and, therefore, less truly electro-osmotic ejection will occur; see Ch. 1, Pt. I).

IV.1 Effect of drug concentration

It has been seen that at the usual levels of current used for microiontophoresis, and for solutions of between about 20 mM and 1 M solute concentration, the amount of compound released theoretically by iontophoretic current alone is essentially independent of solution concentration, and this is probably approximately true for *any* drug concentration likely to be studied (that is in the range of about 2 mM to 3 M). However, this will patently not be so for electro-osmotic efflux since the amount ejected by this means will be directly proportional to the solution concentration. In practical terms the amount of compound ejected electrically from a micropipette will show clear dependence on concentration.

PART V EJECTION BY PRESSURE

Even in some of the earliest studies of the pharmacology of single neurones it was realized that the ejection of substances from micropipettes by the application of pressure presented a viable alternative to the ejection by electrical means, and pressure ejection was sometimes used as a means of totally eliminating potential artefacts due to iontophoretic current (Krnjević and Phillis, 1963a). The method has been largely neglected, however, in favour of iontophoresis, probably because the latter presents a more controllable ejecting force. With increasing interest in the single-cell responses to drugs, many of which are poorly soluble or are poorly ionized in aqueous media, and in the effects of peptides which tend to have a low ionic mobility some investigators have begun a closer examination of the possibilities offered by 'micropressure ejection' (Palmer, 1982).

Suitable electrodes (Ch. 2) and equipment (Ch. 3) for pressure ejection have been considered earlier.

The amount of material released by pressure can be determined by the same methods that have been used in conjunction with iontophoresis: chemical assay, radiolabel counting, electrochemical measurement and so on, but in addition there is the distinct advantage that the volume ejected can be *seen*. Thus microscopic observation of the formation of an aqueous droplet at the tip of a micropipette allows a direct measurement of release which can be checked easily and rapidly before, after or at any appropriate point during an experiment, and without the need for sophisticated electronic hardware.

However, it is not easy to assess the comparability of release between different laboratories as the measurements are often different, the tips may be very different in size or no information is provided, and the time-scale of ejection pulses may vary from milliseconds to minutes. Representative results are shown in Figures 21, 22 and 23.

Several conclusions may be drawn nevertheless from published studies. Firstly, release is almost invariably a linear function of applied pressure, or of the time for which a constant pressure is applied (Figures 21, 22, 23) (McCaman *et al.*, 1977; Sakai *et al.*, 1979; Palmer *et al.*, 1980; Poulain and Carette, 1981; Dray *et al.*, 1983). The volumes ejected from tips about 1 μM in diameter appear to range from about 0.5 femtolitres s^{-1} p.s.i.$^{-1}$ (Sakai *et al.*, 1979) through several hundred picolitres s^{-1} p.s.i.$^{-1}$ (Krnjević *et al.*, 1963a; Obata *et al.*, 1970; Poulain and Carette, 1981; Palmer, 1982) to 1.5 nanolitres s^{-1} p.s.i.$^{-1}$ (McCaman *et al.*, 1977).

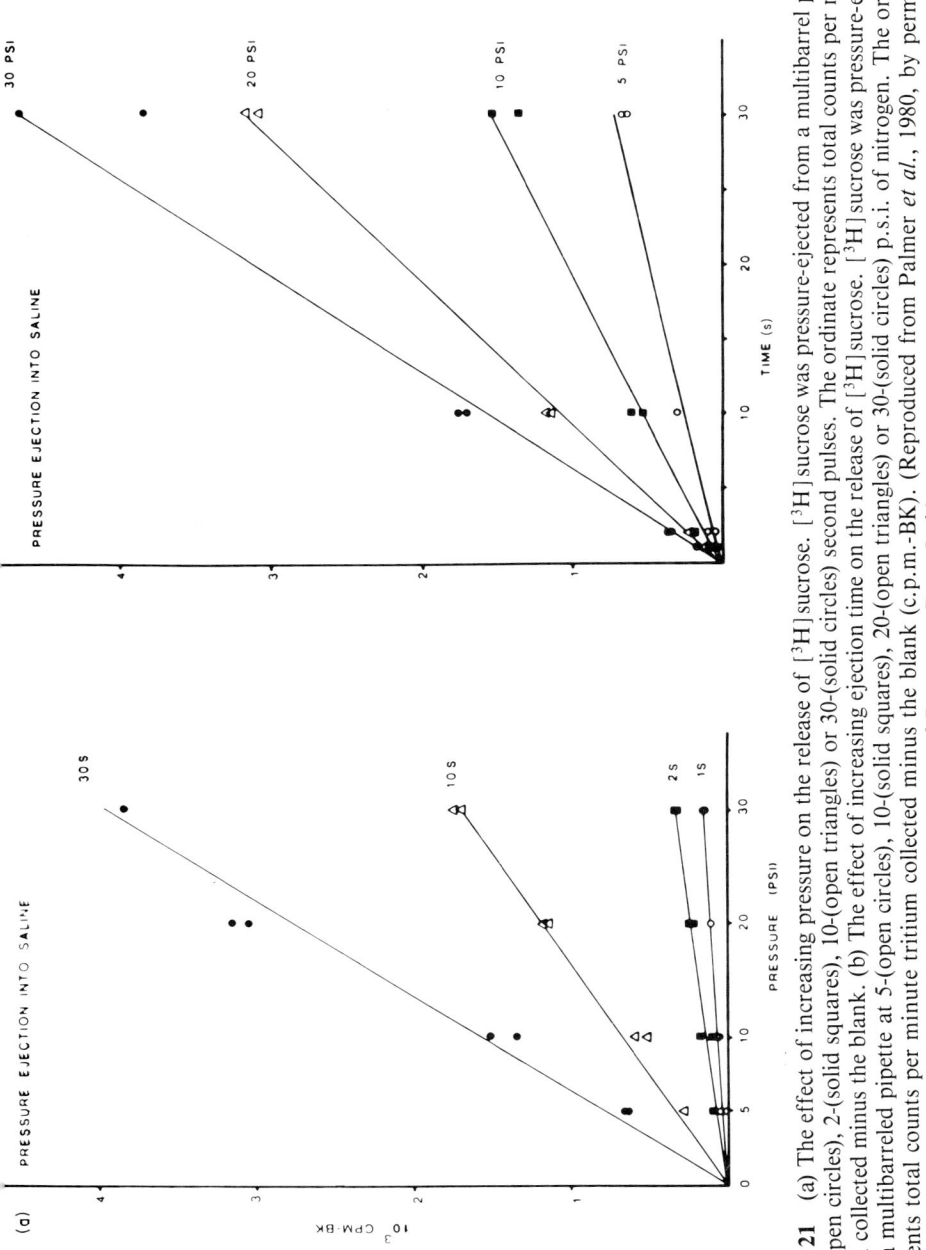

Figure 21 (a) The effect of increasing pressure on the release of [^{3}H] sucrose. [^{3}H] sucrose was pressure-ejected from a multibarrel pipette in 1-(open circles), 2-(solid squares), 10-(open triangles) or 30-(solid circles) second pulses. The ordinate represents total counts per minute tritium collected minus the blank. (b) The effect of increasing ejection time on the release of [^{3}H] sucrose. [^{3}H] sucrose was pressure-ejected from a multibarreled pipette at 5-(open circles), 10-(solid squares), 20-(open triangles) or 30-(solid circles) p.s.i. of nitrogen. The ordinate represents total counts per minute tritium collected minus the blank (c.p.m.-BK). (Reproduced from Palmer et al., 1980, by permission of Pergamon Press Ltd.)

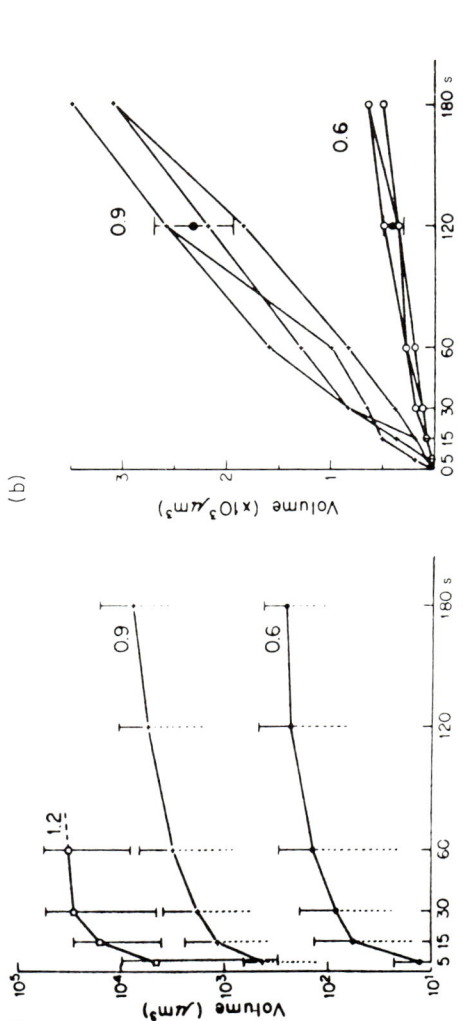

Figure 22 (a) Differences in volume of 1 M KCl solution ejected from electrodes of different tip size. Ejections from three groups of electrodes with 0.6, 0.9 or 1.2 μm tip size are shown. Each curve represents the average obtained from five electrodes within one group. The vertical bars at each point indicate standard deviation. Abscissa indicates duration of pressure application. Ordinate indicates volume in logarithmic scale. (b) Reproductivity of repeated ejection. Results of serial experiments from two different electrodes are plotted (tip size 0.9 μm above, tip size 0.6 μm below). Vertical bars at 120 s indicates error range (SD) of measurements of diameter of the droplets; filled circles indicate the means. Some of the measurements overlapped. (Reproduced from Sakai et al., 1979, by permission of Pergamon Press Ltd.)

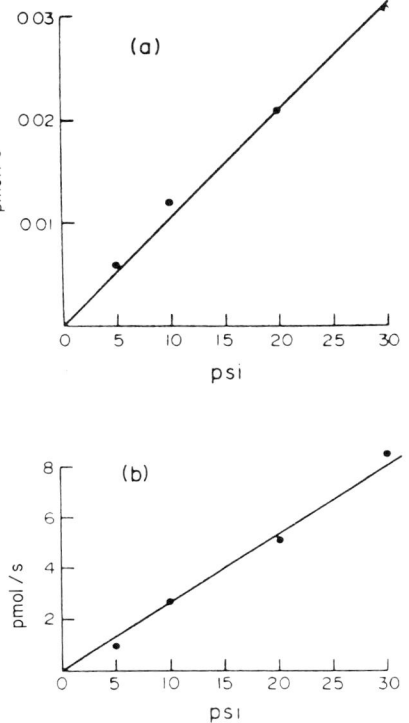

Figure 23 (a) Mean rate of release of substance P (0.01 mM) by pressure from four pipettes. Rate of release was in the 0.005–0.04 pmol/s range. (b) Mean rate of release of substance P (1.0 mM) by pressure from four pipettes. Rate of release was in the 0.5–10 pmol/s range. (Reproduced from Dray et al., 1983, by permission of Pergamon Press Ltd.)

Secondly, the volume of solution ejected is markedly dependent on tip size. As seen in Figure 22a there can be a ten-fold difference in the volume ejected by a given pressure (in this case 80 p.s.i.) from pipettes which differ in tip diameter by only 0.3 μm.

Thirdly, even using pressure application it cannot always be assumed that the ejectate is a drop of solution of exactly the same composition as the fluid placed into the micropipette or that the solute is not affecting in some way the volume ejected. Thus in Figure 23a it is clear that the amount of substance P ejected from a solution of 0.01 mM peptide was only about one-third of that predicted from an examination of the release from a 1 mM solution (Figure 23b). The authors interpreted this as indicating that proportionately less *solution* was ejected at the stated concentrations, but it is also possible that the same volume was ejected in both cases, but containing proportionally less peptide from the weaker solution (Dray et al., 1983). However, it would be easier to understand this perhaps if the peptide were held at the glass surface trapped by the electrical double layer, as this would cause a disproportionate depletion of the weaker solution.

Dray *et al.* (1983) also made the observation that less material was ejected into brain tissue than into saline, an effect which was attributed to a simple restraining effect of tissue on the flow of solution out of the pipette.

The variability which occurs between different micropipettes and even different barrels, for iontophoretic ejection does not seem to arise for pressure microejection. Pipettes are much more consistent in their behaviour. In addition, pressure ejection may often mean that, provided high enough pressures are used for long enough, substances which only dissolve to concentrations of less than 1 mM, or which are un-ionized (Poulain and Carette, 1981) can be applied to single neurones whereas that would be almost impossible by microiontophoresis.

It should be noted that there is no single means of reducing the spontaneous leakage of compound (diffusional and hydrostatic) from the pipette tip. Although this also means that the problems of solution depletion are less in the tip, the leakage of very potent compounds may present serious difficulty. It may be possible though, with such compounds to reduce the solution concentration to only a few micromolar, at which this efflux is no longer significant, but responses are retained.

PART VI IONIC MOVEMENTS AND TISSUE CONCENTRATIONS AFTER IONTOPHORESIS

Curtis *et al.* (1960) were among the first to point out that since the electrical resistance of the external medium was normally substantially lower than that of an iontophoretic micropipette, there would be a very small gradient of potential in the medium between the pipette tip and a distant indifferent electrode. Any movement of ejected ions due to electrical factors would thus be restricted to the immediate vicinity of the micropipette tip, whereas the main factor determining the distribution of compound in the medium would be diffusion. Therefore an attempt was made to estimate the concentrations attained in tissues during iontophoresis by developing the equations for heat conduction from a continuous source (Carslaw and Jaeger, 1959).

Regarding the micropipette tip as a point source of material located in a homogeneous medium the concentration C of substance achieved at a distance of r μm from the tip at T seconds after beginning ejection at a rate of Q mol s^{-1} would be (del Castillo and Katz, 1955; Carslaw and Jaeger, 1959; Curtis *et al.*, 1960; Herz *et al.*, 1969; Curtis, 1964; Kelly, 1975):

$$C = \frac{Q}{4\pi rD} \, erfc. \, \frac{r}{2(DT)^{1/2}} \qquad \text{(VI.1)}$$

where D is the diffusion coefficient and erfc. refers to the complementary error function (Carslaw and Jaeger, 1959). After modifying this equation to take into account the finite duration of iontophoretic ejections, Curtis *et al.* (1960) then

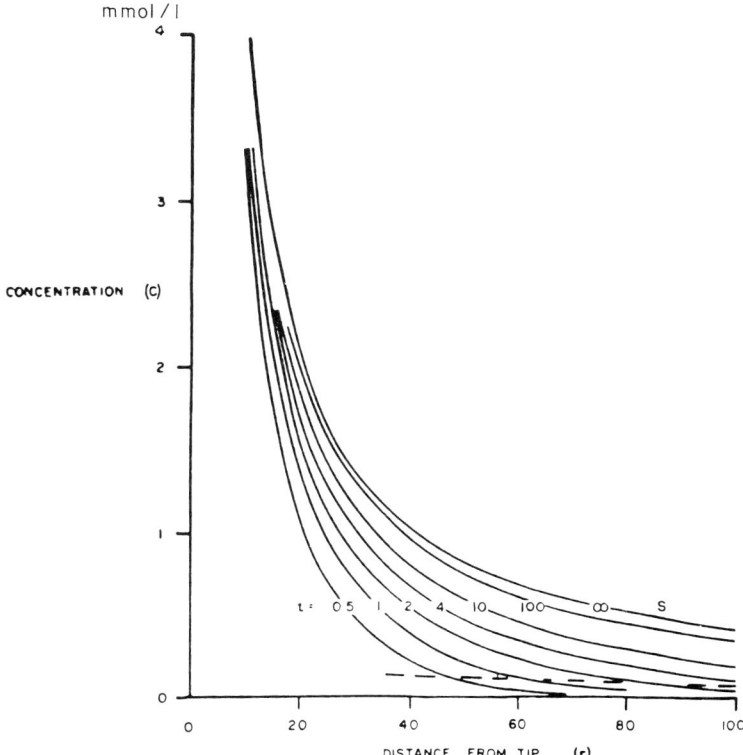

Figure 24 Concentration (ordinate), in millimoles/litre, of a univalent ion of diffusion coefficient 1×10^{-5} cm^2/s and transference number 0.5 at a distance $r\mu$ (abscissa) from the tip of an electrode when passed by an ionophoretic current of 100 nA. The different curves indicate concentration–distance relationships at the indicated times after the beginning of the ionophoretic current. (Reproduced from Curtis et al., 1960, by permission of the International Society of Neurochemistry.)

derived a series of curves estimating the concentration of material at different distances from a micropipette produced by an iontophoretic current of 100 nA (Figure 24). A transport number of 0.5, valency 1 and diffusion coefficient of 10^{-5} cm^2 s^{-1} were assumed. If it is considered that most responsive neurones lie at distances of between 20 and 100 μm from the micropipette tip, and that responses to most compounds would occur with iontophoretic currents of 100 nA applied for between 1 and 100 seconds, then the effective concentration required for those responses should according to Figure 24 be in the range of 0.4 to 2 mM.

If a compound is ejected as a relatively brief pulse such that the micropipette tip approximates an instantaneous point source, the concentration achieved at time T is given by:

$$C = \frac{Q}{8(\pi DT)^{1.5}} \exp(-r^2/4DT) \qquad (\text{VI.2})$$

(del Castillo and Katz, 1955; Carslaw and Jaeger, 1959) and the maximum concentration at distance r will be

$$C_{max} = \frac{0.0736\ Q}{r^3} \qquad (VI.3)$$

Further, since the time at which this maximum will occur is

$$T_{max} = \frac{r^2}{6D} \qquad (VI.4)$$

a value of r can be calculated from the time of maximum response. This value can then be used in equations (VI.2) and (VI.3) to estimate C and C_{max}. By assuming a diffusion coefficient D of $5.10^{-6} cm^2 s^{-1}$ for glutamate and estimating a quantity of 50 fmol of glutamate released from a micropipette Krnjević and Phillis (1963a) used this approach to calculate that most neurones studied lay several tens of microns from the pipette tip and that the concentration of glutamate effective in causing excitation was usually about 0.1 mM.

Several experimental studies have also examined the spread of ions within brain tissue and the concentrations achieved by iontophoresis. Herz *et al.* (1969), for example, used pairs of multibarrelled micropipettes in the cerebral cortex and caudate nucleus to show that the activation of neurones by glutamate released at various distances could be accounted for by the theoretical model of diffusion discussed above (Carslaw and Jaeger, 1959). The authors were also able to estimate a distance of approximately 20 μm for the mean tip to neurone distance of satisfactorily recordable cells. Herz *et al.* (1969) proceeded to calculate a mean value of 0.25 mM for the threshold concentration of glutamate required to activate cells at that distance.

More recently Misell and Richards (1979) have made estimates of the threshold concentration of glutamate required to activate neurones in a brain slice preparation as between 0.2 and 0.4 mM, in excellent agreement with the conclusions of Krnjević and Phillis (1963a) and Herz *et al.* (1969).

Candy *et al.* (1974) chose to eject α-methylnoradrenaline or noradrenaline using realistic iontophoretic parameters of 50 nA for up to 5 minutes, doses which are sometimes used for amines and peptides, particularly if plateau responses are studied, and which are almost always needed for the application of antagonists. The ejections were made into the brain stem of anaesthetized animals and the area subsequently examined using fluorescence techniques. It was found that after ejection for 30 seconds a spot 200 μm in diameter could be detected, increasing to 400 μm after 2 minutes and 600 μm after 5 minutes. Comparable experiments using radiolabelled noradrenaline ejected from a 1% solution gave comparable results with the additional observation of a 1000 μm spot after 10 minutes. By comparing their results with perfusion experiments, these authors note that the concentrations attained in the brain stem after only 4 μC of charge (50 nA for 80 seconds) would be adequate to produce EEG and blood pressure changes. This conclusion must have major implications for iontophoretic studies in any area such as hypothalamus and brain stem from which distant changes of cardiovascular or hormonal status might be produced which could affect the results.

Although the preceding paragraphs deal only with diffusional models of drug movement, occasional flirtations have been made with the idea that other factors are involved. In particular, Trubatch and Van Harreveld (1972) have attempted to confirm experimentally their contention that the distribution of ions in brain is represented by the equation:

$$IT = \frac{4\pi r^3}{3S\mu} \qquad \text{(VI.5)}$$

where current I is applied for a time T, r is the distance from the electrode tip, S the specific resistance of the tissue and μ the electric mobility of the ion.

This equation was derived from the premise that ions are carried through the external tissue (brain) by the potential gradient established by iontophoretic current. This, it will be recalled, was considered an unlikely event by other authors because of the low resistance of brain compared with a micropipette. Trubatch and Van Harreveld (1972) consider that the resistance of brain is not likely to be entirely negligible compared with an iontophoretic barrel.

Experimental support for this notion was obtained by making use of the observation that the iontophoretic application of glutamate in the cerebral cortex produces a lesion characterized by a light spot (Methylene Blue II stain) in which were grossly distorted neuronal and glial elements. Forming an annulus around this spot was an area containing shrunken cell bodies. Trubatch and Van Harreveld (1972) examined the size of the area of damaged brain cells after applying glutamate from a micropipette with a current of 250 nA for 1 hour. The glutamate solution was 150 mM. Figure 25 shows the linear relationship found between the diameter of the damaged tissue sphere and the cube root of the applied current. This plot is thus consistent with equation (VI.5).

However, these authors also noted that a charge of 1.5 mC produced different sized lesions whether applied as 5 μA for 5 minutes (spot of 596 μm diameter) or 0.42 μA for 1 hour (spot of 370 μm diameter). This they explained on the assumption that the slower ejection parameters would allow uptake processes and metabolism to lower the glutamate concentration below the threshold for observable toxic effects, towards the periphery of the sphere of glutamate ejection.

Similarly it was found that lowering the pipette concentration of glutamate from 150 to 10 mM by diluting with Ringer's solution produced a reduction in the size of the damaged tissue spot from 300 to 80 μM (following ejection with 250 nA for 1 hour). In this case much of the iontophoretic current would be carried by chloride ions, again effectively reducing the tissue concentration of glutamate, the authors suggested, below the threshold for causing morphologically detectable cell toxicity. Trubatch and Van Harreveld (1972) boldly suggested that the concentration of glutamate in the micropipette which

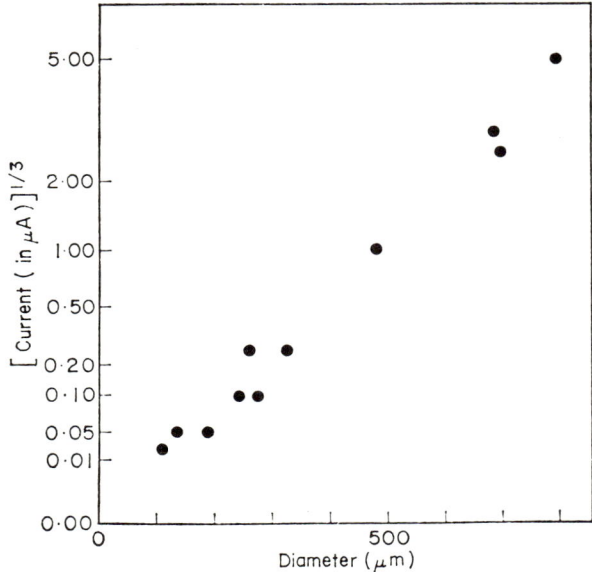

Figure 25 The cube root of the current (in μA) used for the iontophoretic deposition of glutamate in the rat's cerebral cortex was plotted on the ordinate, the diameter (in μm) of the area in the glutamate lesion characterized by grossly swollen tissue elements on the abscissa. A micropipette filled with 150 mM glutamate was used and the current was applied for 1 h. (Reproduced from Trubatch and Van Harreveld, 1972. With permission from the Journal of Theoretical Biology, **36**, 355–366. Copyright 1972 by Academic Press Ltd.)

would yield a threshold observable change in the tissue was 'of the order of 8 mM'. The authors concluded that the difference in concentration of glutamate in the pipette and that causing observable tissue damage was insufficient to explain the movements of glutamate entirely by a diffusion gradient. Conversely, by calculating the electric field which probably occurred across the region of damaged tissue (50 mV cm^{-1}) they showed reasonably good agreement between the calculated radius of glutamate movement in that field (290 μm) and the size of the spot actually observed (250 μm). Therefore, although these authors did not, unfortunately, perform any calculations on diffusion for comparison they concluded that 'the linear relationship of the dimensions of the glutamate effects and the cube root of the applied current indicate that under the conditions of these experiments electrical forces are dominant in transporting glutamate through the tissue'.

In spite of the undoubted utility of Trubatch and Van Harreveld's experiments and calculations in some very specialized cases (for example tissue marking) these authors themselves emphasize that their glutamate iontophoresis was made with high intensity and very prolonged (1 hour) duration currents, and with the observable result of the ejection being a destructive lesion for the production of which a threshold concentration of about 8 mM is required in the tissue.

Routine iontophoresis of substances on to nerve cells usually entails ejection with currents of the order of 50 nA, rarely for longer than a few minutes and with a resulting response which has a threshold of 0.1 to 1 mM. It is impossible as yet to try and assess the relative contributions of diffusion and electrical field to ionic movements under these circumstances.

Szabadi and Bradshaw (1973) have indeed argued that in the vast majority of cases where iontophoresis is being used to study neuronal responses the results are readily explicable on the basis of diffusion only. Further, these authors claim that many of the discrepancies between observed and predicted results, which required Trubatch and Van Harreveld (1972) to invoke uptake processes, could be adequately explained by a purely diffusional model for glutamate distribution.

The same conclusion was also reached by Norman (1975) who undertook a more quantitative analysis of the problem and concluded that the influence of electric field on ionic movement would become negligible compared with diffusional considerations whenever the voltage gradient falls below about 50 mV. Norman (1975) points out that potentials of this size would themselves cause changes of neuronal excitability. Since results are normally discarded when neurones appear to be affected by iontophoretic current it is unlikely that electrically induced movements are of any significance in practice.

Although Herz *et al.* (1969) attempted to correct their calculations for the complexity of brain tissue most of the above discussion has been based on the rather naive assumption that the receiving medium during iontophoretic experiments is homogeneous. This may be approximately true for some invertebrate preparations and *in vitro* systems (e.g. cell cultures) where compounds are being effectively ejected into the saline medium. However, homogeneity is not an outstanding feature of the mammalian brain and Nicholson *et al.* (1979) have attempted to take this into account by introducing into the diffusion equation (VI.1) terms which reflect the tortuosity (λ) and available volume fraction (α) of brain tissue. The latter term refers simply to that fraction of tissue (e.g. extracellular space) which is accessible to the penetrating molecule. The tortuosity factor, λ, is a correction for the increase of path length followed by a molecule diffusing through a complexly organized available volume fraction. Equation (VI.1) should be accordingly modified as:

$$C = \frac{Q}{4\pi r D^* \alpha} \operatorname{erfc} \frac{r}{2(D^*T)^{1/2}} \qquad (VI.6)$$

where D^* is the modified diffusion coefficient D/λ^2.

Nicholson *et al.* (1979) also tested the validity of this treatment by ejecting tetraethylammonium ions by microiontophoresis into brain (anaesthetized rats) and agar and measuring the concentrations achieved 35–200 μm away using ion-selective electrodes. The authors were thus able to derive a value of 8–29% for the available volume fraction α in the cerebellum, a value consistent with recent estimates of the extracellular space in brain, and a value of 1.6 for the tortuosity

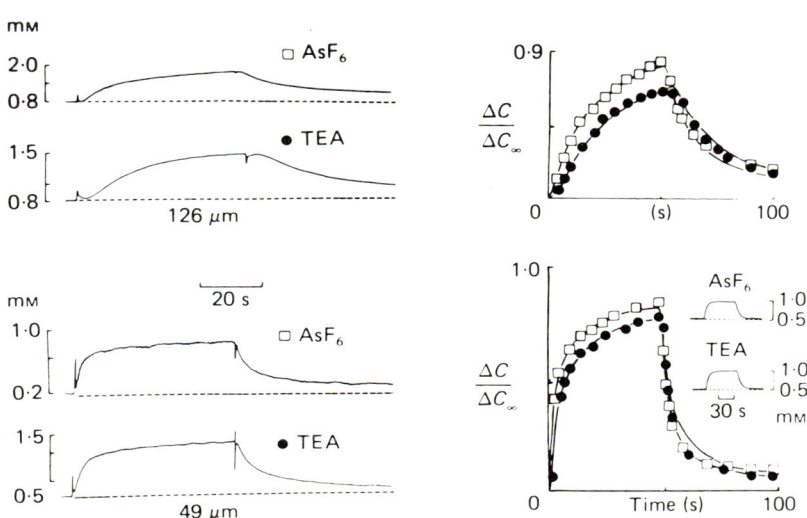

Figure 26 Test of charge discrimination using double ionophoresis. Arrays were made with pairs of ion-selective micropipettes, the reference barrel of each contained the ion that could be sensed by the other one; in this way the reference barrels could be used for iontophoresis and direct comparison of cationic and anionic diffusion could be made without any spacing error. Two such experiments are shown, using AsF_6 and TEA at 126 μm and 49 μm. The graph on the right shows that the experimental data points closely fit the theoretical curves; The curves were calculated with the same λ for cations and anions. For the upper data $\lambda = 1.45$; for the lower data $\lambda = 1.55$. The inset shows the responses of the ion-selective micropipettes to pulses of calibrating solutions in the cup above the brain. (Reproduced from Nicholson and Phillips, 1981, by permission of The Physiological Society.)

factor λ. The authors noted that this latter figure agreed well with values obtained following the intraventricular instillation of radiolabels.

Nicholson and Phillips (1981) later expanded this treatment to an examination of two cations, tetramethylammonium and tetraethylammonium, and two anions, α-naphthalene sulphonate and hexafluoroarsenate. Essentially similar results were obtained, though the authors in addition looked at the homogeneity of the cerebellum to diffusion of these ions at different depths, and to factors such as the effect of charge. Figure 26, in which experimental data points have been superimposed on to theoretical curves, shows that diffusion is effectively the same for anions and cations. Of course all the ions used in this study remain in the extracellular space: the effect of cellular uptake must be taken into account for biologically relevant ions.

Waud (1968) has derived an electrical circuit analogue of the diffusion process and published a set of curves computed from this system to illustrate the changes of drug concentration to be anticipated at various distances from a micropipette tip (Figure 27). It is interesting to note the relatively slow rate of rise of concentration at distances of 16–32 μm since many cells are probably situated

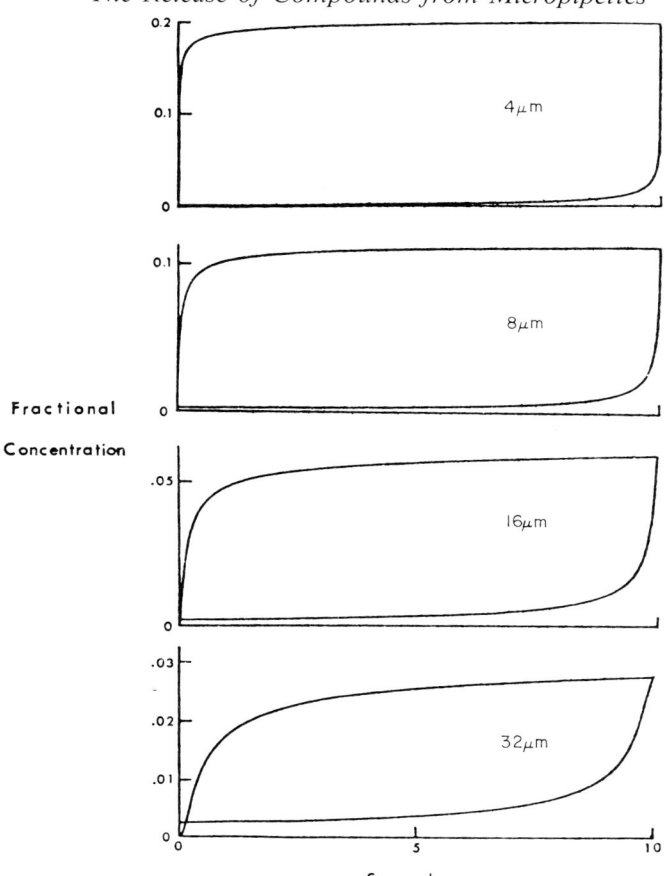

Figure 27 Computed concentration at various distances from a point source of 10 s duration. $D = 10^{-5}$ cm^2/s. Panels from above downward represent events 4, 8, 16 and 32 μm from origin. Ordinate: concentration relative to that at origin; abscissa: time in seconds. Rise of concentration was recorded from left to right (upper curves); then point source was terminated and fall in concentration was recorded from right to left. (Reproduced with permission from Waud, 1968; copyright 1968 The American Society for Pharmacology and Experimental Therapeutics.)

at around that distance (Krnjević and Phillis, 1963a; Herz et al., 1969). It is one of the many advantages of studying plateau responses to compounds for quantitative analysis that the steeply rising phases of the curves in Figure 27 can be largely avoided: within the first second or so of ejection small changes in electrode position could have a significant effect on drug concentration at the cell surface. Similarly a slight distortion of the tissue produced by the electro-osmotic or pressure ejection of a putative antagonist in several picolitres of solution could cause a change of a few microns in the tip to cell distance and thus alter apparent sensitivity to the agonist.

CHAPTER 5

Analysis of Results

I QUALITATIVE PRESENTATION	76
I.1 Gating or Window Discrimination	78
I.2 Ratemeters	80
I.3 Histograms	81
I.4 Microcomputers	82
II QUANTITATIVE ANALYSIS	84
III THE PROBLEM OF DOSE	84
IV THE PROBLEM OF RESPONSE	88
V DOSE-RESPONSE CURVES	90
VI USES OF QUALITATIVE MICROIONTOPHORESIS, AND THE RESPONSE CRITERIA EMPLOYED	96
VI.1 Spontaneous or Evoked Baselines?	98
VII USES OF QUANTITATIVE MICROIONTOPHORESIS	99
VII.1 Antagonism	99
VII.1.a Measures of Antagonism	99
VII.1.b Baseline Fluctuations	99
VII.2 Comparisons of Potency or Sensitivity	100

PART I   QUALITATIVE PRESENTATION

In reports of the earliest iontophoretic experiments in the CNS the results were presented as photographic records of the oscilloscope screen (Curtis and Eccles 1958a,b; Krnjević and Phillis, 1963a,b). Very few authors today content themselves with such a simple qualitative illustration of results and, in parallel with the general trend towards an increasingly sophisticated treatment of scientific data, they analyse (some would say massage) the raw information into a form which can be dealt with mathematically and statistically. Although a measure of cautious scepticism about the manipulation of data is always advisable there are many experimental situations where some form of quantitative analysis is essential. Such situations would include a comparison of neuronal sensitivity in different strains of animal, or after the destruction of input pathways (McLennan, 1980) or after chronic treatment with drugs (Jones and Olpe, 1984). It would also be necessary in comparative studies of agonist potency (Perkins and Stone, 1983a,b) or antagonist potency and selectivity (Perkins et al., 1981).

Nevertheless, if a series of observations are being reported which are largely qualitative statements of the action of a compound, agonist or antagonist, oscilloscope traces of raw spike trains (Figures 28 and 29) possess many valuable features for the sceptical reader:

1. The size, duration and polarity of the spikes give a feeling for the proximity of the recording tip to the cell membrane. Spike size of course will also depend on the size of the neurone being studied, since the recorded spike is a reflection of current flow in the extracellular space and the greater the area of active neuronal surface the greater will be the net current flow. However, if an electrode presses on to the outer membrane of a neurone sufficiently to cause damage, the duration of the spike may increase considerably from its normal value of 0.5–1 ms to a value of 2–5 ms. Similarly a spike recorded from a distance of about 10 μm or more from most cells will appear as a wholly negative potential, but with closer approach, especially when sufficient to press on and inactivate a small patch of membrane this potential will become positive–negative or more unusually negative–positive, as the local membrane begins to act as a passive current source for the spike-generating mechanism.
2. It is immediately clear whether a single cell was being studied, whether several cells were responding to the drug or whether several cells were recorded but only one was responding, etc.
3. The passage of electrophoretic current can cause a substantial increase of electrical noise. If small spikes are being recorded, and a gated output (see below) is being monitored, it is possible for the noise to generate gated pulses and give a misleading idea of potency. Presentation of the spike record eliminates this doubt.
4. It is immediately apparent whether or not a compound produces a change of spike height. This may be of paramount importance when studying the host of pharmacological agents with membrane-stabilizing properties (atropine, propranolol, phenothiazines, etc.), particularly if they are being tested against agonists causing excitation.

   It is also useful to know the effect on spike height of excitatory compounds themselves, particularly those belonging to a related group of agonists, such as the excitatory amino acids. Some members of this group such as kainate cause overdepolarization (Figure 28a) with a loss of spike height quite readily whereas others, such as homocysteate and quinolinate are reluctant to do so. This distinction may well correlate with a difference of receptor type and mechanism.
5. The precise time-course of drug responses can be seen from a spike record. When using potent substances such as excitatory or inhibitory amino acids applied close to the cell surface, onset latencies can easily be less than 1 second. Yet this is obscured in all processed records of firing rate by

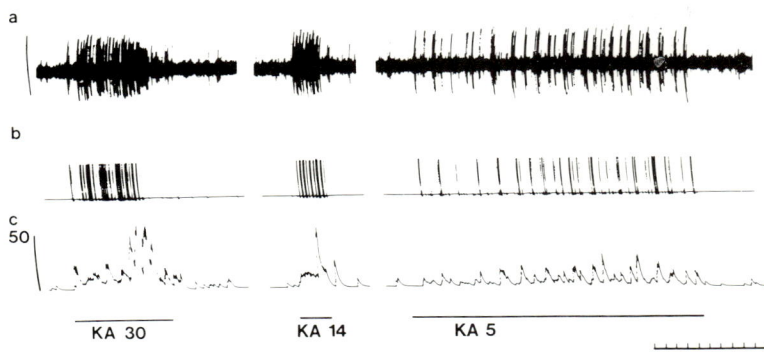

Figure 28 The use of a window discriminator to monitor spike activity. Panels (a) show a spike record replayed from magnetic tape on to a pen recorder at 1/16 original speed. The firing rate is greatly increased by kainate (KA) 30 nA. (b) Shows the constant sized output pulses from a window discriminator. (c) The effect of placing a 1 μF capacitor across the recorder input. Note that the first kainate application produces overdepolarization, with a loss of spike height, but the discriminator cannot show this and indeed with a high gate threshold does not even detect the declining spikes. Information on the time-course and pattern of firing of gated spikes is, however, retained

the time constant of the integrator used. Again using the example of excitatory amino acids, some members of the group (L-glutamate, L-aspartate) with short response latencies can be readily differentiated from analogues with a slower onset such as *N*-methylaspartate.

In the case of intracellular work photographic records (or playback from magnetic tape on to a chart recorder) are the norm rather than the exception, since the interest is usually less in the rate of firing and more in the associated changes of membrane potential and conductance, and the shape of the action potential. In extracellular work, however, spike records are rare and the data are processed in one of the ways to be described.

I.1 Gating or window discrimination

The most common first stage in processing spike data is to convert those spikes of interest into a uniform pulse size. A number of instruments are available commercially, including the Digitimer Spike Processor, the Window Discriminator from WPI and modular items from Haer, Colbourn, Neurolog (Digitimer), Dagan and many others.

All these units generate an adjustable voltage level, such that any component of the recorded signal which crosses that level will generate an output pulse which is constant in size and duration. If two or more voltage levels are available then output pulses may be selected for signal voltages greater than the larger of those voltage levels or for signal voltages lying between the two. Hence the term 'voltage window' or 'gate'. It is thus theoretically possible to select any single spike from a multi-spike signal for further processing. In practice the size of window used must take into account any variations of spike size due to movement artefacts (electrode movement, cardiac or respiratory pulsation, etc.) or drugs used (atropine, propranolol, etc.).

A circuit design was published by Freeman (1971) for a spike discriminator capable of distinguishing one to six voltage levels simultaneously.

The gated output pulses can be recorded directly on a chart recorder to give a continuous unquantified record of neuronal activity (Figure 28b; Stone, 1972a, 1973b; Moss *et al.*, 1978). This is certainly simpler and cheaper than photographic recording and in the absence of a calibrated integrator may be an acceptable experimental record. However, simply placing a capacitor across the input terminals of the chart recording will produce a crude record of firing rate (Figure 28c) which can be calibrated using a frequency generator.

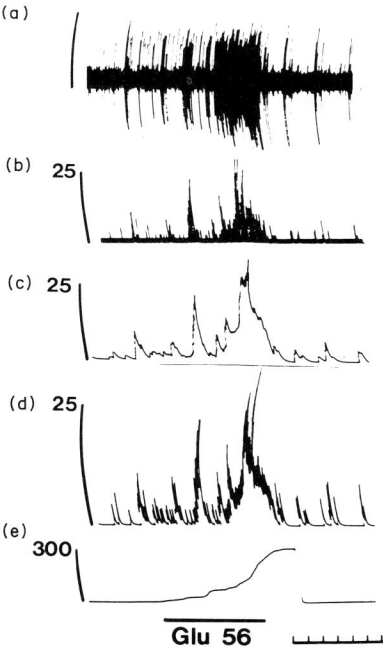

Figure 29 Different methods of monitoring neuronal firing rates. Panel (a) is a spike record, replayed from magnetic tape on to a pen recorder at 1/16 original speed. The firing rate is greatly increased by glutamate, 56 nA (bottom centre bar). (b) A record of the same activity processed though a window discriminator on to a resetting integrator, reset time 1 s. (c) and (d) Displays of the discriminator output on an instantaneous ratemeter using time constants of 2 s and 0.5 s respectively. In panel (e) a cumulative record of spike count was begun at the time of starting the glutamate application and continued until the response had clearly ended. The height of this record is thus proportional to total spike count. Calibrating scales 400 μV in (a), spikes/second in (b)–(d); total spike count in (e). Time marks are 16 s playback time, 1 s real time

While records of gate output pulses do not provide information on spike size, noise level, non-specific effect of drugs on spike size or shape, etc., they do retain the valuable feature of indicating the precise time-course of drug action. Thus in cases where photographic facilities are not available, or when cells are being studied whose spikes are sufficiently small to make photography very difficult, these records present a reasonable alternative.

I.2 Ratemeters

There are basically two kinds of ratemeter. The resetting integrator simply accumulates input pulses (from a discriminator) until it is reset to zero, when accumulation begins again (Figure 29b). Most resetting integrators have an internal programme which can be used to reset automatically at a selection of popular intervals (such as 1 or 10 seconds) and provision for an external resetting pulse to provide other time intervals. Although virtually all the raw spike information has, of course, been lost it is still possible to retain much information on the time-course of responses by selecting a suitably short reset time. A 1 second reset time is, however, adequate for most extracellular situations because the unknown contributions of ejection delay and diffusion to receptors make hazardous any attempt to draw conclusions about onset latencies of that order. Certainly a second reset is more than adequate for slowly acting compounds such as some amines and peptides.

The provision of a manual reset button on accumulating integrators of this type (e.g. Grass 7P 10) is an extremely useful feature for quantification purposes. Thus if the integrator is reset to zero coincident with the start of a microiontophoretic ejection pulse, allowed to accumulate throughout the response and is then reset to zero as the response finishes (or the firing rate returns to the baseline firing level for a spontaneously active cell) a record is obtained of which the peak height is a direct reflection of the total spike count during the response (Figure 29e). This method can be applied to both excitatory and inhibitory responses for either quiescent or spontaneously active cells, if baseline firing is measured for total count over the same period of time used for the response.

The instantaneous ratemeter is so-called because the indicated rate is allegedly an indication of firing frequency at that instant in time. In fact, of course, this is only true for phenomena in which the frequency is constant over a period several times greater than the time constant of the ratemeter. That is, the meter only gives a true indication of frequency under equilibrium or plateau conditions. Unless one is lucky enough to be working with neurones which show a very regular firing pattern (or applying substances into the medulla and observing changes of heart rate) the instantaneous ratemeter will provide only an indication of mean firing rate over successive epochs determined by the time constant. For extracellular studies involving response latencies greater than 1 second and response durations of several seconds or longer a time constant of 1 to 2 seconds is usually convenient (Figure 29).

I.3 Histograms

Arguably the most satisfactory method of recording iontophoretic responses is the cumulative histogram (Figure 30). Here, gated output pulses are accumulated into successive bins of the histogram, in much the same way as seen with the resetting integrator. By recycling the programme several times to coincide with repeated iontophoretic ejection cycles a summed or averaged histogram is generated. This clearly facilitates any attempts at quantitation of the data by reducing the number of measurements to be made several-fold. The bin width can be set to any suitable period, although an external clock may be required to generate bin widths of 1 second or more suitable for study compounds whose responses are measurable in minutes rather than seconds. Most histogram generators provide 256 bins for data accumulation.

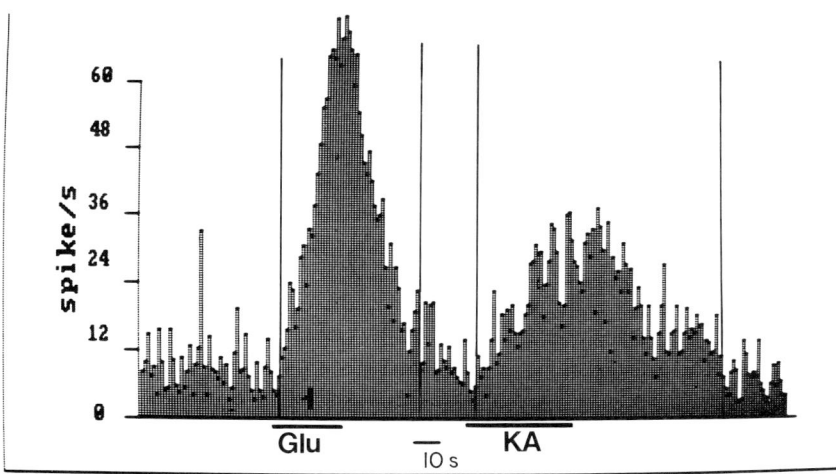

Figure 30 A cumulative histogram composed of three successive responses to glutamate, 40 nA and kainate, 15 nA. Note that the total spike count between cursors 3 and 4 was 2020, and between 1 and 2 was 1903. These figures exclude baseline firing and indicate that peak height cannot be used to reflect total activity if the response profiles are appreciably different

The equipment needed for such histograms need not break the bank. Several excellent averager/histogram modules are available from various manufacturers (Neurolog from Digitimer; Ortec; Haer; Dagan; Coulbourn). There is much to be said for having a modular system which includes amplifiers, filters, gating and histogram generation from the same manufacturer. These systems also have the advantage that pulse generator modules can be included which can be used to increase bin width over the range provided, as noted above.

I.4 Microcomputers

Currently, of course, there is a strong appeal towards obtaining more sophisticated microcomputer systems to do the work, and several companies have specifically aimed at the market for processing neuronal spike data (e.g. Medical Systems; Bio Data; Coulbourn).

The Computer Institute, for example, has developed the Cambia II Data Acquisition System as a stand alone data processing package. The system can perform signal averaging, auto-correlation, rate analysis, spike interval histograms and response time histograms. The software can also be purchased separately for use in conjunction with an Apple microcomputer.

Along similar lines RC electronics produces a package of hardware and software which converts an Apple II into a data analysis system. The Applescope package hardware include A/D converter, memory and triggering facilities and a Direct Memory Access module which permits real time data handling. The basic Applescope package also includes software which converts the display monitor into the equivalent of a digital storage oscilloscope, with four lines of text appearing below the displayed waveform. This allows direct readout of the axis parameters as well as the numerical magnitude of any desired point, indicated by means of a movable cursor.

An array of separate software is also available including programs for signal averaging and histogram generation. The histogram program copes with two channels of information, includes automatic scaling of axes and the readout of number of events in any desired bin.

Biodata Limited manufactures a modular system of signal conditioning units known as Microlink. The modules available include A/D converters, clocks, multiplexer, analogue output and switching units which interface the experimental data with Sirius, Commodore or Hewlett-Packard microcomputers.

An excellent package including Waveman and Dataman programs to run on Apple IIe systems is available from Stoelting.

A final example of commercially available Spike processing equipment is the Neurograph (Medical Systems Corp.). This microcomputer system carries the considerable advantage in the present context that it is specifically designed for use in conjunction with microiontophoretic studies. The Neurograph will use pulses from a suitable window discriminator to generate interspike interval histograms or post-stimulus time histograms with a total sweep duration of 250 ms to 250 s (or longer if an external timer is used). Histogram generation includes autoscaling (i.e the ordinate is initially set to a scale of 0-25 but if the counts per bin exceed this limit the scale is immediately and automatically doubled). The count number is 64K in any one bin. A most useful feature of the Neurograph is that the same input data can be accumulated simultaneously into histograms with two different time bases (Figure 31). Thus one can observe, for example, the effects of an iontophoretically applied synaptic antagonist on the early and late components of an evoked neuronal response at the same time.

Analysis of Results

The supreme advantage of the Neurograph over other commercially available data acquisition systems is in the manipulation of the accumulated data which can be performed. As illustrated in Figure 31 a number of cursors are available on the Neurograph: three pairs are provided for establishing a control low, control high, average 1 low, average 1 high and average 2 low and high. The alphanumeric display to the right of the histogram then indicates the average value of counts per bin between these pairs of cursors. The cursors can be set independently for the upper and lower histograms, and reproducibility between successively generated histograms can be obtained by noting the time at which the cursors have been positioned (penultimate line of text).

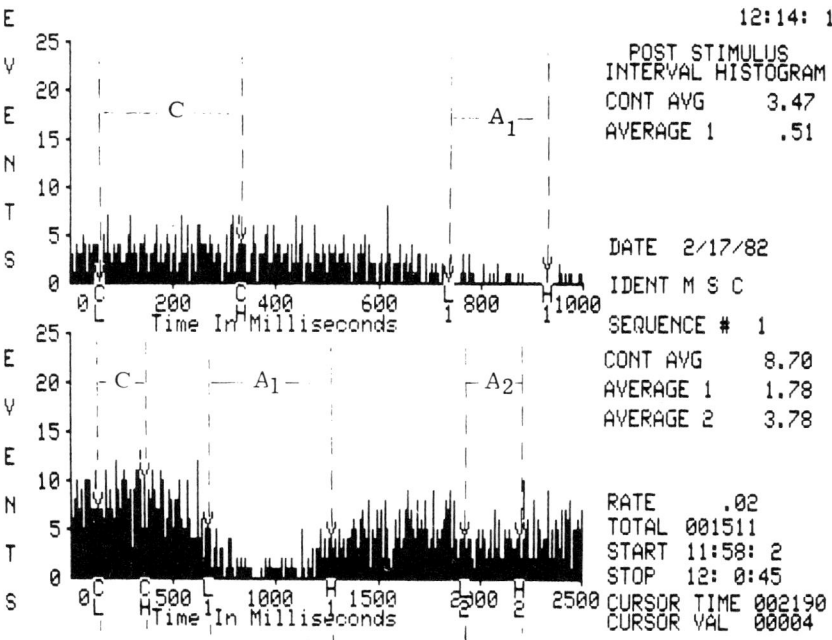

Figure 31 A representative rate/time histogram generated on the Neurograph (Medical Systems) spike processing system. Using a time-scale of seconds the system is well suited to iontophoretic applications in order to calculate total spike count in user-defined control and response periods. (Reproduced by permission of Medical Systems Corp.)

The Neurograph will also generate signal averages and superimpose 95% confidence limits at the press of a single key.

For those laboratories without money to spend on commercial apparatus, but with the time and expertise to build their own equipment, several designs for spike processing equipment have recently been developed (Leendertz and Wright, 1983).

PART II QUANTITATIVE ANALYSIS

If the intention is to produce a qualitative analysis of drug effects, it may be perfectly adequate to provide a verbal description accompanied by suitable representative illustrations. Indeed the majority of iontophoretic studies are of this kind, and are most impressive when clear changes are involved. For example the reports that morphine but not naloxone will potently suppress neuronal firing in locus coeruleus but that after chronic administration of opiates the morphine effect is much weaker, and naloxone now causes a large increase of firing (Aghajanian, 1978) are of this type.

It is also frequently obvious when a compound is acting as a selective antagonist (see Figures 45 and 53) without the need for constructing dose–response curves and assessing statistical differences. However, there will certainly be instances where some form of quantitative analysis is desirable to compare the sensitivities of different neuronal populations, or a similar population under different conditions, or to obtain some statistical indication of the selectivity of an antagonist compound.

So, either we have a chart record of neuronal firing rate with time, or we are sitting at our computer terminal. What do we measure or what do we instruct the computer to measure and what do we do with those measurements? These questions are addressed in the following sections.

PART III THE PROBLEM OF DOSE

In most pharmacological systems there is a clear distinction between the terms dose and concentration, although it has to be admitted that many authors ignore that distinction. The term 'dose' refers to the amount of compound administered into a system. That is all. There are no implied assumptions concerning the 'concentration' of that compound which may exist as a result at any particular site. Indeed following any given dose, the concentration of compound will usually be different at different sites and will vary with time, the instantaneous level depending not only on the dose administered but also lipid solubility, non-specific binding, uptake, metabolism, excretion, etc. In reality a number of factors such as these may determine drug concentration at its receptors even in an isolated organ bath. The term 'concentration' should ideally be reserved for those instances where all such factors are at equilibrium in the face of a perfusion at constant drug concentration and an unvarying tissue response can then be measured at that (bath) concentration.

Viewed in this way an iontophoretic 'dose' of compound is not substantially different in concept from a systemic or bath-applied 'dose'.

However, whereas the administration of a systemic dose occupies usually only a very small fraction of the time taken by the subsequent response, which may be measurable in hours, an iontophoretic administration may occupy a very large proportion of the response time. For this reason it is not adequate to express iontophoretic dose simply as current passed; the time domain must be considered also, as if the ejection were an infusion (Simmonds, 1974) and dose expressed as charge passed (nanocoulombs = nA × seconds).

The importance of this point may be illustrated by example. The very disparate response profiles of Figure 32a, for example, resulted from ejections using similar currents, but it would be naive to suggest that the two compounds were equipotent. There are clearly other factors, probably physical and biological, to take into account but it is likely that the tissue concentration of noradrenaline will be substantially greater than that of GABA. The use of charge passed, in this case 7520 nC of noradrenaline and 480 nC of GABA, to produce responses of similar peak size instantly conveys to the reader that a smaller amount of ejected GABA was probably needed than noradrenaline. To be certain of this, of course, one would also have to determine the transport numbers of the two compounds to rule out major differences of ejection characteristics.

A possible problem with the use of charge, however, arises if responses are being compared on very different time-scales. In Figure 33 for example the open circles represent neuronal responses to quisqualate applied for 10 second periods. The closed circles indicate responses at appropriately adjusted current strengths applied for only 50 ms. Clearly there is an element of reciprocity failure here, with responses of similar magnitude being produced by a much smaller total charge at the shorter ejection duration. The reason for this is not entirely clear, but the phenomenon is discussed again in Part V of this chapter.

For many compounds whose relative potencies might be required, the responses may be sufficiently similar in profile that applications of the same duration may be made, and only the ejecting current varied to provide responses of comparable size. Such is the case for instance with excitatory and inhibitory amino acids (Figure 32b). It would then be more acceptable to quote current as a measure of dose for the calculation of relative potencies or in the generation of dose–response curves.

A second situation in which ejecting current alone may be an adequate reflection of dose is when the time domain has become irrelevant, that is when the responses being studied reach a constant level, or plateau (Figure 32d). The assumption here is that the various factors contributing to the response such as ejection delay, diffusion through tissue, uptake, metabolism, etc., have reached an equilibrium. It can then be stated with modest conviction that ejection currents of 80 nA of glutamate and 5 nA of quisqualate are sufficient to maintain a plateau excitation S spikes s^{-1} or of $P\%$ of the spontaneous firing level.

Indeed this last method of estimating iontophoretic dose by taking the ejecting currents needed for plateau responses is to be preferred over all others for several reasons. Firstly, all time-dependent factors become irrelevant. It has been seen in Chapter 4 that the use of retaining currents can severely prejudice the onset latency of a response and this would clearly be reflected in the total ejection charge needed to induce a response. Reference to Figures 16 and 17, for example, clearly reveals that due to the retaining currents a given ejecting charge will expel less compound: the greater the retention the smaller the ejection.

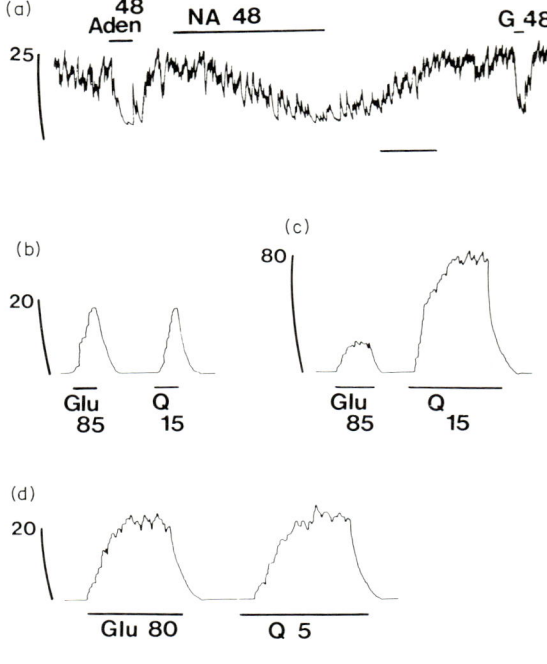

Figure 32 (a) A record of firing rate of a neurone in the cerebral cortex in response to the iontophoresis of adenosine (Aden) 48 nA, noradrenaline (NA) 48 nA and GABA (G) 48 nA. The record emphasizes the impossibility of using current alone as a means of comparing sensitivity to different agents. Time bar 1 min. (b)–(d) Illustrate the need for plateau responses. In (b) responses to glutamate (Glu) 85 nA and quisqualate (Q) 15 nA applied for the same period of time, appear comparable, suggesting a possible potency ratio of 5.7. However, if the ejecting currents are continued so that a plateau is reached, it becomes clear that the glutamate response is near maximal but quisqualate is not. (c) (Note the change of scale.) Taking into account the difference of response size implies a potency ratio nearer $4 \times 5.7 = 22.8$. This is supported by (d) in which plateau responses of similar size are obtained using a dose ratio of 16. This is probably a more reliable figure than the 23 obtained from (c) as there are no problems of interpretation which arise from the use of greatly different firing rates in (c). Time bars 1 min; ordinates, spikes/second

Curtis *et al.* (1971a) have attempted to circumvent this particular problem by determining for each iontophoretic barrel the size of retaining current which would just prevent leakage of the test drug from the barrel, and subsequently calculating the *effective* ejection current as actual ejecting current plus preceding retaining current. However, since retention appears to be a continuing, time-dependent process it may not be the case that a retaining current which is just adequate at one time point will remain so indefinitely (Bradshaw and Szabadi, 1974). In the author's experience most moderate retaining currents (in the range 5–15 nA) can appear to be just adequate for long periods of time, presumably

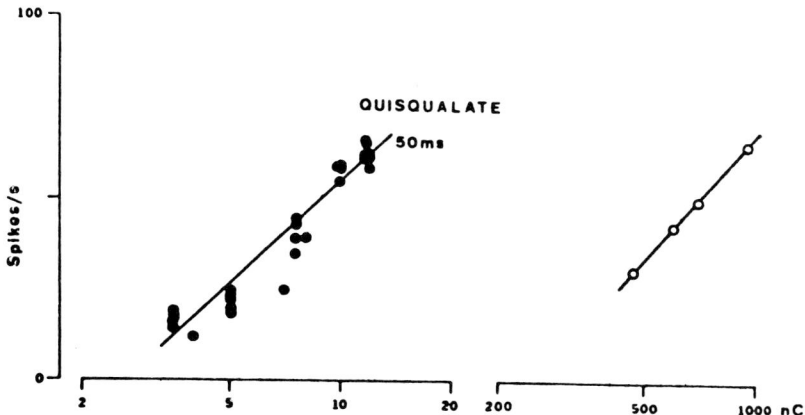

Figure 33 Dose–response curves for quisqualate in which the agonist was applied in pulses of 50 ms duration (closed circles) or 10 s (open circles) at currents adjusted to produce comparable responses. (Reproduced from Nistri and MacDonald, 1978, by permission of Plenum Publishing Corp.)

as an equilibrium is established between ion withdrawal from the tip and diffusion back into it. However, the time taken for such an equilibrium to be achieved, often several tens of minutes, is an order of magnitude greater than the usual period elapsing between ejection pulses.

The second reason for preferring plateaux is that responses can then be made truly comparable. In Figure 32b, for example, there is no way of knowing where either of the responses would lie on a dose–response curve. In fact the quisqualate response proved to be about 25% of the maximum attainable at the same ejection current while the glutamate response proved to be nearly maximal (Figure 32c). This is clearly unsatisfactory for a comparison of potency which in this case would change with the ejection parameters. In conventional pharmacology dose–response curves are constructed wherever possible from measurements of responses which have reached an equilibrium. In the specific example of Figure 32 the potency ratio of quisqualate to glutamate, approximately 16 : 1 from panel D could only be approximated by a combined examination of B and C, yielding a ratio of 23 (5.7 × 4).

By using plateau responses then, the ratio of ejecting currents alone needed to maintain those responses may be used as an index of relative functional potency. The word 'functional' is important because it emphasizes again that many factors such as tissue uptake and binding, metabolism, desensitization, indirect effects, etc., may still contribute to the observed response. It should also be remembered that the substance of interest will be carrying only a proportion of the ejecting current (Ch. 4) and that to eliminate micropipette characteristics as thoroughly as possible from estimates of potency, the transport numbers for the compounds must be assessed and used as multipliers of the ejection parameters.

PART IV THE PROBLEM OF RESPONSE

The following parameters are available for quantification of response size.

1. Meaasurement of peak height. This may be achieved by a simple manual measurement of the response size in ratemeter recordings (Figures 29 and 32) or the hard-copy output from a computer-generated histogram (Figures 30 and 31). It may be derived from microprocessor systems either by taking single cursor readings at the response peak and during the control period or, with the more sophisticated systems such as Neurograph, using the cursors to obtain a mean firing rate during control and peak periods (Figure 31).
2. Measurement of total spike count during the response. This may be relatively easy to obtain from a computer analysis but is more difficult to read from a chart record. However, measurement of the area occupied by a response would be a satisfactory reflection of total spike count and may be obtained using a planimeter.

    Alternatively, although old-fashioned, non-programmable, inexpensive methods of analysis are often regarded with suspicion and some dismay, particularly by newer generations of microprocessor-educated students, there is nothing wrong with cutting out (or photocopying and cutting out) the area of interest and weighing it.

    If a resetting integrator with manual reset is being used a record can be obtained on-line of total spike count as described earlier (Figure 29). A simple electronic counter, operated manually, could also be used to the same purpose. Most modular systems of electrophysiological equipment include cheap and suitable digital counters.
3. Measurement of a temporal parameter, such as latency from the start of ejection to start of response, latency from the start of ejection to peak of response or the rise time to half peak response ($t_{1/2}$). Any of these may be obtained from computer analyses or measured directly from hard copy.
4. In some cases it may be feasible to study the size of a field potential as an indication of the behaviour of a population of cells. The usual way to quantify these is simply to measure the amplitude of the potential, but the problems with this will be deferred to Chapter 6, Part XII.

In comparing the relative validity of these parameters it is perhaps best to begin by considering exactly what any particular experiment is designed to study. In the case of intracellular recordings, of course, interest is normally focused on the amount or direction of membrane conductance changes and the associated movements of membrane potential. In the study of antagonist compounds it may also be possible to compare directly the blockage of synaptically evoked potentials with responses to iontophoretically applied transmitter in order to distinguish presynaptic and postsynaptic actions.

In extracellular work, on the other hand, it would be foolish to pretend that one is looking at depolarization. While it is true that in several systems the rate of action potential production is related directly to membrane depolarization, it is probably dangerous to assume this as a universal generalization in the CNS. The measurement of firing rates should be considered to provide information only on the ability of a neurone to produce action potentials. Little can be meaningfully said about the underlying depolarization or ionic mechanisms. Indeed in many respects it may be said that intracellular studies are concerned primarily with the input to neurones and the factors which affect synaptic integration whereas extracellular studies are concerned more with the output consequence of that integration.

Returning to a comparison of measurement parameters (1) to (3), then, it is likely that under most circumstances the best indication of response size would be the total spike count or equivalent. As long as the response height is a reliable, and at least proportionate, reflection of the total spike count this too would be acceptable. The major problem here is in determining whether response height does bear such a reliable relationship to total spike count. If responses to different agonists are comparable in profile then this is likely to be so as in the case of glutamate and quisqualate responses in Figure 32. It will not be the case, however, when the response profiles are dissimilar, as for the glutamate and kainate responses of Figure 30. Here, because of the long duration of the kainate excitation, the same total spike number is encompassed by a lower peak ratemeter record than for glutamate.

However, it may not always be possible to adjust the responses so that they are comparable in profile — responses to a wide range of compounds from amines to some peptides are slow in onset and of long duration irrespective of the amount ejected. On a shorter time-scale, quinolinic acid almost invariably shows a latent period of several seconds to its excitatory action and the rate of increase of firing is relatively low while compounds such as quisqualic acid produce a much faster onset response. If the quisqualate ejection current is reduced or the solution in the micropipette diluted, the latency may be increased, but the rate of increase of firing from the start of the response will still usually be greater than for quinolinate. As the current is reduced further, even if applied for long periods of time (several tens of seconds), there may be no response at all, presumably due to either neuronal accommodation or desensitization to the agonist or a balance between rate of ejection and neuronal uptake. In cases such as these the responses would be better described in terms of total spike count for the ejection parameters used since this would make clear to the reader that a fundamental difference existed in the character of the responses.

Temporal parameters have been used relatively rarely for quantitative analysis, but persuasive arguments for their use have been put forward by Hill and Simmonds (1973) and Simmonds (1974). These authors advocate the measurement of time taken for a response to reach 50% of its maximum, the T_{50} value. The basis for this procedure is the supposition that each individual response to an agonist may be considered as a cumulative dose–response relationship reflecting the gradual increase in tissue concentration of drug during the ejection period. If a series of such responses are obtained, reaching the same maximum amplitude, they can then be readily characterized by the T_{50} value. This will be discussed again in the next section, but for now it may be noted that the method has two marked advantages over measurements of response size. Firstly, a single figure is obtained which, if it is regarded as truly equivalent to the ED_{50} value in conventional pharmacological work, is more representative of the drug-cell system than any measure of a single response size. Conversely, to generate an equivalent figure from measures of response size would require an examination of several responses produced by different doses. The T_{50} value thus implicitly requires less work.

The authors also claim that the T_{50} value is easier to measure accurately than a response size. Certainly it can be very difficult indeed to obtain reproducible graded response amplitudes to some very potent compounds such as amino acids. Any changes of firing rate during a response which ideally should be of the plateau variety may further complicate any assessment of the response size, whereas in the determination of T_{50} values all responses increase to the same maximal level, which may be 100% inhibition, (Hill and Simmonds, 1973) or a clear maximal plateau of excitation tending towards overdepolarization, (Clarke *et al.*, 1974).

PART V DOSE-RESPONSE CURVES

Armed with a measure of the iontophoretic 'doses' of compounds together with convenient and reproducible indicators of the responses induced it would be perfectly possible to generate a numerical statement of their relative potency or of the specificity of blockade by an antagonist from a very small number of data points. However, this procedure would be generally unacceptable in conventional pharmacological studies, since the relationship between dose and response may have a different slope for each of the agonists tested; their relative potency or degree of antagonism would then depend on which part of the dose-response curve was being examined.

Curtis *et al.* (1971a) and Kelly and Renaud (1973) were among the first to draw attention to the fact that the same problem exists in iontophoretic experiments and that meaningful pharmacological conclusions can only be drawn from studies in which full dose-response curves are constructed. In their study Kelly and Renaud (1973) observed that 'it is not difficult to select isolated parts of the ratemeter records . . . which show bicuculline to antagonise some of the responses to glycine'. The construction of full dose-response curves, however, clearly revealed the greater specificity of bicuculline for GABA (equipotent dose ratios around 2) compared with glycine (equipotent dose ratios around 1.1). The difficulty in interpreting individual responses was due to a two-fold greater slope of the dose-response curve for glycine than for GABA.

In most dose-response studies (Kelly and Renaud, 1973; Curtis *et al.*, 1971a) the dose is plotted as log current, to produce a log current v. response curve. The almost linear nature of the curves (Figure 34) clearly deserves comparison

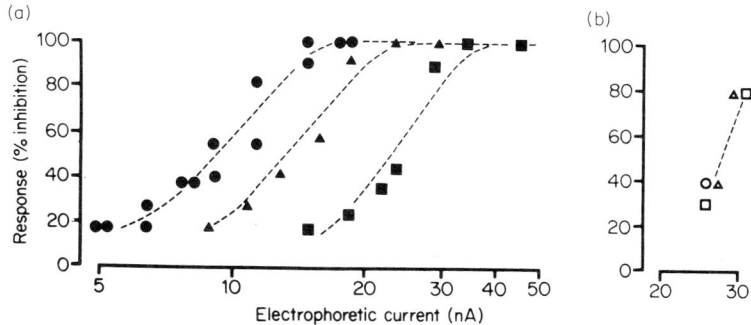

Figure 34 The effect of strychnine on the sensitivity of a spinal interneurone to glycine and GABA. The firing rate of the neurone was maintained at a frequency of approximately 60 spikes per second by continuously administered DLH and the dose–response curves relate percentage inhibition of firing (ordinate) to the electrophoretic current (logarithmically plotted as abscissae) used to eject the depressant amino acid. Filled symbols (a) glycine, corresponding hollow symbols (b) GABA. Circles, control observations; triangles, during the electrophoretic ejection of strychnine (+ 5 nA, 2 mM in 165 mM NaCl); squares during the administration of strychnine with a current of 10 nA. (Reproduced by permission of Springer-Verlag from Curtis *et al.*, 1971a.)

with the log dose v. response curves of classical pharmacology and, on the assumption made by these and other groups that drug release by iontophoretic ejection was linearly related to ejecting current (Ch. 4) the log current/response curve may well reflect the pharmacological behaviour of the test system just as much as a log dose/response curve derived from an organ bath experiment. Various factors such as uptake, metabolism, desensitization, lipid solubility, diffusional access, non-specific effects, etc., will contribute to the final curve in both situations.

The curves of Figure 34 were constructed from measurements of apparent plateau responses obtained at different ejecting currents but, as noted earlier in this chapter, there are several problems with this method, including the need for extremely stable recordings throughout the entire process of obtaining a full dose–response curve (since any movement of cell or electrode may change the drug's access to its receptors), the fact that many compounds exhibit very steep dose–response relationships, and the difficulty of identifying a true plateau response. Even the smallest doses of GABA may produce total inhibition if the application is sufficiently prolonged (Hill and Simmonds, 1973). In addition it was pointed out by Kelly *et al.* (1975) that the generation of such sequential dose–response curves can easily occupy several minutes, and it is impossible to be certain that the antagonist concentration in the tissue is constant over that period, i.e. that it has reached an equilibrium.

The use of individual responses as mini-cumulative dose–response curves reflecting the gradual increase of tissue concentration during an ejection period (see this chapter, Pt. IV) overcomes some of these problems since the question

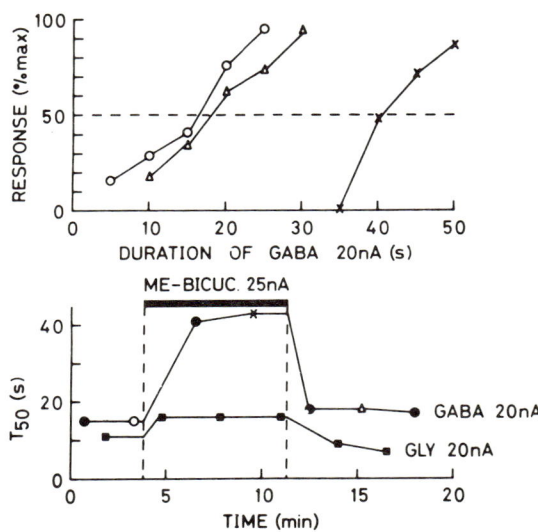

Figure 35 Effect of methylbicuculline (ME-BICUC) on the depressant responses to GABA and glycine (GLY) of a spontaneously active single neurone in the cuneate nucleus of a cat anaesthetized with halothane. Microiontophoretic applications of GABA 20 nA and glycine 20 nA were made alternately. Response curves to three of the applications of GABA before (O), (during (x) and after (Δ) the continuous microiontophoretic application of methylbicuculline are shown at the top. The values of time to 50% inhibition (T_{50}) measured from each response are plotted against elapsed time throughout the experiment. Note the marked increase in GABA T_{50} in the presence of methylbicuculline, indicating antagonism. The responses to glycine were much less affected. (Unpublished results of Hill and Simmonds. Reproduced from Simmonds, 1974, by permission of Pergamon Press Ltd.)

of generating a series of plateau responses does not arise. Furthermore, by measuring T_{50}, the time taken to reach a half-maximal response, equivalent in many respects to a classical ED_{50}, the time course of antagonism can be followed simply by examining successive responses (Figure 35). It is certainly the case that parallel shifts of the response v. time plots can be observed by altering the amount of material ejected from a pipette (Figure 36).

It is interesting to note, however, that plots of response v. time appear to be more meaningful than plots of response v. *log* time (Hill and Simmonds, 1973). This assertion is made on the basis of the finding that displacements of the time–response curve for GABA by antagonists such as bicuculline and picrotoxin are more nearly parallel to the control curve than are displacements of log time–response plots. On theoretical grounds, assuming the existence of spare receptors, displacements of log concentration–response curves should remain parallel (Stephenson, 1956). The authors, therefore, concluded that the concentration of GABA outside the pipette tip must increase in approximately exponential fashion with time, the 'log' component of the concentration axis becoming implicit in the use of linear time in the dose–response relationship.

Analysis of Results

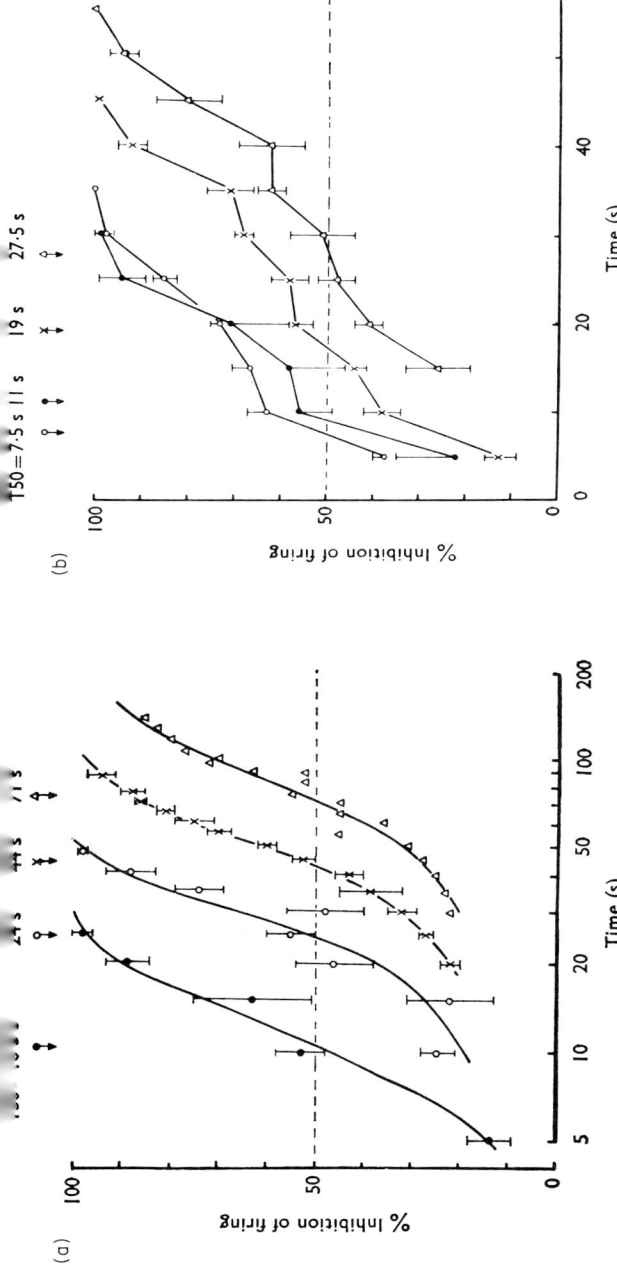

Figure 36 (a) Time-courses of inhibition of neurone firing due to microiontophoretic application of γ-aminobutyric acid (GABA) with four different currents, 20 nA (●), 10 nA (○), 5 nA (×) and 2 nA (△). Each curve was obtained from the same neurone at a depth of 957 μm in the middle suprasylvian gyrus of cat cortex. The neurone was driven by continuous microiontophoretic application of L-glutamate 20 nA. Each of the points for the 20 nA, 10 nA and 5 nA applications of GABA is the mean ± SEM of three values obtained from three separate applications of the same current of GABA. The values of T_{50} shown are the times taken to achieve 50% inhibition of neurone firing. (b) Effect on the γ-aminobutyric acid (GABA) response-linear time relationships of four different retaining currents applied to the GABA barrel between expulsions. Each point is the mean + SEM obtained from four separate applications of GABA 10 nA following passage of a retaining current of 5 nA (●), 10 nA (○), 25 nA (×) or 50 nA (△). The responses were obtained in a 4 × 4 latin square sequence from a single neurone driven by continuous application of L-glutamate 15 nA at a depth of 1062 μm in the middle suprasylvian gyrus. The control firing rates of the neurone (spike/s) during passage of a retaining current through the GABA barrel were 42 ± 2.8 at 5 nA, 48 ± 2.9 at 10 nA, 53 ± 3.7 at 25 nA and 59 ± 3.1 at 50 nA (means ± SEM of four values). (Reproduced from Hill and Simmonds, 1973, by permission of the British Pharmacological Society.)

Such an exponential rise of drug concentration can be readily understood from the effects of retaining current discussed in detail in Chapter 4, Part II. The efflux of compound from a pipette tip, both diffusional and induced by iontophoretic current, will increase during at least the early part of an iontophoretic ejection as the diluted fluid in the pipette tip is recharged by mobile ions. If potent compounds such as GABA are being used, where ejection periods are relatively short, this exponential phase may occupy the whole of the ejection pulse (Clarke *et al.*, 1973).

As yet there seem to have been few studies designed to determine whether the observations discussed above are more generally applicable to compounds other than inhibitory amino acids. This particular group of substances, of course, carries the clear advantage of an easily defined maximum response (complete suppression of firing). The situation is less satisfactory for excitatory amino acids where the maximum attainable response may be either the achievement of a plateau of firing which cannot be increased by higher ejecting currents, or the onset of overdepolarization (Clarke *et al.*, 1974). These two parameters do overlap, however, with some compounds to an extent which makes interpretation difficult. Thus, even as the plateau level is approached there may already be some noticeable decline of spike height. In spite of these problems Clarke *et al.* (1974) have been able to demonstrate parallel shifts of the time–response curves for acetylcholine but not glutamate by atropine, and of glutamate but not acetylcholine by 1-hydroxy-3-amino-pyrrolidone-2 (Figure 37).

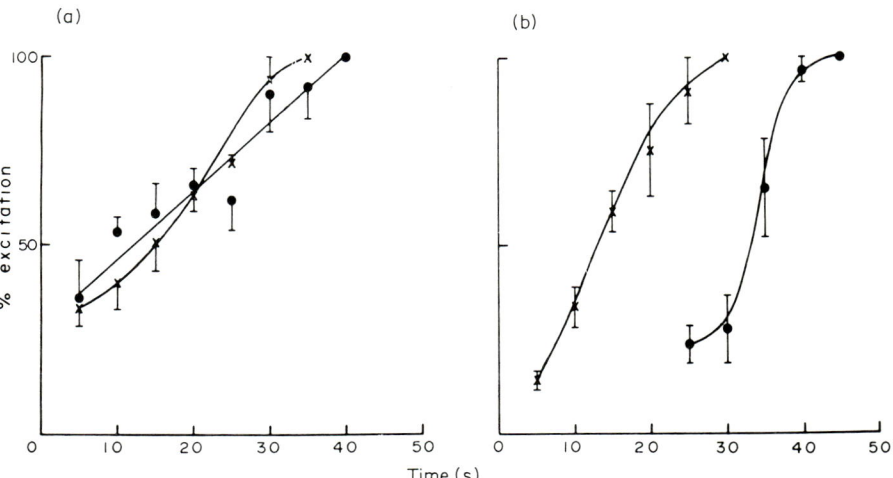

Figure 37 Effect of microiontophoretic HA-966 on the time-courses of excitation of a neurone to acetylcholine (a) and L-glutamate (b). Each curve is the mean + SEM of three responses. Acetylcholine was expelled with a current of 100 nA (×) and L-glutamate with a current of 50 nA (×). The two test curves (●) were 150 s after starting to apply HA-966, 50 nA. Range of maximum rates: acetylcholine, 40–45 Hz; L-glutamate, 55–60 Hz. (reproduced from Clarke *et al.*, 1974, by permission of Pergamon Press Ltd.)

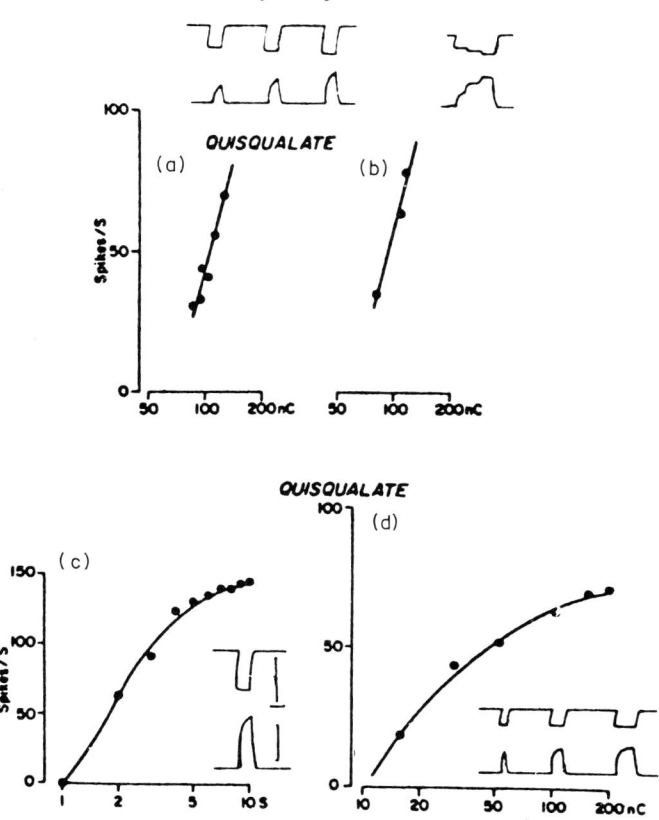

Figure 38 Different methods of obtaining dose–response relations. Some original tracings (currents, top; spike activity, bottom) are shown above (a) and (b) and beside (c) and (d). In (c) calibration bars (also valid for all the other tracings): current 15 nA; time (horizontal bar) 10 s; response 100 spike/second. Abscissa (log scale): nc for (a), (b) and (d); seconds for (c). Ordinate: spikes/second. Same neurone for each method. (Reproduced from Nistri and MacDonald, 1978, by permission of Plenum Publishing Corp.)

Similarly there have been few studies designed to pursue the question of whether time–response, log time–response, current–response or log current–response plots have particular respective advantages for the estimation of drug potency or antagonism.

Nistri and MacDonald (1978), however, have attempted a comparison of different types of dose–response curve for excitatory amino acids. Those results relevant to the present discussion are illustrated in Figure 38. A plot of response against log current or log charge reveals the very steep relationship noted above and in studies of inhibitory amino acids. The lines obtained are very similar whether the responses are measured sequentially (Figure 38a) or cumulatively (Figure 38b). When the responses are measured with respect to time, however, either using single responses (Figure 38c) or a fixed ejection current applied for varying periods of time (Figure 38d), the dose–response relationship is much more tranquil (Note that if Figure 38c were plotted with linear time on the abscissa, as discussed above the curve would assume a shape almost identical to Figure 38d.)

Clearly the dose–response relationships of Figures 38a and b are not comparable in position or slope with those of Figures 38c and d and the reasons for this require some investigation if dose–response curves obtained from microiontophoretic studies are to be acceptable and meaningful. One possible explanation of the difference may lie in the rapidity with which responses are produced using the different methodologies. When measuring response size produced by sequentially increasing doses (Figures 38a and b) for example, it is necessary to obtain stable, preferably plateau responses. But at the lower doses which would be necessary to obtain responses at the lower end of the dose–response relationship the responses are also delayed (Figures 16 and 17) so that the period over which the agonist concentration is rising becomes increasingly extended as the ejecting current is reduced. Therefore, the possibility of desensitization of receptor mechanisms, or of accommodation of the neuronal spike-generating mechanism becomes correspondingly greater and the chances of obtaining clear reproducible responses correspondingly less (see Ch. 6, Pt. I). At the lower doses too there will be a more delicate balance between tissue concentration and uptake for many agonists, and saturation of the uptake mechanism may result in unexpectedly large responses.

In the case of higher doses it is still necessary to allow responses to develop relatively steadily towards an equilibrium value and one might postulate a balance existing between the drive for depolarization and the tendency for desensitization, accommodation or uptake saturation which could account for the steepness of the upper part of the curve.

The problem of inactivation would presumably not apply to measurements used in Figures 38c and d because relatively high ejecting currents are being used and the entire response is completed in about 10 seconds, i.e. a low rate of firing can be achieved within 1 or 2 seconds.

An extension of this argument might lead to the prediction that as the duration of application is progressively reduced (but using higher currents), thus reducing the effect of uptake, inactivation, etc., still further, a smaller total charge might be required to produce a given response. This is indeed what is found experimentally (Figure 33).

PART VI USES OF QUALITATIVE MICROIONTOPHORESIS, AND THE RESPONSE CRITERIA EMPLOYED

In common with many other fields of biology qualitative microiontophoresis attracts its share of criticism from those who denigrate purely phenomenological research. It remains nevertheless an exceedingly useful method for the determination of whether neurones respond, or do not respond, to a suspected neurotransmitter or drug, and for a crude assessment of whether any responses can be blocked by antagonists known to be effective in peripheral systems. It can be used to assess whether antagonists show a clear selectivity of effect towards different agonists or whether there is sufficient doubt that only a more detailed quantitative analysis can decide the issue. It can be used to compare the nature of responses to supposedly related agonists or to determine whether sensitivity to a compound is restricted to one particular type of cell. Even at this level, though, there are complications in any analysis which require careful consideration.

The first of these is the decision of what constitutes a response. It is relatively rare to encounter neurones which fire at a sufficiently regular rate that small deviations of, say, 10%, from that rate can be readily detected. Many authors have, therefore, defined a response as a change of 25% or 30% of the mean baseline firing rate, but the value chosen as the criterion may require modification depending on the type of firing pattern and the type of response being considered.

Nagler et al. (1973) have used the concept of Critical Ratio (CR) to define a criterion response. The CR is a function of the resting spontaneous firing rate S, and that evoked by drug application E, the relationship being of the form:

$$CR = (E - S)/(E + S)^{1/2}$$

Values of CR of $+1.96$ or greater are considered significant, and correspond to an approximately 30% change of baseline firing. This criterion has been used recently by Mandelbrod et al. (1983) in a study of neuronal sensitivity to sodium ions.

An alternative definition of a response might take into account that a change in the pattern of firing could occur, even without a change in the overall firing rate. Such a change of firing pattern would be most easily detected as a shift in the frequency or interspike interval histograms for the neurone. Various statistical analyses of such histograms are available, but a simple indicator of a shift would be to express the number of spikes in the main control histogram bin as a proportion of the total number of spikes in the histogram (Nagler et al., 1973).

Perhaps even more difficult is the definition of a 'non-response'. Unlike most other areas of pharmacology the experimenter can never be certain that his iontophoresed compounds are gaining access to the relevant receptors, or indeed that the compounds are being ejected at all (Ch. 4). If initial experiments suggest that a high proportion of cells do not respond to an agent it may well be a sensible precaution to include two barrels containing the substance in each pipette. It is unlikely that both will work or fail in parallel.

Certainly if a compound has a clear action on a high proportion, say 50%, of a population of cells it is probably reasonable to assume that those effects represent a real sensitivity to the substance. It would be wrong on the other hand to conclude that a compound is inactive because it acts on only 5% or

10% of the population. There may be many substances for which specific receptors exist on only a small fraction of neurones. However, no one is likely to become overexcited about responses in 5% of a cell group unless the validity of the effects can be supported by firm evidence of physiological or pharmacological specificity or relevance.

It is undoubtedly misleading, however, to obtain for example a complete (100%) suppression of firing on 2 of 10 cells and then to conclude that the substance produces a mean depression of 20% of baseline firing. It becomes particularly important, if a low incidence of responses is obtained, to list, individually, all the cell responses (Stone, 1983b). On the one hand it is impossible to be categoric about the significance of an absence of iontophoretic responses, while on the other hand the potentially high significance of two 100% responses should not be submerged in attempts at pseudo-quantification.

VI.1 Spontaneous or evoked baselines?

Almost all of the preceding discussion relates to that large majority of investigations in which study is made of changes in spontaneous firing rate. There are others in which quiescent cells are aroused from their inactivity by an excitant compound, frequently an amino acid, in order better to examine the effects of supposedly inhibitory compounds. There is an increasing realization, however, that such a procedure requires the possible interaction between excitant and depressant compounds to be taken into account, and that the efficacy of the depressants will depend partly on the ionic changes induced by the excitant. This procedure is, therefore, falling out of fashion.

When artifical baseline firing is induced, the possibility must also be considered that the size, or even direction of agonist responses may depend on the background firing level chosen (see this chapter, Pt. VII. 1b) (Szabadi *et al.*, 1977).

Posing even greater problems for interpretation and the definition of a response are comparisons of the effects of compounds on spontaneous and neurally evoked activity. As a clear example, the effects of noradrenaline iontophoresed in the cerebellum have usually been found to inhibit spontaneous firing (Hoffer *et al.*, 1971b; Siggins *et al.*, 1971a) but when tested against activity evoked by stimulation of afferent neurones or iontophoretically applied amino acids that activity was enhanced (Freedman *et al.*, 1977; Moises *et al.*, 1979). Analogous observations of potentiated excitatory or inhibitory responses have since been reported on neurones in the cerebral cortex (Waterhouse and Woodward, 1980; Waterhouse *et al.*, 1980).

Similarly dopamine is usually considered to have a depressant effect on the spontaneous activity of neostriatal cells, whereas it is said to facilitate activity induced by local electrical stimulation in 80% of the cells tested (Norcross and Spehlmann, 1978a).

Clearly in cases such as these where a compound has opposite effects on different parameters a simple statement of excitation or inhibition is not possible.

It is likely that in the future the effects of substances applied by microiontophoresis will be more rigorously characterized in terms of their effects on a range of synaptic and exogenous chemical stimuli as well as on spontaneous firing.

PART VII USES OF QUANTITATIVE MICROIONTOPHORESIS

VII.1 Antagonism

Probably the most frequent attempts to quantify microiontophoretic data pertain to the selectivity or otherwise of antagonists (e.g. Curtis *et al.*, 1971a). Methods of constructing dose–response curves have been discussed above but it may be useful at this point to re-emphasize the unknown extent to which the choice of a particular method may influence the conclusion. For example early descriptions of the use of bicuculline as a selective antagonist of GABA were largely qualitative (Curtis *et al.*, 1971b). However, the group of Hill *et al.* (1973) using measurements of T_{50} (this chapter, Pt. IV and Pt. V) reported that tubocurarine was a far better antagonist of GABA than was bicuculline (subsequently disputed by Curtis *et al.*, 1974) and that bicuculline frequently *enhanced* responses to GABA. It should be emphasized though that it is still not entirely clear whether these differences of opinion are wholly attributable to the different parameters used for measurement. The differences could also reflect the use of cortical neurones by Hill *et al.* (1973) or the fact that in all these early studies bicuculline base, which hydrolyses rapidly in solution, was used and different methods of filling the micropipettes, or the frequency with which new electrodes containing fresh solutions were used could have contributed to the discrepant observations.

VII.1.a Measures of antagonism

A numerical descriptor of antagonism is readily obtained from log dose–response curves as an equipotent dose ratio of the agonist, usually calculated from the mid-point or ED_{50} level of the dose–response plot. In the T_{50} method of Hill and Simmonds (1973) each individual response is regarded as a cumulative dose–response curve and the T_{50} becomes equivalent to the ED_{50}. However, ratios of T_{50} cannot be used as equivalent to the conventional dose ratio as the value obtained would depend on factors peculiar to iontophoresis such as the use of retaining currents, which impose a delay on the responses. Equally the value T_{50} (test-control) would vary depending on the absolute levels of ejecting current used. The ratio T_{50} (test-control)/T_{50} (control) was, therefore, developed as a means of minimizing the variation introduced by both these factors (Hill and Simmonds, 1973).

VII.1.b Baseline fluctuations

A problem frequently encountered in drug interaction studies is that the potential antagonist or potentiating drug itself produces changes of the baseline firing rate (this chapter, Pt. VI.1) (Hill *et al.*, 1973). The effect which such a change might have on agonist responses has been the subject of disagreement; Szabadi *et al.* (1977) have reported that the probability of observing excitant responses to monoamines was greater in slowly firing cells whereas the likelihood of obtaining inhibitions was lessened. Conversely, depressant responses were more likely on rapidly firing neurones. Curtis *et al.* (1971a), however, noted that depressant amino acids became *less* effective with elevations of basal firing rate.

Clearly it is essential to try and take into account fluctuations of baseline firing rate if meaningful assessments of potentiation or antagonism are to be made. One theoretical possibility would be to eject a compensatory excitatory or inhibitory compound to maintain a constant background firing. This would raise additional questions regarding the interaction of the substance of interest with the compensatory compound (this chapter, Pt. VI.1).

A more realistic solution in cases where a putative antagonist depresses background firing may be to use a histogram summation method which accumulates a sufficient number of sweeps that the background firing levels become comparable. Examples of this procedure for excitatory and inhibitory agonists are illustrated in Figures 39 and 40. In Figure 39 the effects of atropine against excitant responses to acetylcholine and cyclic GMP are being studied (Stone and Taylor, 1977) whereas Figure 40 illustrates the use of the same technique to compensate for the marked depressant action of manganese ions which became problematic in investigating their reported antagonistic action against monoamines (Freedman *et al.*, 1975). In both these cases the computer summation technique allows sufficiently clear responses to be seen that calculations of percentage depression, and thus an assessment of antagonism can be performed.

It must always be considered, of course, that, as noted earlier, the depression of background produced by the antagonist may itself alter the efficacy of the agonist, or its reversibility by the antagonist, i.e. the computer summation technique can only compensate for the observability of a response, not the effect which the antagonist depression itself may have on those responses. It is always desirable to perform suitable control experiments in which the spontaneous firing is artificially suppressed or raised by an unrelated substance.

VII.2 Comparisons of potency or sensitivity

A neurone might, perhaps naively, be expected to exhibit a greater sensitivity towards a compound which is used as a transmitter on to that neurone, than to a related substance. Attempts to demonstrate such a difference of sensitivity between glutamate and aspartate will be discussed in detail in Chapter 7 but here it is sufficient to note the following points. Firstly, log current–response curves can be used to reveal differences in neuronal sensitivity (Gent *et al.*, 1974; Gent and Wolstencroft, 1976a; Norcross and Spehlmann, 1978b). Gent and Wolstencroft (1976a), for example, have used dose ratios taken from such curves

Analysis of Results

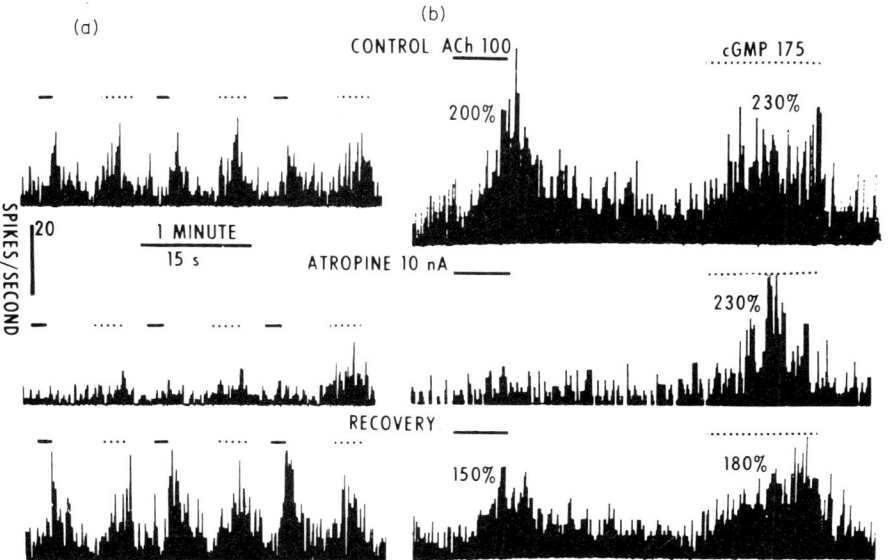

Figure 39 (a) Ratemeter records of the responses of a pyramidal tract neurone to acetylcholine, 100 nA (continuous bars over record) and cyclic GMP, 175 nA (interrupted bars). The duration of drug ejection and the time between pulses was accurately controlled by a Devices Digitimer as described by Freedman et al. (1975). The upper trace is the control record. During the application of atropine, 10 nA (middle trace) the spontaneous rate was markedly reduced, making the determination of responsiveness to the agonists difficult. During the post-atropine recovery period (lower trace) the cell again clearly responded to acetylcholine and cyclic GMP. (b) Post-stimulus time histograms derived from summed responses of the cell shown in (a) (Freedman et al., 1975). Percentage of excitations was calculated by comparing the mean number of counts per bin for the period of drug response with the mean number of counts per bin during the periods before and after the drug applications (see Methods). The upper trace shows the firing pattern before, middle trace during, and lower trace 3 min after the iontophoresis of atropine, 10 nA. During the atropine application, cyclic GMP produced the same degree of excitation as in the control periods, while acetylcholine responses were completely blocked. Time bar is 1 min for (a), 15 s for (b). (Reproduced from Stone and Taylor, 1977, by permission of the Physiological Society.)

to reveal a correlation between relative sensitivity to glutamate and aspartate and vibrissal input in the rat thalamus.

Dose–response curves have also been used to follow changes of amine sensitivity. Norcross and Spehlmann (1978b) obtained significant displacements of their dopamine log current–response curves in the striatum after dopamine depletion, and Haas et al. (1978) were able to demonstrate significant changes in the currents needed to produce both threshold and maximum plateau responses to histamine after lesions of the medial forebrain bundle. Although there was a four-fold decrease of threshold response current and a two-fold drop in maximum responses current for histamine, there was no change of GABA sensitivity.

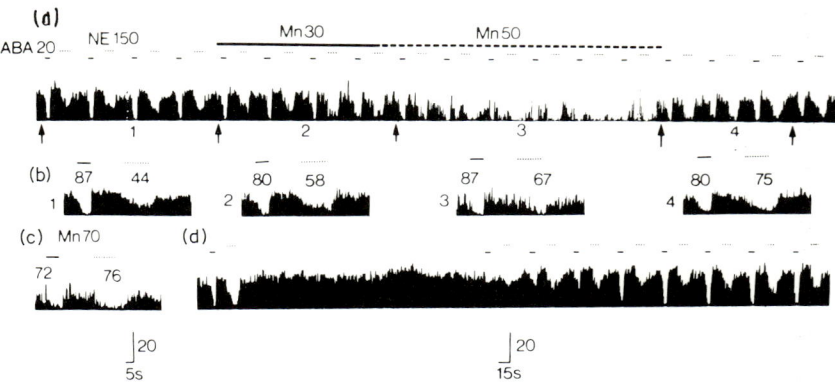

Figure 40 Ratemeter and drug response histograms showing effect of manganese (Mn) and interruption of agonist pulses on inhibitory responses to GABA (solid line) and noradrenaline (NA) (dotted line). (a), (b), (c) and (d) all from the same Purkinje cell, recorded over a period of 6 h. (a) The continuous ratemeter record of the effects of periodic application of GABA and NA. The numbers and arrows beneath the record show the regions used to construct the associated drug response histograms in (b). Note that despite the large reduction of spontaneous activity produced by 50 nA of manganese, there is no decrement in noradrenaline-induced inhibition during (b3) or after (b4) manganese. An even larger dose of 70 nA of manganese (c) reduced spontaneous discharge rate to 0.3 spikes/second but did not reduce NA-induced inhibition. (d) The differential effect of pulse interruption. At the resumption of pulsing, both GABA- and NA-induced inhibition are diminished. However, the GABA response recovers by the 4th cycle whereas the NA inhibition is still only 50% recovered by the 8th cycle. The calibrations bars under (c) and (d) are for histogram (counts per address) and ratemeter (spike/second) records, respectively. (Reproduced form Freedman *et al.*, 1975, by permission of the British Pharmacological Society.)

In a cautionary paper Gent *et al.* (1974) emphasized the need to take into account variations between pipettes, particularly with regard to transport numbers, before drawing conclusions about relative potencies. By measuring transport numbers for glutamate and aspartate before and after a sampling of neurones in the brainstem these workers noted that differences of sensitivity could appear, disappear or even be reversed when the transport characteristics were taken into account.

While such considerations are undoubtedly important when a random sample of cells is taken, they may be less important when, as in the later study of Gent and Wolstencroft (1976a) a clear correlation emerges with some anatomical, physiological or pharmacological parameter unrelated to the iontophoresis technique. The random variations of sensitivity observed by considering pipettes individually are then presumably swamped by biological factors.

The existence of large variations of ejection characteristics between barrels and between micropipettes makes it difficult to compare the potencies of individual compounds in absolute terms in different experiments and in particular between different laboratories. One way round this is to compare the relative apparent potencies of two compounds—that ratio would not be expected to vary greatly as a result of purely technical differences provided a sufficiently large and homogeneous population of cells is studied (Perkins and Stone, 1983a).

Another trick to minimize the contribution of electrode differences to apparent differences of sensitivity is to use the *same* electrode in both areas of CNS or both animals under consideration, in the same experiment, testing two or three cells alternately in the two test tissues (Perkins and Stone, 1983a). Ideally, following a central lesion, it may be possible to alternate between the control and lesioned areas on the two sides of the brain.

Various aspects of the problem of comparing neurotransmitter sensitivity before and after chronic drug treatment have been discussed by Bloom *et al.* (1981).

CHAPTER 6

Limitations and Problems of Interpretation

I	EFFECTIVE DRUG CONCENTRATION	105
	I.1 Extrajunctional Receptors	110
	I.2 Chronic Changes	110
II	RETAINING CURRENTS	110
	II.1 Antagonist Studies	112
	II.2 Current Instability	112
III	CURRENT ARTEFACTS	113
	III.1 Sodium	114
	III.2 'Electrical Diversion'	115
IV	INTERBARREL COUPLING	116
V	INDIRECT DRUG EFFECTS	117
	V.1 Neurones and Terminals	117
	V.2 Blood Vessels	119
	V.3 Glial Cells	119
	V.4 'Non-Specific' Effects	120
VI	pH EFFECTS	120
	VI.1 pH and Pressure	123
VII	COUNTER ION EFFECTS	123
VIII	TEMPERATURE EFFECTS	124
IX	OSMOTIC EFFECTS	124
X	CONTAMINATION	124
XI	INFLUENCE OF ANAESTHETICS	125
XII	FIELD POTENTIALS	129
XIII	PRESSURE EJECTION	132

This is *not* a pharmacology textbook, and many of the most serious problems of experimental design and interpretation in iontophoretic studies are peculiar to the project concerned and relate directly to the pharmacology involved. If examining the sensitivity of neurones to a neurotransmitter after lesioning an input pathway or following drug treatment, for example, it is just as important to assess the relative contributions of altered uptake, metabolism or access to a change in sensitivity as it is in organ bath studies.

In this chapter an attempt will be made to catalogue some of the recognized problems which need to be considered when interpreting specifically microiontophoretic and pressure ejection data. A superficial glance might give the impression that the number of problems is so large that it is surprising anyone bothers with the technique. In its defence, it is the author's opinion that this catalogue is a healthy reflection of 25 years of use, and thoughtful discussion. In the case of some other techniques for looking at transmitter receptors, such as radioligand binding, it is difficult to escape the feeling that a certain promiscuity of practice has outstripped any realistic fundamental theoretical appraisal.

PART I EFFECTIVE DRUG CONCENTRATION

This subject will not be dealt with here again in detail since a theoretical discussion of the amounts of drug ejected and their distribution in the target tissue has been presented in Chapter 4. Also, the problems which a lack of knowledge of drug concentration presents for the analysis of results have been discussed in Chapter 5. The topic is mentioned again here mainly to re-emphasize that this absence of information on the concentration of drug at its receptor is usually considered to be one of the primary disadvantages of the microiontophoretic technique. Although the concentrations of drug present in the brain may be equally uncertain, for example, after systemic administration (and one has the potentially greater problem of distinguishing direct from indirect effects), those concentrations do not vary along a space–time continuum as they do after iontophoretic administration.

For the same reason it is not necessarily adequate to know the amount of drug ejected from a pipette, or its concentration at a single point in the tissue. Thus the use of suitably calibrated micropressure ejection allows the experimenter to know with reasonable accuracy how much drug has been ejected, but that measurement provides no information on the access of drug to the cell or cells being recorded, which may be several tens of microns distant, or on the distribution of the drug to different parts of a cell such as dendrites or soma: in most parts of the brain this will depend primarily on the relative orientation of electrode and cell. This is undoubtedly one of the reasons why regularly oriented cell layers such as those in the hippocampus are becoming increasingly attractive for iontophoretic studies, especially *in vitro*.

The same limitations apply to the use of carbon fibre measurements of drug concentrations (see Figures 15 and 68); they can provide little information on the distribution of drug at the cell surface, only on its concentration during ejection in the immediate environment of the tip. Of course, both pressure ejection and carbon fibre measurements during iontophoresis represent distinct advantages over blind iontophoresis in that they remove the additional uncertainty of variation between pipettes and their ejection characteristics. The carbon fibre technique in particular confers the signal advantage of being able to adjust the iontophoretic current to maintain a constant ionic concentration around the tip for a relatively extended period of time (Figure 68) during which the same concentration would presumably become distributed over an appreciable volume of tissue, including the recording site. Used especially under equilibrium conditions, therefore, the use of carbon fibre analysis would represent substantial advantages for quantitative iontophoresis.

Without electrochemical measurements of concentration, however, such an equilibrium cannot be claimed and the electrode/cell relationship becomes critical. A small cell, for example, must be approached more closely than a larger cell in order to obtain a suitable signal-to-noise ratio, and this may result in a higher drug concentration at the surface of the smaller cell. The problem is not solved merely by approaching all cell bodies as closely as possible: in the case of cells with extensive dendritic arborizations damage to those dendrites may preclude close access. Also with such cells an electrode near the cell soma for recording may be several hundred microns from a receptive area on the dendrites. It may then become necessary to take into account other parameters of the drug response such as onset delay, which may provide clues as to the tip-to-membrane distance.

It is clearly totally unacceptable to conclude that two entirely different cell populations have different sensitivities to a compound if no consideration is given to their geometric characteristics. One partial solution is to compare the sensitivities of both cell types when ejection is performed at different distances from the cell body using combination electrodes as described in Chapter 2, Pt. VI. Another solution would be to compare the sensitivity to the test compound with sensitivity to a control substance which would have a predictable and perhaps non-specific effect on the cell membrane. Thus the sensitivity of a cell to a local anaesthetic, or veratridine for example, might be a useful indicator of the distance of the ejection pipette from the cell (soma) surface.

Problems of this kind can be substantially reduced by studying a clearly identified population of neurones rather than the randomly encountered cells used in the majority of iontophoretic studies (Bloom, 1974). Cells may be identified *in vivo*, for example by stereotaxis in the case of large regularly organized cells such as hippocampal pyramids, though preferably confirmed by stimulation of an appropriate synaptic pathway. Alternatively these cells as well as corticofugal cells in the neocortex, Purkinje cells, motoneurones, hypothalamo-hypophyseal projection neurones and many others can be identified by antidromic stimulation of their axons or terminal fields. Some cells may be best identified by their short latency responses to an orthodromic input. In all these cases the result of identification is the selection of a population of neurones which is likely to be relatively homogeneous in terms of size and geometry (though not necessarily orientation). The experimenter can, therefore, be reasonably satisfied that to a first approximation the size of a recorded spike will provide an indication of the distance between electrode and cell soma.

In some cases an excellent correlation can be demonstrated between functionally identified neurones (for example neurosecretory versus non-neurosecretory, warm-sensitive versus cold-sensitive, etc.) and their responses to locally ejected compounds (Ch. 7). While these correlations may indeed be an indication of the functional pharmacology of the respective neuronal populations, the possibility also exists that the differences are in part a reflection of a different surface geometry.

Herz et al. (1969) have discussed another facet of this problem. This group was interested in the threshold concentration for activation of neurones by iontophoretically applied glutamate but they concluded that the threshold for activation of more distant cells was relatively lower than that for cells closer to the pipette tip. The authors' explanation of this was that a relatively large volume of damaged tissue would exist around the tip of a multibarrelled pipette, so that the released glutamate would be effectively diluted at the surface of a cell situated only a few microns away. More distant cells might however, experience a relatively higher concentration of glutamate due to its being restricted to the extracellular space. Another and perhaps more probable explanation of the results could be that more distant cells are likely to receive glutamate over a larger proportion of their total surface area than cells whose soma is situated close to the pipette tip, and summation effects could lead to the apparently decreased threshold of the distant cells.

Undoubtedly the greatest perils presented by a lack of knowledge of drug concentration are encountered in studies of drug interactions. The subject was first discussed in detail by Curtis et al. (1971a) and summarized by Curtis (1976). In conventional pharmacological work an increased drug dose (systemic or bath applied) is assumed to affect an increased number of receptors distributed throughout the entire area of a given membrane. This is not so for a compound applied from a point source as in microiontophoresis. Increasing doses of the substance will in this case activate not only a greater density of receptors on the membrane closest to the micropipette but will also gain access to receptors on previously virgin portions of the membrane (Figure 41). The concentration of agonist (E) decreases from the centre to the periphery of the affected area in each case. This immediately places a limitation on the value of dose–response curves and clearly means that they should never be compared with dose–response curves obtained from systemic or *in vitro* studies.

However, this leads on to even greater difficulties of interpretation when antagonists are tested. As illustrated in Figure 41b an antagonist A may be ejected so as to block responses to the agonist, but increased doses of E may appear to overcome that blockade, not because the antagonism is competitive, as would be concluded in conventional pharmacology, but because new receptors are being reached. Equally a compound D which only acts on receptors some distance away from the pipette tip may appear to be unaffected by the antagonist at concentrations which block E.

Because of the diminishing concentration of compounds from the centre to periphery of the affected membrane patch, iontophoretic (or pressure) application of compounds may result in interference with responses by non-specific effects of drugs in a high proportion of tests. Thus an agonist may reach a sufficiently high concentration at one part of the membrane to cause desensitization or inactivation before a large enough area of membrane has been reached to give rise to an observable depolarization or discharge.

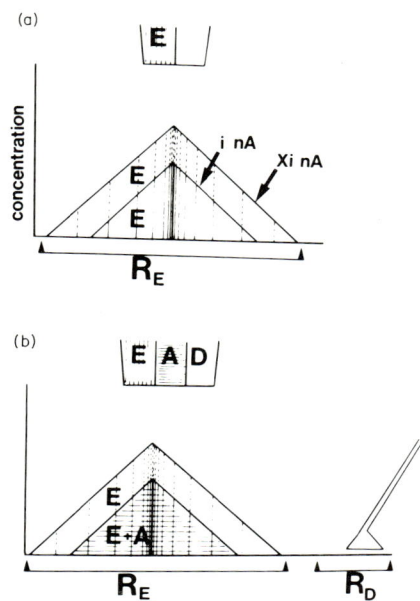

Figure 41 (a) An agonist compound, E, applied with a current of i nA will reach an effective concentration over an area of membrane covered by the inner triangle. The concentration of E will decrease from the centre to the edge of this area. A larger dose of E using Xi nA of current will not only increase the concentration at all points within the original area, but will also reach new regions of cell surface. The change of response between i and Xi nA doses will depend, for example, on whether any parts of the i nA membrane area received maximal concentrations, whether there is any desensitization, etc. (b) An antagonist A may block completely a low dose of agonist E but be overcome by a larger dose not because the antagonism is competitive, but because of the recruitment of new receptors. A compound D may appear to be unaffected by the antagonist because it only acts on relatively distant receptors not reached by doses of A which completely block E. R_E and R_D indicate areas of cell surface bearing receptors for E and D respectively

This point has been raised in connection with the construction of dose–response curves (Figure 38; see also Ch. 5, Pt. V).

Similarly when an antagonist is applied the concentration reached at the centre of the receiving membrane area may be sufficient to cause non-specific effects which preclude an assessment of potency or selectivity.

Clearly all these problems will be most severe when studies are being conducted of relative sensitivity, or the selectivity of antagonism, using agonists which act on different regions of the cell membrane. As long as all compounds are ejected from the same micropipette, however, and iontophoretic currents are comparable for all the agonists, the problems of interpretation can be contained. This may not be so for comparisons between locally ejected compounds and synaptic input, since the latter may well be situated hundreds of microns away. In order to reach a concentration at that distance sufficient to reduce the action of the transmitter an antagonist would almost certainly exist at concentrations several orders of magnitude greater near to the pipette tip, concentrations which may well cause a non-selective blockade of a range of agonist substances. Conversely, the application of antagonist at a dose which discriminates between a series of agonists but does not affect a synaptic input cannot be used as an argument that the synapses do not use the antagonized compound: this result may merely imply that the synapses, releasing the locally antagonized substance are located too far away to be accessed by the antagonist. Curtis *et al.* (1971a) and Curtis (1976) have argued that the most reliable way of examining the effects of antagonists is to administer them systemically so that the concentration is more evenly distributed over the neuronal surface.

Since the concentrations of agonists and antagonists will be changing in time and space after microiontophoretic application it is most important that experiments are designed very carefully. It is often tempting, for example, to apply an antagonist just as long as needed to block selectively one of a pair of agonists and turn off the ejection before the next pulse of the other agonist. This would be misleading since the local concentration of antagonist will begin to decline as soon as ejection is terminated so that the second agonist will be competing with less antagonist, giving a false impression of the selectivity of the antagonist. The experiment is likely to be biased the other way, of course, by maintaining the antagonist ejection through the 'control' agonist response, but since the concentrations of iontophoretically applied compounds increase more slowly during the ejection phase than they decrease on termination (Figure 17) this would still be a more satisfying and meaningful experimental design.

Adams (1976) working at the neuromuscular junction has emphasized that similar problems of interpretation apply to studies of desensitization using compounds applied by microiontophoresis. Thus the application of increasing maintained background (conditioning) doses of agonist will lead to activation of an increasing area of membrane by regularly repeated pulses of agonist, as more distant receptors are recruited on to the dose–response curve. There will be relatively little change in the degree of activation of membrane nearest the pipette tip, however, as the response there will be near maximal, while the contribution to the observed response of the more distant areas will become relatively much greater as those areas will be functioning on the rising phase of their dose–response curves. Conversely the areas closest to the pipette tip will tend to desensitize more rapidly due to their high concentration of agonist whereas distant sites will desensitize very little. A complex interaction between these opposing tendencies (increased response and desensitization) will be established which can explain the surprising observations that increasing conditioning applications of agonist may initially *decrease* the overall rate of desensitization of the postjunctional membrane (Adams, 1976).

I.1 Extrajunctional receptors

A further corollary of the uncertainty of drug concentration and distribution on the neuronal surface is that the extent to which different receptor populations are contributing to a response may be unknown. Where junctional and extrajunctional receptors can be studied independently, as at the neuromuscular junction, it is clear that such receptors have different pharmacological properties both in vertebrate and invertebrate preparations (Ch. 7). In the CNS there is little information available on the possible existence of such receptor variations but if the phenomenon does occur the possibility must be considered that the responses to exogenous agonists are being mediated largely via extrajunctional sites and that there may be fundamental differences of pharmacology between these and synaptically activated sites. Although the selective antagonism of one of a series of agonists in parallel with blockade of a synaptic input is powerful evidence for the identity of a synaptic transmitter the converse is clearly not true: negative results give little useful information.

I.2 Chronic changes

If changes of neuronal sensitivity are being studied after chronic administration of drugs or after lesions of neuronal pathways it is essential to consider the possibility that the imposed treatment has not altered the uptake or removal processes for the compound being tested since this will result in a different effective concentration at the receptors. As noted in the opening of this chapter this problem is not peculiar to microiontophoresis and this and related problems of a purely pharmacological nature should never be overlooked.

PART II RETAINING CURRENTS

The physics of retaining currents and their effect on drug ejection has also been treated in depth in Chapter 4. The reason for mentioning them again here is that the use of retaining currents probably provides a greater source of misinterpretation than any other facet of microiontophoresis.

The problem, it will be recalled, is that any retaining current will tend to draw appropriately charged particles away from the barrel tip. This will be partly a time-dependent phenomenon, as the ions will be withdrawn along an ever-widening diameter barrel until an equilibrium is reached where the cross-sectional area has caused the charge density to fall to a level which only just counteracts the net diffusional forces carrying ions towards the tip. The greater the retaining current, the greater and more rapid will be this withdrawal.

Of course, this dilution of solution in the barrel tip is the reason why retaining currents are used in the first place: with many potent compounds the absence of such a holding current will lead to a gradual change of firing rate or responsiveness as the compound diffuses from the tip. It is then essential to use a retaining current, the appropriate magnitude of which can be estimated by increasing its strength until an additional increment causes no further change of firing rate. (It is not sufficient that the current be increased until a constant, stable firing rate is seen, as this could still represent an equilibrium or plateau firing rate maintained by drug leakage.) It may be necessary to use retaining currents of 10–20 nA with potent neuroactive compounds.

Responses to some monoamines, particularly excitatory responses, may be prone to desensitization (Roberts and Straughan, 1967; Boakes *et al.*, 1971; Stone, 1973b). In these cases any hydrostatic or diffusional efflux of amines from a micropipette tip could result in the loss of responses or indeed failure to observe them at all. The problem should be surmountable by the use of low concentrations of agonist in the barrel and the use of high retaining currents, e.g. 25 nA (Johnson *et al.*, 1969a).

In the author's experience the use of a small retaining current (5–8 nA) often improves responses even to excitatory amino acids, presumably by reducing desensitization of the receptors, or by reducing a background of subliminal depolarization which can lead to rapid overdepolarization on ejection.

The main difficulty with using a retaining current is that the subsequent ejection period begins with a phase in which the drug ions are being pushed back into the barrel tip, i.e. there is an ejection delay. The physics of this interaction have been discussed in Chapter 4, but there are also biological and technical considerations. If the retaining current is very large, then in order to eject an effective amount of compound a large ejecting current may be needed. But once the drug ions have started to reach the barrel tip their rate of ejection may rapidly become so great that the response cannot be controlled, i.e. the cell's firing may be totally depressed by a potent inhibitory compound, or the cell may be overdepolarized by an excitant. In other words, in order to have a controllable response it is necessary to have a milder rate of ejection and in order to use a mild ejecting current, and get a response within a reasonable space of time, it is necessary to go easy on the retaining current. In the author's laboratory retaining currents of about 5–8 nA are found sufficient to eliminate detectable leakage of amino acids such as glutamate, and this allows good responses to be produced by 30–40 nA within about 5 seconds.

Since retention is also time dependent an increase of retention time may also lead to smaller responses subsequently unless ejection charge is increased to compensate. (This assumes that the retention parameters are not such that equilibrium is achieved during the retention period.)

Unfortunately it is often not realized that the same principle which requires such attention to retaining currents also applies to ejection currents. Consider for example the ejection of an agonist in the *absence* of any prior retaining current. By promoting the movement of ions towards the pipette tip an ejecting current will cause some concentration of the compound within the tip. After the ejection pulse the concentration in the tip will start to fall as the ions begin to diffuse away (into less concentrated solution above as well as into the tissue). If the next ejecting pulse is delivered before this process has reached equilibrium there will still be more drug in the tip than during the preceding pulse and, therefore, more will be ejected. Thus, even in the absence of retaining current an improvement in response may be seen over several ejecting pulses — (the 'warm-up' phenomenon (Freedman *et al.*, 1975). Furthermore, any change in ejection current or duration, or of the interval between ejection, will provoke gradual changes in the amount ejected over several ejection periods.

II.1 Antagonist studies

The greatest howlers in iontophoretic studies are undoubtedly committed during the examination of antagonist effects due to an inadequate consideration of retaining currents. It is not uncommon to see reports in which a series of agonist responses are followed by an antagonist application and the agonist ejection then recommenced with no regard given to the greater intervening retention time, which will tend to cause a decrease in the first responses following the 'antagonist', with, of course, a gradual apparent recovery. It cannot be emphasized enough that when studying drug interactions, such as selective antagonism, it is absolutely essential to have *regular* pulses of agonists applied with exactly the same ejection parameters each time (Figure 40d). After *any* change of ejection or retention parameters at least two and preferably three or more complete cycles of agonist responses of the same size must be obtained in order to ensure that equilibrium has been re-established. When using potent compounds in particular, the effect of a 1 nA change of retaining current or a 1 second change of retention time should never be underestimated. Automatic ejection cycles are always to be preferred to manual procedures in order to eliminate variations in the timing of ejection and retention periods.

If for some reason it is not desirable or practicable to deliver a putative antagonist simultaneously with a continuous series of agonist pulses then control tests must be performed in which the agonist pulses are stopped for the same period of time used for the antagonist, in order to assess the effect of the time interval *per se*.

II.2 Current instability

A technical problem associated with retention currents results from the fact that their magnitude may be approaching the stability or accuracy limits of the iontophoretic apparatus. Some commercially available apparatus provides the set current only to within ± 0.5 nA. However, it should be clear from the previous paragraph that a fluctuation of this size can greatly influence the subsequent ejection of a compound. As the proportionality effect of retaining current on subsequent ejection decreases as retention is increased, so it is better to use the largest, rather than the smallest retaining current possible, compatible with the factors discussed above, if it is necessary to obtain consistent reproducible responses. These considerations do not apply to equipment whose output is claimed to be accurate to 1% or less (Dagan, WPI).

Limitations and Problems of Interpretation

PART III CURRENT ARTEFACTS

The current strengths used for the microiontophoretic ejection of drugs are small, ranging usually from 10 to 200 nA. Nevertheless these currents are large enough to cause marked changes in the firing rate of some cells. Usually cells susceptible to the effect of current have been slightly damaged by the descending electrode, and the recorded spike potentials have a large initial positive component as a result. This is not always so, however, and wholly negative extracellular spikes may be recorded from a cell which is easily excited by anionic current and/or depressed by cationic current (see Krnjević and Phillis, 1963a).

In the author's experience cells in some areas of the CNS, such as hypothalamus, ventral striatum and cerebellum are far more sensitive to current flow than cells in other areas, this being consistent with the observations of others (e.g. Aleksanyan *et al.*, 1972 in hypothalamus and Crossman *et al.*, 1974 in striatum). This sensitivity could be related to the small size of cells in these regions.

Changes of firing induced by current can usually be distinguished by the extremely rapid onset and ending of the response as seen in Figure 42. This is not, however, an entirely reliable criterion for deciding whether a change

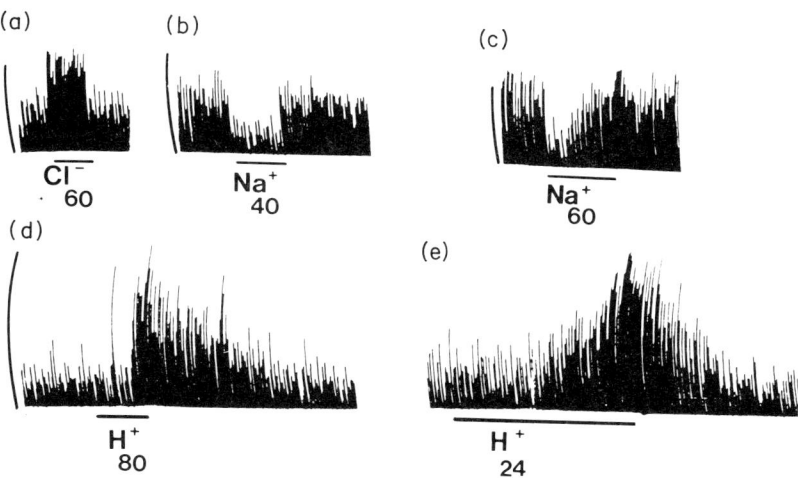

Figure 42 Examples of current and pH effects encountered during microiontophoresis. (a) and (b) Illustrated 'classical' current artefacts in which the cell is activated by inward iontophoretic current and depressed by outward current. Note the virtually instantaneous onset and offset of the effect. (c) A cautionary example to illustrate that cells can be recorded, particularly in areas such as cerebral cortex, where the firing rate recovers during the current application. This may be due to disinhibition of inhibitory cells or similar interneuronal effects. Note the small rebound excitation. In (d) an outward current is passed through a solution of NaCl containing HCl to a pH of 2. After a latent period the cell exhibits a sharp increase of excitability which can take several minutes to decay. In (e) the solution in the micropipette is at pH 4. The excitation is still seen but shows a much longer latency and is less abrupt in onset

of firing rate is caused by a drug or the ejecting current. A cell in which firing is initiated by an ejecting current could, particularly in a lightly anaesthetized or unanaesthetized animal (*encéphale isolé*), excite inhibitory neurones which could reduce the cell's firing rate before the cessation of the current. Also difficult for interpretation would be the recruitment of cells which re-excited the cell under study, thus prolonging the cell's activity beyond the current application.

It is necessary, therefore, to perform specific controls for such current effects. To this end, one barrel of a multibarrel pipette is always filled with an 'inert' solution such as sodium chloride, potassium acetate, potassium citrate, etc., through which the effect of current alone on a cell can be tested. Thus if a cell were depressed by the ejection of a drug ion D^+, then an ejecting current of equal magnitude would be used to eject Na^+ or K^+ from the control barrel. (There still remains, however, the problem that the mobility of Na^+ and a large drug ion may be very different.) This type of routine differential testing of drug and then current is a technique employed by many current authors.

Interpretation may still be difficult, however, in relatively few instances where cationic currents cause excitation of cells, and anionic currents depression, even when there is no evidence of cellular damage (Krnjević and Phillis, 1963a).

In an attempt to reduce these difficulties, the technique of current balancing was introduced (Salmoiraghi and Weight, 1967). In this modification an appropriate current is passed continuously through the control (usually sodium chloride) barrel so that the algebraic sum of current at the tip of the whole multibarrel pipette is always zero. That is, at each instant in time the control barrel current is of equal magnitude but opposite polarity to the sum of the retaining and ejecting currents in the other barrels of the pipette. The result of using this technique should be that the only factor acting on a particular cell is the drug under study. Technical aspects of current balancing have been considered in Chapter 3.

III.1 Sodium

The combined routine use of the current balancing method and subsequent testing of the current alone is probably adequate to eliminate potentially confusing current effects from the many difficulties of iontophoretic interpretation. However, the experimenter should also be aware that a 'current control' in effect usually means the expulsion of Na^+ or Cl^- by iontophoresis. Such ejections are undoubtedly irrelevant in a vast majority of tests, but Mandelbrod *et al.* (1983) have clearly shown that some cells in the hypothalamus are very sensitive to the ejection of Na^+. The problem appears to be particularly marked when glutamate or potassium are also present in the iontophoretic or recording pipettes, since Mandelbrod *et al.* (1983) reported that both of these ions would greatly potentiate the (excitatory) effects of sodium ions. Far fewer responses to sodium were also seen when ejections were performed from solutions more dilute than the molar solutions initially employed in these experiments. Presumably sodium-sensitive units in the hypothalamus are specialized units concerned with ionic balance in the body, but one should be alert to the possible existence of analogous cells elsewhere in the CNS.

III.2 'Electrical diversion'

A further source of confusion due to current balancing arises from the fact that the movement of ions as they exit from a barrel tip may be affected by the currents passing through the other barrels. Thus Lambert and Flatman (1981) have described the possibility that ejected glutamate ions may be 'sucked up' into a barrel through which an outward current is passing. There is little hard evidence for this possibility although it has been noted in the author's laboratory that, when using substances which are ejected using current pulses lasting only a few seconds, the responses are frequently smaller in size when the ejecting current is balanced than if the ejection is made unbalanced. Similarly Herz *et al.* (1969) noted that the latency of glutamate responses was increased when ejections were made balanced rather than unbalanced. These observations would clearly be consistent with Lambert and Flatman's (1981) suggestion, although it may not be necessary for ions to be drawn into another barrel: it may be sufficient that local current flow restricts the diffusion of the ejected ion away from the multibarrel tip to its site of action.

Lambert and Flatman (1981) have drawn attention to this possible confusion in terms of the movement of an ejected ion into a NaCl barrel used for balancing that ion. On this basis the authors attempted to control for the phenomenon by placing the glutamate balance barrel immediately adjacent to the glutamate barrel itself. In this way any diversion of ejected glutamate by local outward current was expected to be near maximal. Thus the influence of pentobarbitone or its outward current balance barrel, which was situated at a distance from the glutamate barrel, should have been relatively small. Even so, some depression of glutamate responses was seen during the ejection of NaCl, which was attributed to this electrical diversion effect.

If this phenomenon is indeed real, however, it is very difficult to control it adequately under all experimental situations. The possibility is raised that the size of retaining currents and, of course, of the net balance current, which will be continually changing with each agonist pulse, may affect the amount of a test compound reaching its site of action. Even when a series of constant agonist pulses are obtained with no retaining current and in an unbalanced mode, the current used to eject a potential antagonist may cause diversion of the agonist ions and thus a diminution of responses.

It is not intended to labour this particular point excessively, but it is the author's view that this is a seriously underestimated source of confusion in microiontophoretic studies which is probably at the root of a good many conflicting reports and surprising, inexplicable or unrepeatable observations. We have ourselves obtained pharmacologically nonsensical drug interactions which have disappeared when the test was repeated using different current conditions.

Suspicions should be aroused in a microiontophoretic experiment if a drug interaction appears and/or disappears very quickly. If doubts do arise about an interaction the only way to be sure is to repeat the tests under as many different current carrying conditions as possible: balanced, unbalanced, using a reasonably high constant inward and outward current respectively through the balance barrel, with retaining currents, without retaining currents, etc. This is indisputably tedious, but infinitely preferable to publishing meaningless rubbish.

An additional approach which we have adopted in some cases is to apply a putative antagonist intermittently *between* agonist pulses so as to minimize the electrical diversion problem (Stone and Perkins, 1979).

PART IV   INTERBARREL COUPLING

This heading covers a multitude of problems which stem from the fact that near the tips of micropipette barrels the solutions are separated by a film of glass only 1 μm or so in thickness. In the vast majority of cases this layer is able to maintain an efficient mechanical and electrical barrier between barrels (unless several hundred volts are being applied for several minutes in which case some breakdown of the layer may be anticipated). However, unless very carefully prepared a 1 μm layer of glass is unlikely to be homogeneous, and instances are to be expected where mechanical or electrical leakage can occur across thinner areas of the glass membrane (Curtis, 1964). Examples of the former are easily detected because the ejection of a compound will cause an uncharacteristic response. The effects of electrical leakage are much more difficult to detect during an experiment and are more likely to cause confusion. For example the passage of current through one barrel may increase or decrease the effect of current passed through an adjacent barrel containing an active ion, or may even cause unwanted ionic ejection, especially if the adjacent barrel has a lower tip resistance. Conversely the passage of current through a barrel of high tip resistance containing an active ion may be shunted through the barrel wall into an adjacent barrel of lower resistance. This kind of phenomenon may also contribute to the observation that quite high currents can be passed into barrels containing normally active substances without any apparent response (see Ch. 4, Pt. III). If interbarrel coupling of this nature is suspected it should become routine practice to measure the resistance between barrels *before* beginning an experiment. Coupling can be easily detected then and rogue trodes discarded.

A particularly insidious way in which artefacts such as these can create havoc with iontophoretic studies is when they involve the balance barrel. Several tens of nanoamperes may be passing through a balance barrel throughout an experiment, and if any current leakage occurs from here to an adjacent barrel causing continuous ejection or excessive retention, extremely erratic and confusing results may be obtained. Note that the effect may not be readily obvious merely by performing a current control. The effect of balance current may be to increase the retention of a compound. The current-balanced administration of a putative antagonist would then increase that retention even further, leading to an apparent selective antagonism. But passing balance current alone would have little observable effect on the cell.

Whereas the artefacts described above (Ch. 6, Pt. III) may occur between any two barrels, interbarrel coupling necessarily involves only adjacent barrels, and systematic errors may, therefore, be eliminated by changing the relative positions of the solutions. The only way to be reasonably sure of not studying artefacts, however, is to use as large a number of pipettes as possible and discard, or at least check out very thoroughly and cautiously any unusual or infrequent observation.

If it is possible electrodes should be used in which problems of contamination or interbarrel coupling are minimized such as those in which a glass rod is used to separate the individual barrels (Curtis, 1964; Large, 1983).

PART V   INDIRECT DRUG EFFECTS

The main advantage of the microiontophoretic technique for the study of drug action is usually said to be the localization of response which the method affords. Following parenteral administration, for example, a drug may affect an area of CNS by acting on that area, on a distant but connected area, on neuroglia, local vasculature or even on various areas of the periphery by altering afferent activity or hormone release. However, it is at least possible to obtain an idea of the contribution of some indirect actions by means of blood flow and pressure measurements, cross-perfusion experiments between animals, measurement of hormonal levels, etc. When using microiontophoresis, however, although the effects of a drug are certain to be *relatively* localized, it is very difficult at present to assess the contribution to an observed response of indirect effects.

V.1   Neurones and terminals

The action of any iontophoretically applied compound in the central nervous system may be exerted directly on the postjunctional surface of the cell, on those presynaptic endings which synapse on to the cell, or on the cell bodies of neurones which in turn synapse on to the cell being studied. In intracellular recordings it may be relatively easy to distinguish between these possibilities *in vitro* or *in vivo* by applying tetrodotoxin, and *in vitro* by perfusing with low-calcium high-magnesium solutions. Tetrodotoxin could not be used for extracellular work as the action potentials would be blocked. Equally it may be difficult to modify local calcium and magnesium concentrations adequately, and even if it were possible, some compounds (tyramine, for example) can produce a calcium-independent efflux of transmitters by displacement.

The problem of differentiating direct from various indirect actions, therefore, represents a major difficulty for microiontophoresis. The only answer is to perform appropriate physiological and pharmacological tests, for example comparing the effects of a drug on a synaptic pathway with effects on cell firing rate or on antidromic potentials, in an attempt at distinguishing presynaptic and postsynaptic actions. This may still leave major problems of interpretation, however, as the relevant synapses may lie on dendrites some distance away from a recording electrode located at the cell soma, and larger iontophoretic currents would, therefore, be required to block the former (see above, Ch. 6, Pt. I). This could lead to an erroneous impression that the drug acted preferentially on the cell soma.

A method for partly overcoming this problem has been proposed by Sawada *et al.* (1983). Slices of guinea-pig hippocampus were incubated in a low-calcium high-magnesium medium in order to suppress synaptic transmission, but calcium was then ejected from one barrel of a multibarrel assembly during stimulation of an afferent pathway. This ensures that the only active synapses contributing to the observed response are within reach of any compound ejected from the same multibarrel. The method was used to study the effects of amino acid antagonists on the mossy fibre input to CA 3 pyramids.

It is also conceivable that in cases where firing is being maintained by a tonically active synaptic input an applied substance would act primarily on the nerve terminals so as to produce a secondary change of cell firing by increasing or decreasing that action. With the demonstration in recent years of a variety of presynaptic receptors for the transmitter itself (autoreceptors) as well as substances released from other cells in the vicinity, the presynaptic terminal has become increasingly recognized as a site of drug action and one accessible to iontophoretically applied agents.

Axons are unlikely to contribute to iontophoretic drug responses. Indeed Fries and Zieglgänsberger (1974) and Millar and Armstrong-James (1982) have advocated the use of glutamate ejection to differentiate between recordings of somatic activity (which is increased by glutamate) and axonal firing (which is unaffected).

It will be clear from Chapter 4, Part VI that compounds can reach targets several tens, perhaps hundreds of microns distant from the point of application. A volume of tissue can, therefore, be affected which includes a large number of cells and it would be naive not to consider the possibility that the effects of a compound might be mediated indirectly by disinhibition or by activating an interneurone.

A particularly salutary example of an iontophoretically applied drug acting in this way is provided by experiments in the olfactory bulb. Here it was thought for a time that noradrenaline depressed the mitral cells of the olfactory bulb, correlations being made between the time-course and pharmacology of this depression and that resulting from lateral olfactory tract stimulation (Salmoiraghi *et al.*, 1964). Further evidence, however, suggested that noradrenaline could be exciting inhibitory cells lying adjacent to the mitral cell being recorded, and the former could then cause inhibition of mitral cell activity by releasing γ-aminobutyric acid as the transmitter (Nicoll, 1971).

V.2 Blood vessels

The possibility that cells may be affected indirectly by drugs acting on nearby blood vessels must be considered since many of the substances which cause changes in cell firing in the CNS when applied iontophoretically are also active in altering the tone of small vessels in the periphery.

This is a particularly serious possibility when some vasoactive peptides, or amines such as noradrenaline and 5-hydroxytryptamine are being considered, which cause changes of cell firing with long latencies of the order of 10–40 seconds. It has been shown that the microiontophoresis of noradrenaline on to arterioles of the rat intestine and mesentery causes a constriction of those vessels with a latency of this order (Stone, 1971, 1972b).

It is unclear at present whether or not there is an important adrenergic innervation of cerebral vasculature, but many studies, including histochemical studies, physiological studies of the changes of blood flow following nerve stimulation and pharmacological studies suggest that this is so. In this case, the iontophoretic application of noradrenaline in, for example, the cerebral cortex could cause a localized constriction of a small arteriole as has been observed in the periphery (Stone, 1971, 1972b). This action could reduce the availability of oxygen to a cell, and this in turn could cause excitation of that cell. Evidence for the latter statement comes from three sources. Firstly, Lorente de No (1947) in his classic studies of nerve physiology, noted that slight hypoxia could depolarize a nerve fibre. Secondly, Edwall and Scott (1971) have shown that constriction of the microvasculature of the tooth pulp following stimulation of sympathetic innervation to that vasculature, caused an excitation of the sensory unit of the dental pulp. Thirdly, Speckmann (1970) has attempted to separate the effects of hypoxia, hypercapnia and asphyxia on an animal, and finds that hypoxia alone causes an initial excitation of units in the cerebral cortex. Li and McIlwain (1957) in their studies on brain slices *in vitro* have also noted a depolarization of units to a membrane potential of approximately zero during the administration of a low oxygen gas mixture.

These various lines of evidence are suggestive of a possible relationship between a local hypoxia and neuronal excitation.

Without wishing to dwell on this controversial area it is also interesting to note the evidence that a large proportion of central noradrenergic neurones arising from the locus coeruleus may innervate blood vessels rather than neurones. It has also been proposed that many neurones situated midway between cerebral capillaries are delicately poised with respect to oxygen diffusion such that a small change of oxygen availability could alter the neuronal firing rate (Halgren *et al.*, 1977). Such cells would clearly be affected by amines causing a local change of vessel diameter and thus oxygen availability.

V.3 Glial cells

One of the main functions of neuroglial cells is probably to regulate the ionic environment of neurones, particularly with regard to potassium ions. If this is so, then damage caused by a penetrating microelectrode or changes of glial permeability and metabolism produced by locally ejected drugs could indirectly affect neuronal firing by compromising that regulation. There is no doubt that glial cells have receptors and uptake mechanisms which would allow them to interact with a variety of neurotransmitters and drugs (Henn and Henn, 1980).

There is also evidence that the neuroglia possesses some contractile ability which can be affected by a variety of compounds. For instance it has been shown in isolated cultures of glial cells that the number of pulsation-like movements made by these cells is greatly increased in the presence of minute amounts of 5-hydroxytryptamine (Benitez *et al.*, 1955; Woolley and Shaw, 1957). Such an effect, were it to occur *in vivo* as a result of the microiontophoretic administration of 5-hydroxytryptamine, could conceivably distort the cell under study or some of the presynaptic endings impinging upon it sufficiently to alter the pattern of input affecting that cell. This might be seen as an apparent excitation or inhibition of the cell by 5-hydroxytryptamine.

V.4 'Non-specific' effects

Related to the question of indirect drug effects is the problem of assessing the contribution to a drug's action of direct depressant effects of a non-specific nature on neuronal membranes. For example, a number of substances such as atropine and propranolol have quite potent local anaesthetic properties which may cause blocking of the regenerative electrical properties of the membrane, and an apparent reduction of firing rate (Curtis and Phillis, 1960). These changes are, however, accompanied by a broadening of the soma spike, together with a reduction in amplitude and frequently an increase in the positive phase of the spike due to the locally inactivated membrane becoming a current source for more distant parts. Continuous oscilloscope monitoring of the action potentials should allow these changes to be detected easily and taken into account.

Very few attempts have been made to assess the disturbing effect of electrode insertion on ongoing neuronal activity. One such study was performed by Stopp and Whitfield (1963) who reported that the introduction of even a small, 0.5 μm single electrode into the auditory cortex could cause an increase of spontaneous activity of up to 20%. Presumably the effects of a multibarrel pipette with a tip size ten times greater than that could cause very substantial changes indeed of neuronal activity.

PART VI PH EFFECTS

As described earlier (Ch. 2, Pt. VIII.3) the pH of most drug solutions is adjusted to improve the chemical stability of the drug, and/or to increase its ionization. On this account amines such as noradrenaline are often used at the relatively low pH of 3.5–4.0. There is, therefore, a possibility that during the cationic ejection of ionized noradrenaline the simultaneous ejection of hydrogen ions may significantly influence the behaviour of the neurone under study. Before 1971 most authors performed some sort of control experiments to eliminate the possibility that the ejection of H^+ or OH^- was not contributing to the drug responses recorded (Krnjević and Phillis, 1963a; Johnson et al., 1969a). Krnjević and Phillis (1963a) concluded that H^+ significantly affected cell firing only when ejected alone with currents of the order of 60 nA. Johnson et al. (1969a) performed a particularly rigorous set of controls to eliminate the possibility that the responses they observed to noradrenaline were due to hydrogen ions. These results were subsequently challenged by Frederickson et al. (1971) and Jordan et al. (1972) who reported respectively that noradrenaline and 5-HT would cause primarily excitation of cortical units if ejected from solutions of pH about 3, but primarily depression if applied from solutions of pH 4 or 5. However, not only was this in conflict with Johnson et al. (1969a), but these results could not be confirmed by Stone (1972c) or Bevan et al. (1973b).

Furthermore the pH hypothesis overlooks the finding that amine responses can be blocked in some cases by conventional antagonists. It is, therefore, unlikely that the responses are produced directly by hydrogen ions, but the possibility has never been explored that H^+ could interfere with membrane channels or produce subthreshold changes of membrane potential such that the direction of amine responses is changed while their pharmacology remains unaltered.

There is even some disagreement about the effects of hydrogen ions themselves on neuronal firing, as Bevan et al. (1973b) could observe little change of firing in response to H^+ ejection. Other authors, however, obtain marked increases of neuronal excitability by ejecting H^+ (Krnjević and Phillis, 1963a; Hewes and Frederickson, 1974). In the author's experience pure H^+ effects can be produced easily only by ejection from solutions of pH 2.5 or less. The responses have a characteristic profile, taking 10–15 seconds to become apparent using a current of about 80 nA, and then consisting of a rapidly developing excitation which decays very slowly after ending the ejection (Figure 42). When ejecting from solutions of pH greater than 2.5 hydrogen ion responses may still be obtainable, but with more difficulty. It may be necesssary to eject with 60 nA for 1 or 2 minutes.

It is important to note that merely ejecting H^+ from a solution of HCl or acidified NaCl at a pH equivalent to the test material is not necessarily an adequate control for pH interference. Curtis (1964) pointed out that when an ion is ejected into a medium of pH significantly different from that of the parent solution, the ion can either release or take up an H^+, depending on the nature of the ion and the relative pH values. This could lead to a localized change of pH much greater than would be expected to result purely from the ejection of the H^+ originally present in the solution.

This concept, of course, makes it very difficult to devise good control experiments. One of the most satisfying approaches is that employed by Boakes et al. (1971) in the brain stem, showing that (−)noradrenaline produced (excitatory) responses on cells where (+)noradrenaline had little such effect.

Both isomers were ejected from solutions of the same pH, and since they have identical physico-chemical properties, including presumably their ability to release hydrogen ions in contact with an alkaline solution, the different responses could not be due to pH. The use of stereoisomeric pairs may have a similar utility in other situations.

Another method of assessing the effects of pH is to apply a compound as a cation and an anion from solutions of the appropriate pH (Curtis *et al.*, 1959). This method is certainly applicable to a wide variety of a small molecular weight substances.

It has been reported that a change of pH can alter the transport number of noradrenaline (Bevan *et al.*, 1973a). When filled with solutions of noradrenaline

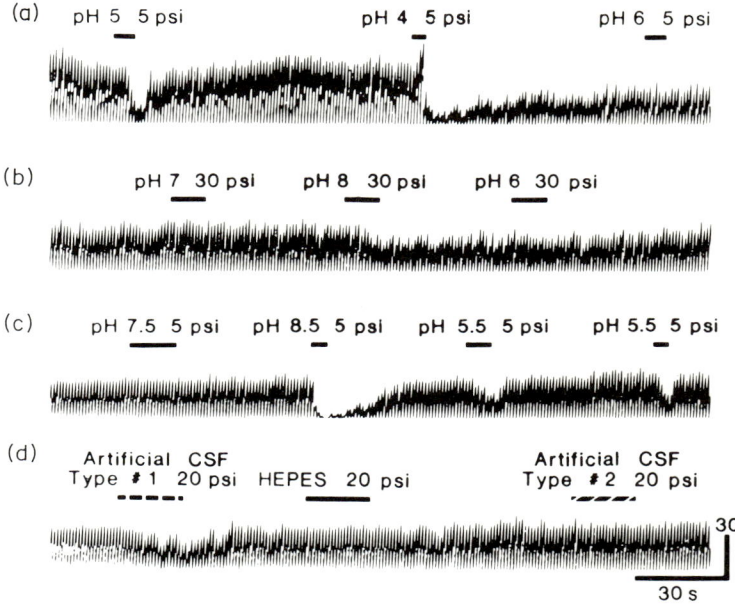

Figure 43 Ratemeter records from four cerebellar Purkinje cells illustrating the effects of various potential drug solvents on neuronal activity. In this figure and all succeeding ratemeter figures, the numbers after the drug show ejection pressure in pounds per square inch (lb/in^2); the duration of ejection is indicated by the underlying bar, and the ratemeter ordinate is expressed in spikes per second. (a) The 5 lb/in^2 pressure ejection of 165 mM NaCl at pH 4 and pH 5 but not at pH 6 cause marked changes in neuronal activity. Both pH 4 and pH 5 cause apparent inhibitions associated with decreases in spike height. However, an increase in neuronal firing rate was obvious from oscilloscope tracings during applications of these solutions. (b) Neither pH 6 nor pH 7 alters neuronal activity at 30 lb/in^2, while a similar application at pH 8 caused a small inhibition. (c) Pressure application of 165 mM NaCl at pH 7.5 did not alter neuronal activity, while pH 8.5 and pH 5.5 caused marked effects. (d) Artificial CSF Type No. 1 caused a small depression of spontaneous neuronal activity, while no effects were observed of relatively large doses of 50 mM HEPES in 165 mM NaCl or of artifical CSF Type No. 2 (see this chapter, Pt. VI.1). (Reproduced from Palmer, 1982, by permission of Pergamon Press Ltd.)

at pH 5 pipette barrels were found to have 50% lower resistances than at pH 3.5, and the transport number for noradrenaline was increased from the range 0.02–0.18 at pH 5 to 0.18–0.43 at pH 3.5 Over this pH range, however, there is little change in the concentration of noradrenaline present in the cationic form and the authors consequently explained these observations on the basis of the Na^+OH^- which had to be added to raise the solution pH from 3.5 (bitartrate salt in distilled water) to 5. The authors calculated that the Na^+ concentration at pH 5 would be about 100 mM, enough to carry a significant proportion of any iontophoretic charge.

Clearly the possible effects of H^+ on iontophoretic responses are complex and adequate control experiments may require careful planning, but it is clear that possible contributions of H^+ or of the ions which are added to adjust pH (Na^+, Cl^-), must always be carefully considered, particularly when excitatory responses are studied, or compounds in low concentrations or of relatively low mobility (such as peptides) are being tested.

Much less is known about effects of OH^{-1} ions on neurones than H^+, but the author has observed increases of firing of cortical units following the ejection of OH^{-1} alone from solutions of pH 10 or greater. Undoubtedly, however, the same kind of complexity applies to ejection from high pH as from low pH and such simple controls should probably be considered inadequate.

VI.1 pH and pressure

The inability of neurones to tolerate appreciable changes of pH is revealed most clearly by pressure ejection. The application of solutions at pH 5.5 or less and 8.5 or greater, for example, causes profound changes of spike height and firing rate (Palmer, 1982) (Figure 43). Similarly Henderson (1983) has noted that pressure ejection of a solution of even pH 7.0 may cause responses of cultured leech neurones.

PART VII COUNTER ION EFFECTS

The use of retaining currents means that the supposedly inactive ion in a solution is in effect being ejected for long periods by iontophoresis, and it is, therefore, necessary to check that the ion is not having any effect on the cell. For example, if a cell appeared to be excited by a cation X^+, this excitation could be due to the removal of the retaining current, which was in effect ejecting the associated, but unsuspectedly *depressant* anion Y^- in the periods between iontophoresis of X^+.

A similar difficulty may be encountered with organic complexes. For example, the ejection of aminophylline which is a complex of theophylline and ethylenediamine, has been shown to cause a profound depression of neuronal firing, but it is likely that this is primarily due to the GABA-mimetic properties of the ethylenediamine component (Stone and Perkins, 1984).

PART VIII TEMPERATURE EFFECTS

It could be that the ejection of a small volume of solution which accompanies iontophoresis may cause a local change of temperature sufficient to alter neuronal firing particularly when micropipettes are stored at 4 °C. The minute size of a micropipette tip, however, is probably such that the temperature of the contained solution rapidly reaches that of the surrounding neural tissue and such an effect becomes insignificant.

The suggestion has also been made (Spehlmann, 1963) that the passage of current across the quite high resistance of the electrode tip may generate enough heat energy to distort or alter the metabolism of neuronal membranes locally. Rush *et al.* (1968) have calculated that the passage of more than 1 μA of current could cause a significant change of temperature across a microelectrode tip, and that 10 μA could probably cause the boiling of solutions in electrode tips. Microiontophoretic currents, however, are usually less than 100 nA. Since, in addition, most ejecting currents are applied for less than 60 seconds, and usually at several microns distance from a cell membrane this effect, if it occurs, is unlikely to be significant. It may become significant during the ejection of dyes and other markers (Ch. 8).

PART IX OSMOTIC EFFECTS

The 'concentrated' solutions of several substances used for microiontophoresis (acetylcholine, amines, amino acids), particularly in the early studies, would be about 3 or 4 molar. Since a solution which is iso-osmotic with body fluids has a concentration of around 165 mM the use of such high drug concentrations represents a potential source of error due to the osmotic withdrawal of fluid from the immediate vicinity of the tip. Besides producing a dilution of the solution in the pipette tip, changes in the size of synaptic terminals or cell bodies, or their spatial relationship, could be caused. This problem may be minimized by using solutions of around 165 mM, and by using small tip diameters. Both these factors would also, of course, reduce the problem of diffusional leakage of drug from the tip.

The ejection by pressure of solutions, with osmotic pressures substantially different from physiological (e.g. distilled water or 330 mM NaCl) causes depressions of firing rate (Palmer, 1982).

PART X CONTAMINATION

Artefacts may also arise due to contamination of solutions in different barrels. This might, rarely, occur through the glass membrane separating barrels near the tip as mentioned above but a more serious source of contamination is movement of solution at the ends of the barrels. The problem is greatest for the non-splayed pipettes in which the barrels are cut flush. Even if it is assumed that the experimenter is not so clumsy as to allow solution to spill directly over from one barrel to the next, it should not be forgotten that solution in an omega-dot type of capillary will track along the entire length of the barrel within seconds of instilling that solution. Then any fluid layer or dust or finger marks on the cut surface may allow the fluid to track across to another barrel. The problem may be diminished by smearing a thin layer of water-repellent grease or siliconizing fluid on the cut surface before filling.

This kind of problem is virtually non-existent for the splayed varieties of micropipettes, but all micropipettes can suffer interbarrel contamination across the tip. Although this is probably the least well recognized form of contamination among people using iontophoresis, we have directly observed fluid movement from one barrel tip to another empty one under the microscope. It seems to occur less with pipettes in which the tip is flat than in which there is an angle or other irregularity.

The same problem has been encountered by Palmer (1982) who consequently injects a few microlitres of solution into each barrel as rapidly as possible. This precludes contamination between the barrel tips. The shanks and stems of the barrels can then be filled at leisure.

In the author's laboratory an attempt is made to reduce the frequency and significance of these problems by filling barrels only to within 1 cm of the top (to prevent spillage), by filling always with an absorbent tissue in contact with the cut surface (to detect leakage as a result of tracking up the capillary) and by filling barrels in a different order each time (to prevent a systematic error due to contamination of barrels by using the same solution first). Problems with the balance barrel can be assessed not only by passing current through the balance barrel alone but also by disconnecting the balance, allowing the electrode and cell time to reach a new equilibrium, and repeating all tests unbalanced.

PART XI   INFLUENCE OF ANAESTHETICS

In view of the fact that experiments *in vivo* ordinarily involve the use of an anaesthetic some thought should always be given to the possibility that anaesthetics may interfere with the sensitivity of neurones to iontophoretically applied substances.

In the past most attention has probably been given to the barbiturates. Phillis and Tebecis (1967) observed that pentobarbitone would depress both the acetylcholine-induced excitation and noradrenaline (norepinephrine)-induced inhibition of thalamic neurones. Crawford (1970) similarly found that pentobarbitone would depress the acetylcholine sensitivity of cortical neurones though he also made the interesting observation that iontophoretic acetylcholine and DL-homocysteate (DLH) were equally susceptible to intravenous barbiturate whereas acetylcholine was more resistant if the anaesthetic was applied iontophoretically. The potential significance of this observation, which the author attributed to possible differences in the spatial localization of acetylcholine and DLH receptors, does not seem to have been explored by subsequent studies. The depression of acetylcholine responses nevertheless seems to be a common finding, occurring not only in the thalamus (Phillis and Tebecis, 1967; Tebecis, 1974) and cortex (Crawford, 1970; Catchlove *et al.*, 1972) but also in the brain stem (Bradley and Dray, 1973) and striatum (Spencer and Havlíček, 1974). In the olfactory cortex slice, however, Smaje (1976) found acetylcholine responses to be largely unaffected by pentobarbitone added to the bathing medium although volatile anaesthetics such as ether, halothane, methoxyflurane and trichloroethylene caused an enhancement of responses (Figure 44).

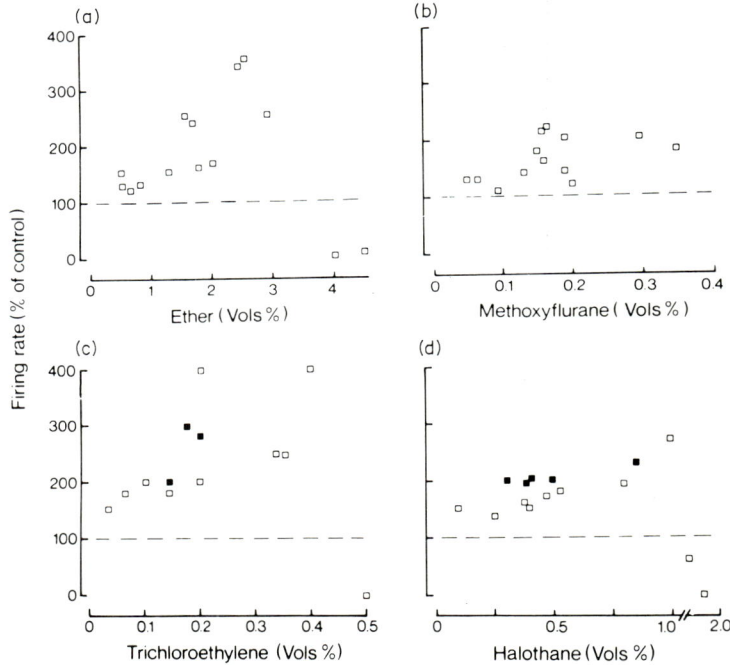

Figure 44 Summary of the relationship between the acetylcholine responses of neurones in the prepiriform cortex and the concentrations of volatile anaesthetics applied. The results are expressed as a percentage of the acetylcholine-evoked firing rate observed in the absence of anaesthetic. (The normalized control firing rate is indicated by the horizontal dotted line.) (□) Experiments in standard saline; (■) experiments in high Mg^{2+}-low Ca^{2+} saline. (Reproduced from Smaje, 1976, by permission of the British Pharmacological Society.)

In a study of the pharmacology of anaesthetic–acetylcholine interactions Godfraind (1979) concluded that at least in the case of lateral geniculate and perigeniculate neurones both chloralose and urethane selectively blocked those components of acetylcholine responses which were mediated by muscarinic receptors. It would be interesting to know whether such selectivity applies also in other areas of CNS and whether it could account for some of the early arguments concerning the presence or otherwise of acetylcholine-induced (muscarinic) depressions of firing in the cerebral cortex.

There is less agreement on the effects of anaesthetics on responses to the monoamines noradrenaline, dopamine and 5-hydroxytryptamine (5-HT). The report of a reduction by pentobarbitone of noradrenaline-induced depressions of thalamic neurones (Phillis and Tebecis, 1967) was followed by a report that the ratio of excitatory to depressant responses to monoamines in the cerebral cortex was much greater during halothane anaesthesia than during barbiturate anaesthesia (Johnson et al., 1969b). However, this report has remained controversial and while similar observations have been made in the striatum when comparing barbiturates and methoxyflurane (Spencer and Havlíček, 1974) a number of authors have failed to obtain more than a handful of excitatory responses to monoamines, whatever the anaesthetic conditions (Frederickson et al., 1973; Nelson et al. 1973; Stone, 1973b). Even in some areas such as the brain stem where excitatory responses to monoamines are more regularly encountered than in neocortex, the responses were said to be unaffected by pentobarbitone, urethane or tribromoethanol administered to decerebrate rats (Bradley and Dray, 1973).

The interactions of amino acids with anaesthetics have also received much attention. Responses to glutamate were found to be relatively resistant to barbiturates in the thalamus (Phillis and Tebecis, 1967) and cortex (Catchlove et al., 1972) although other groups have reported a marked depression of glutamate responses by barbiturates. Lambert and Flatman (1981) have found that barbiturates would diminish the conductance increase produced by glutamate on spinal neurones, while Richards and Smaje (1976) found that at concentrations over 0.1 mM pentobarbitone would depress glutamate responses in the olfactory cortex slice. Barker and Ransom (1978b) also found that barbiturates would reduce glutamate responses of cultured neurones. Richards and Smaje (1976) also noted that several volatile anaesthetics (ether, methoxyflurane and trichloroethylene) reduced glutamate excitation although halothane only did so at concentrations greater than 1%. Catchlove et al. (1972) found that a wide range of volatile anaesthetics did not affect glutamate sensitivity in lightly anaesthetized cats.

It was noted above that DLH responses were more readily depressed by iontophoretically applied pentobarbitone than acetylcholine responses in the neocortex (Crawford, 1970) and this would seem compatible with a detailed intracellular investigation on spinal neurones (Lambert and Flatman, 1981). This group found that DLH depolarizations were invariably depressed by barbiturates, whether administered systemically or iontophoretically to anaemically decorticated cats. As there was no change in the current voltage relationship for DLH, however, the authors postulated an effect of the barbiturates at a site in the receptor–ionophore complex rather than at the receptors themselves.

Interest in the interaction of non-barbiturate anaesthetics with transmitters has been rather limited although the recent discovery that dissociative

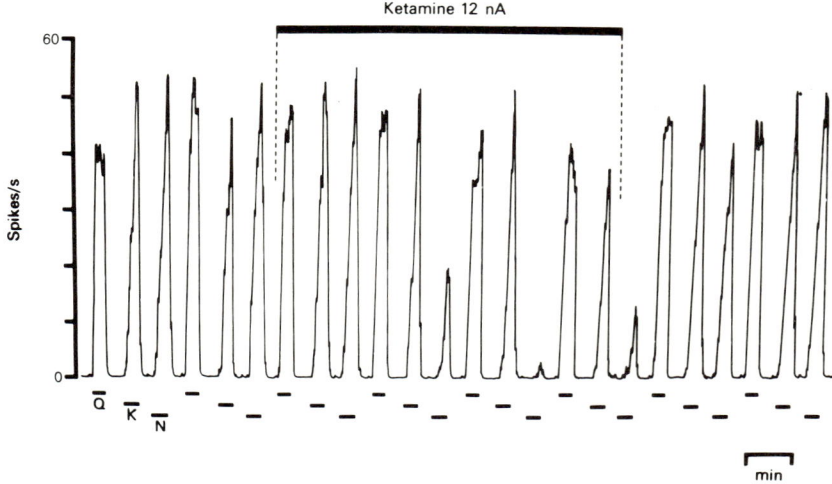

Figure 45 Effect of ketamine on excitation of a cat dorsal horn neurone by quisqualate, kainate and N-methyl-aspartate (NMA). The continuous record shows the firing rate of the neurone in response to the automatically timed electrophoretic ejection of the three excitant amino acids, for the time indicated by the bar beneath the record (Q, quisqualate 56 nA; K, kainate 35 nA; and N, NMA 70 nA). Following control observations ketamine ejected with a current of 12 nA for 7.5 min, as indicated by the bar above the record, selectively reduced the excitant action of NMA. Full recovery of the response to NMA was observed 4.5 min after stopping the ejection of NMA. Ordinate scale: firing rate in spike/second. Abscissa scale: time. Calibration bar = 1 min. (Reproduced from Anis *et al.*, 1983, by permission of the British Pharmacological Society.)

anaesthetics such as phencyclidine and ketamine can selectively block activation of the N-methyl-aspartate receptor (Anis *et al.* 1983) (Figure 45) may lead to a change of this situation. The relevance of the blockade of the N-methyl-aspartate receptor in anaesthesia is still uncertain, however, since the responses are blocked at substantially sub-anaesthetic doses (about one-tenth) of ketamine given systemically.

Halothane and chloralose, but not methoxyflurane may also reduce neuronal sensitivity to DLH and acetylcholine (Crawford, 1970).

The anaesthetic–transmitter interaction for which there is probably most evidence is that between barbiturates and GABA. Barbiturates enhance the conductance increase produced by GABA (see Barker and Ransom, 1978b) and this probably explains the well documented augmentation by barbiturates of inhibitory phenomena in the CNS.

One of the most useful general anaesthetics for iontophoretic experiments is probably urethane (ethyl carbamate, $H_2N \cdot COOC_2H_5$, about 1.5 to 1.8/kg injected i.p. as a 25% w/v solution in water). Holmes and Houchin (1966) were among the first to report that urethane had little effect on the sensitivity of neurones to amines, and that the rate and pattern of firing of CNS neurones were virtually indistinguishable from the firing characteristics of cells in unanaesthetized *encéphale isolé* preparations. Most other anaesthetics, including barbiturates (Crawford, 1970; Dyball and McPhail, 1974) and halothane (Millar and Silver, 1971) depress neuronal firing. The lack of effect of urethane on neuronal responsiveness or spontaneous activity has been confirmed by other groups (Cross and Dyer, 1971; Bradley and Dray, 1973; Dyball and McPhail, 1974).

It is also of interest that urethane may be used as an initial anaesthetic to reduce the trauma of killing in the preparation of *in vitro* systems: Bagust and Kerkut (1981) showed that urethane, in contrast to other anaesthetics, washes out of tissues within a few minutes of their isolation.

Undoubtedly the ideal microiontophoretic experiments are those performed *in vivo* in the absence of anaesthesia. To date this has been achieved only rarely, by training cats to lie quietly for an extended period with the head restrained by means of a perspex block (Frederickson *et al.*, 1973). Although invaluable for settling arguments about the effects of anaesthetic one can sense in their report the authors' frustration with cells lost or electrodes broken when the animal stretched, a factor no doubt contributing to the unpopularity of the method.

PART XII FIELD POTENTIALS

Unfortunately, no matter how many cells are tested with a compound and however rigorous the treatment of the results, one of the major disadvantages of microiontophoresis is the inescapable introduction of sampling bias: the preferential recording of larger or more stable cells, those which show themselves because of their spontaneous activity or which can be detected because they possess receptors for an excitant compound such as glutamate, for example. In attempts to circumvent this drawback several authors have attempted to use field or evoked potentials (Herz *et al.*, 1970; Barasi and Roberts, 1974, 1977; Cherubini *et al.*, 1982; Ropert and Krnjević, 1982; Collingridge *et al.*, 1983; Rovira *et al.*, 1983), since in theory at least a study of the various components of such potentials, produced by a range of different inputs to an area should give a clearer picture of the behaviour of relatively homogeneous populations of cells than could be obtained by single cell recording.

The analytical treatment of such potentials should be relatively straightforward: the size of the potential is a reflection of the number of active cells and thus of the excitability of the neurone pool. A statement of percentage change of response size should, therefore, provide an index of drug action which represents the average of several hundred single unit recording sessions. The use of field potentials in conjunction with microiontophoretic drug ejection should even remove some of the uncertainties surrounding drug concentration in the tissue since the record is of the mean response of a large number of cells, most of which will be experiencing a fairly even concentration of drug at their soma and dendrites and contributing to the mass-evoked response even though they may not individually be distinguishable from background noise.

Herz et al. (1970) had few problems with the demonstration that iontophoretic glutamate would enhance field potentials in the caudate nucleus and that this effect was prevented by GABA. Barasi and Roberts (1974, 1977) subsequently used the antidromically induced field potential to study the excitability of the

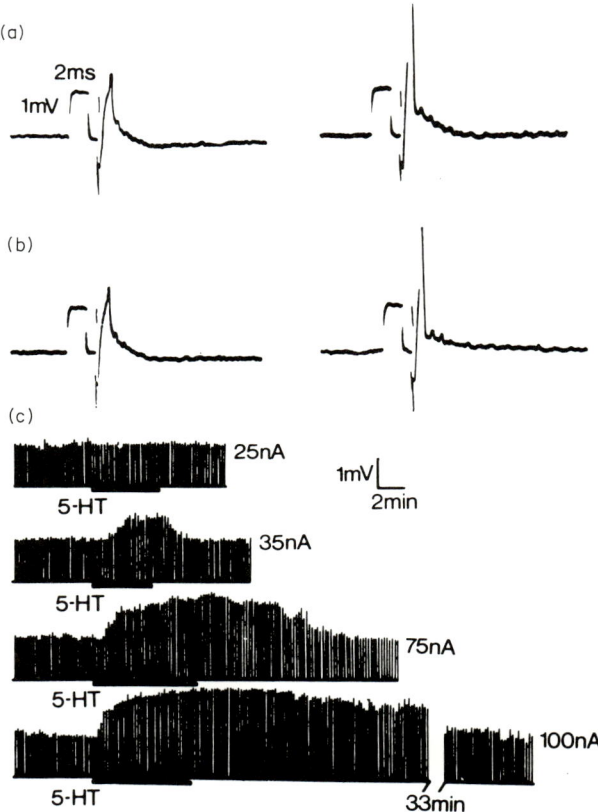

Figure 46 The effect of raphe stimulation and iontophoretically applied 5-hydroxytryptamine (5-HT) on the antidromic field potential. (a) Photographs of the field potential before (left) and after (right) application of 100 nA of 5-HT applied for 2 min. 5-HT more than doubled the amplitude of the field potential. (b) The field potential before (left) and just after (right) conditioning stimulation of the raphe nuclei. Conditioning almost doubled the amplitude of the field potential. (c) Pen writing oscillograph records of the field potential amplitude during iontophoretic application of different currents of 5-HT. 5-HT was applied during the period indicated by the bars under the records with the current shown to the right of the traces. It is apparent that the latency to onset and the maximum amplitude of the response is dependent upon the current of 5-HT. (Reproduced from Barasi and Roberts, 1974, by permission of the British Pharmacological Society.)

motoneurone pool in rat spinal cord, reporting that amines such as 5-HT (Figure 46), noradrenaline and dopamine usually increased the size of the negative field potential while glutamate and glycine usually caused a depression.

However, changes of field potentials have proved singularly difficult to interpret, as discovered by Engberg *et al.* (1979a) who performed a combined intracellular and extracellular analysis of the effects of iontophoretically applied amines and amino acids on antidromic ventral horn activity. This group confirmed the primarily depressant effect of glycine and several excitatory amino acids on the negative wave of the antidromic field potential (Barasi and Roberts, 1974), but amine responses were more variable. Whereas Barasi and Roberts, (1974, 1977) had obtained consistent increases of the negative antidromic potential by 5-HT, noradrenaline or dopamine, Engberg *et al.* (1979a) saw no effect of dopamine and only variable responses to noradrenaline; increase, decrease or no effect in almost equal proportions.

A further major significance of the report by Engberg *et al.* (1979a), however, lies in their analysis of the factors contributing to the ventral-root-evoked field potential. These are perhaps best summarized as follows:

1. Changes in the membrane potential level of individual neurones would cause a corresponding change in the action potential height: depolarization would be associated with a decreased height, hyperpolarization with an increase.
2. Changes in the excitability of a neurone would alter the probability of its being invaded by the antidromic potential.

    In work of this kind, of course, a supramaximal stimulus is used routinely in the expectation that the number of cells invaded will not vary. However, Engberg *et al.* (1979a) point out that there will still be a proportion of cells which will not be invaded unless they are depolarized by preceding synaptic input or by an exogenously applied depolarizing agent. Conversely, a decrease of the field potential could result from applying a hyperpolarizing substance which inhibits antidromic spike invasion.
3. Changes of the rate of rise, or duration of a spike may occur independently of changes of membrane potential and thus factors 1 and 2. The relationship between membrane potential and spike shape will depend on the ionic conductance changes occurring.

The problem then is that these factors can interact in a complex fashion. A drug with a primarily hyperpolarizing action on the motoneurones would tend to increase action potential size and rate of rise, thus increasing the field potential and yet by the same action reduce the number of neurones invaded by the ventral root volley. Indeed interactions of varying complexity were observed by Engberg *et al.* (1979a).

Clearly it becomes exceedingly difficult to draw meaningful conclusions about the effects of substances on neuronal excitability solely on the basis of extracellularly recorded field potentials.

Finally, it should not be forgotten that the same problems of interpretation (drug concentration, pH effects, indirect actions) apply to the use of field potentials with microiontophoretic drug application as apply for single cell work, perhaps more so since more material is usually ejected into a larger volume of tissue.

PART XIII   PRESSURE EJECTION

Clearly much of the foregoing discussion, particularly with regard to drug concentrations and indirect effects (especially pH) as well as pharmacological considerations such as the effects of anaesthetics, will apply to ejection from micropipettes by pressure just as much as to ejection by iontophoresis. However, it is perhaps relevant to emphasize two points. Firstly, although the effects of current no longer need to be considered it is clear that pressure itself can have an effect on neuronal activity. Dunlap and Fischbach (1981) for instance reported that the pressure pulse produced a hyperpolarization of 2–15 mV of chick sensory neurones in culture. The mechanism is obscure although presumably some mechanical distortion of the membrane may conceivably be involved.

During experiments *in vivo* the sudden pressure step of several atmospheres may be sufficient to cause slight movement of the pipette assembly and thus affect neuronal firing (Palmer, 1982; Palmer *et al.*, 1980). The problem may be diminished by including a section of relatively distensible tubing in the pressure line so as to buffer the sharp pressure pulse.

In the study by Poulain and Carette (1981) pressure applications of either water or a physiological medium could 'block' the effects of iontophoretically applied glutamate, although this could not be attributed to mechanical distortion of the tissue since higher glutamate currents still caused excitation. The phenomenon was explained on the hypothesis that the ejected inactive solvent would cause local dilution of the released glutamate below a threshold concentration. The same authors noted that at higher ejecting pressures of saline media a slowing of spontaneous firing could be produced, though a non-specific membrane effect of the applied pressure was postulated to explain this. It has to be remembered that a volume of 1 picolitre represents a cube of side 10 μm. If ejections of several hundred picolitres per second, per p.s.i. are being ejected for many seconds some physical distortion of the tissue is inevitable.

Palmer (1982) has also described depressant effects of distilled water and an artificial CSF on neuronal firing, though modification of the CSF to a medium containing less potassium, calcium and magnesium had no such effect (Figure 43).

CHAPTER 7

Practical Applications: an Introduction to the Microiontophoretic Literature

I	Peripheral Nervous System	134
	I.1 Receptor Localization	134
	I.2 'Noise'	135
	I.3 Desensitization	135
	I.4 Determination of Transmitter Release	137
	I.5 Cooperativity and Receptor Kinetics	138
II	Smooth and Cardiac Muscle	138
III	Myenteric Plexus	141
IV	Central Nervous System	141
V	Excitatory Amino Acids	143
	V.1 Variations of Sensitivity	143
	V.2 Pharmacology	146
	V.3 Synaptic Activation	147
	V.4 Localization of Receptors	149
	V.5 Mechanism of Action	151
VI	Inhibitory Amino Acids	153
	V.1 Pharmacology	154
	VI.2 Synaptic Blockade	156
VII	Acetylcholine	156
	VII.1 Mechanisms	163
	VII.2 Field Potentials	163
VIII	Noradrenaline (Norepinephrine)	163
IX	Dopamine	168
X	5-Hydroxytryptamine	170
XI	Purines	171
XII	Peptides	174
XIII	Opiates and Opioids	176
XIV	Non-Mammalian Central Nervous Systems	177

The purpose of this chapter is not to attempt a comprehensive review of the microiontophoretic literature: this would be out of place in a methodological text. This chapter presents a brief summary of the contribution which microiontophoretic studies have made to current knowledge of neurotransmitter pharmacology, emphasizing the range of preparations and systems where the technique has been used, especially the more recent work, in order to give some feeling for the kind of results which can be obtained by microiontophoresis or pressure microejection. References to the more recent literature have been chosen wherever possible because they include a reasonable selection of references to earlier work. The early studies using microiontophoresis in the cerebral cortex are summarized by Krnjević (1964) while studies throughout the CNS up to 1974 are discussed by Tebecis (1974) and Krnjević (1974). Studies in invertebrates are well covered by Gerschenfeld (1973) and Gardner and Walker (1982). The wide-ranging collection of microiontophoretic papers edited by Ryall and Kelly (1978) may also be a useful source of material. Chapter 5, Parts VI and VII of the present volume also discuss the uses and applications of microiontophoresis in more general terms.

PART I PERIPHERAL NERVOUS SYSTEM

I.1. Receptor localization

Localized applications of suspected neurotransmitters have proved invaluable in demonstrating the specialized features of neuroeffector junctions, since Nastuk (1953) reported depolarization at the neuromuscular junction by acetylcholine applied from his 'electrically controlled microjet'. Indeed some of the first detailed studies using microiontophoresis were attempts to show the localization of acetylcholine sensitivity at the vertebrate neuromuscular junction (del Castillo and Katz, 1955; Kuffler and Yoshikami, 1975b). The same concept has been applied to studies of invertebrate muscle where sensitivity to the probable neurotransmitter glutamate can be shown to be maximal in the region of terminal varicosities (Figure 47) or end-plates of crayfish (Onodera and Takeuchi, 1980; Shinozaki, 1980) or of insect muscle (Cull-Candy, 1978). The ability to apply the putative neurotransmitter in brief pulses, mimicking the synaptically released compound also facilitates a comparison of the electrophysiology (Anwyl, 1977) and pharmacology (Feltz *et al.*, 1977; Shinozaki *et al.*, 1982) of the two substances. Up to three distinct types of glutamate receptor have been postulated at the locust neuromuscular junction (Gration *et al.*, 1979).

In the case of the vertebrate neuromuscular system it has been possible to demonstrate the formation of cholinoceptive 'hot spots' during the development of muscle cells in culture and to show that synapses do not necessarily form at those receptor clusters (Cohen and Fischbach, 1977; Frank and Fishbach, 1979). Similarly iontophoresis has been used to follow the changes of acetylcholine receptor distribution after denervation and during reinnervation by a foreign nerve (Lømo and Slater, 1980) as well as the effects of various types of muscle activity on receptor distribution (Lømo and Slater, 1978). Cull-Candy *et al.* (1982) have recently begun to investigate differences in the distribution of acetylcholine sensitivity in normal and diseased human skeletal

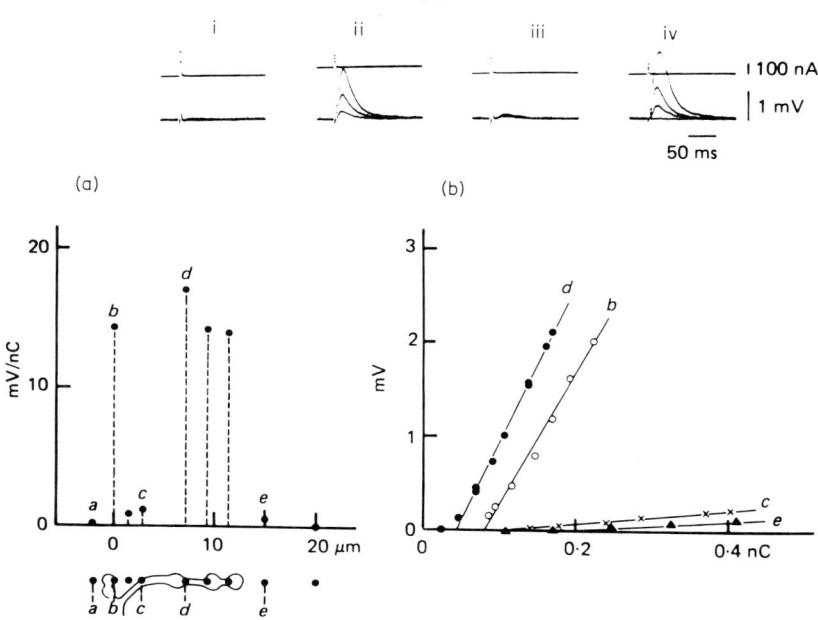

Figure 47 (a) Glutamate sensitivity along a terminal branch, expressed as mV/nC (crayfish neuromuscular junction). (b) The sensitivity was measured from the slope of the dose–response curve. Sample records are shown on the top. (Reproduced from Onodera and Takeuchi, 1980, by permission of the Physiological Society.)

muscle in culture, although the differences found so far seem inadequate to account for the functional pathology of the intact system.

I.2 'Noise'

Since the original description of acetylcholine-induced 'noise' (an increased membrane current amplitude and variance) at the frog end-plate (Katz and Miledi, 1972), noise or fluctuation analysis in response to the application of compounds by microiontophoresis has become extremely popular for the study of conductance and open times of individual receptor operated ionic channels. The technique is still used at the neuromuscular junction (Gage and Hamill, 1980; Magleby and Weinstock, 1980) although the role of microiontophoresis has become threatened by the introduction of the patch clamp technique. Many workers have certainly abandoned intact preparations for noise analysis in exchange for cell or tissue culture systems (Fischbach and Lass, 1978).

I.3 Desensitization

A subject that has received a particularly large amount of attention with microiontophoretic application is desensitization (Anwyl and Narahashi, 1980a,b).

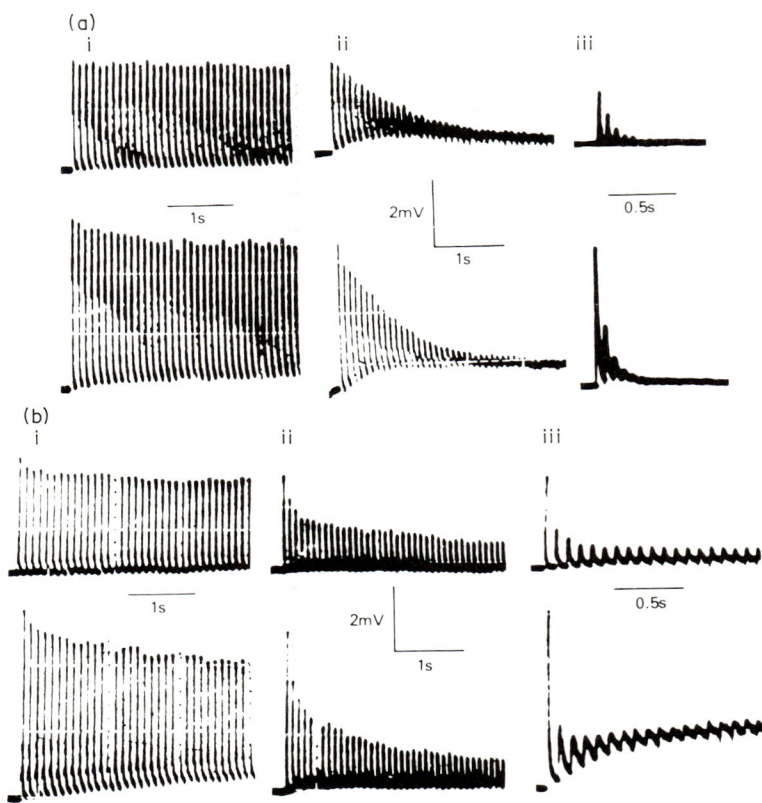

Figure 48 (a)(i) Desensitization of approximately 4 mV (top trace) and 8 mV (bottom trace) acetylcholine (ACh) potentials evoked at a frequency of 10 Hz. The potentials declined eventually to zero amplitude. (ii) and (iii) Time-dependent inhibition of the 10 Hz evoked ACh potentials superimposed on the desensitization caused by Triton X-100 at concentrations of (ii) 0.001% and (iii) 0.005% (b)(i) Desensitization of 4 mV (top trace) and 8 mV (bottom trace) ACh potentials evoked at 10 Hz. (ii) and (iii) Time-dependent inhibition of the ACh potentials caused by chlorpromazine at concentrations of (ii) 1.5 μM and (iii) 3 μM. (Reproduced from Anwyl and Narahashi, 1980b, by permission of the British Pharmacological Society.)

Brief pulses of agonist can readily be applied to a sensitive area of membrane and the time-course of desensitization followed or its pharmacology studied (Figure 48). Recent work has suggested the existence of at least two temporally distinct phases of desensitization which seem to indicate the involvement of two independent underlying mechanisms (Feltz and Trautmann, 1982; Chesnut, 1981) (Figure 49).

Desensitization has also proved a popular subject at the insect (Anis *et al.*, 1981; Clark *et al.*, 1982) and crustacean neuromuscular junction (Shinozaki, 1980; McBain and Wheal, 1984). In the latter study a series of piperidine analogues were found to inhibit the development of the desensitization.

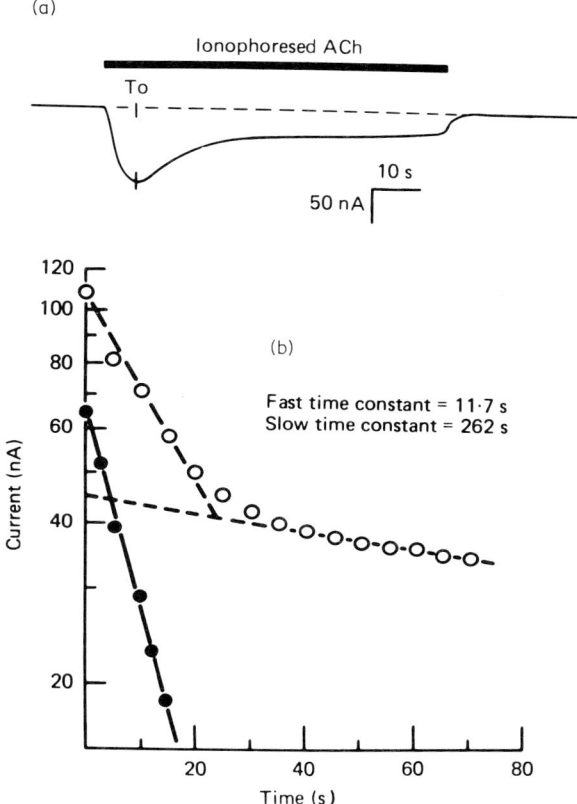

Figure 49 Example of two-component desensitization curve obtained in response to ionophoretically applied ACh. The data in (a) are plotted on semilogarithmic coordinates in (b). The lines were drawn by eye and the line representing the slow component in (b) was used as a baseline for evaluating the fast component (continuous line and dots). The time constant was calculated from the following equation for exponential decay: $I = I_o e^{-t/\tau}$ where I_o is the current (nA) at time zero, I is the current (nA) at time t (s) and τ is the time constant (s). (Reproduced from Chesnut, 1983, by permission of the Physiological Society.)

Previously the only substances known to have this property were compounds such as cytochalasin B.

I.4 Determination of transmitter release

In a model study Kuffler and Yoshikami (1975a) used microiontophoresis to estimate the amount of acetylcholine released in a single quantum at the frog and snake neuromuscular junction. Droplets of 0.6 nl volume containing known amounts of acetylcholine were applied to exposed end-plates and the voltage responses noted. The voltage responses were then determined to similar droplets into which 5000 1 ms pulses of acetylcholine had been passed in order to calculate the release of amine per 1 ms pulse. By then matching iontophoretic responses with depolarization produced by single quanta of acetylcholine (the miniature postsynaptic potentials) it was possible to deduce that the single quantum includes not more than 10 000 molecules of acetylcholine.

I.5 Cooperativity and receptor kinetics

Dudel (1975) reported steep dose–response curves to the iontophoresis of glutamate at the crayfish neuromuscular junction. The curves had a limiting slope of about six implying that six molecules of glutamate would be needed to activate the subsynaptic receptor. This would conveniently allow high sensitivity to locally high concentrations of synaptically released glutamate without much background depolarization by the considerable levels of systemically circulating glutamate.

Peper *et al.* (1975) have applied the same method at the frog skeletal neuromuscular junction to obtain a value of 3 for the Hill coefficient. The same group caution against attempts to draw quantitative conclusions from a comparison of synaptic and iontophoretic responses when the ejecting pipette is very close to the subsynaptic membrane since it is difficult to predict accurately the time-course of responses in that situation.

PART II SMOOTH AND CARDIAC MUSCLE

Parasympathetic nerve stimulation is associated with a substantial delay before a detectable (mechanical or electrical) response in most smooth muscles. Purves (1974) was among the first to address the question of whether this was due to hindered access of transmitter to receptors using iontophoresis. The ejection of acetylcholine even at distances less than 5 μm from smooth muscle cells cultured from guinea-pig taenia coli induced depolarization with latencies in the range 120–500 ms (Figure 50b). When ejected from the same micropipettes on to cultured chick myotubes acetylcholine caused depolarizations with latencies of less than 5 ms. Bolton (1976) subsequently showed that latencies greater than 100 ms were also obtained when carbachol was iontophoresed on to the intact ileum or taenia at distances of less than 20 μm.

It seems likely that these long latencies are physiological, and do not reflect an artefact of the iontophoretic application or of the access of the drugs. Purves (1974) in fact illustrated computer-generated predicted concentration curves for acetylcholine at 8 μM and 32 μM from the iontophoretic pipette regarded as a point source (Figure 50a) to emphasize the discrepancy between the predicted acetylcoholine concentration and the observed membrane depolarizations. He went on to show that if a circular patch of membrane is considered to be the critical area for the response rather than a single point on the membrane, then it can be calculated that in order to produce the time-course of the observed voltage response the iontophoretic pipette would have to lie some 30 μm above the centre of the patch (Figure 50; Purves, 1974).

Practical Applications 139

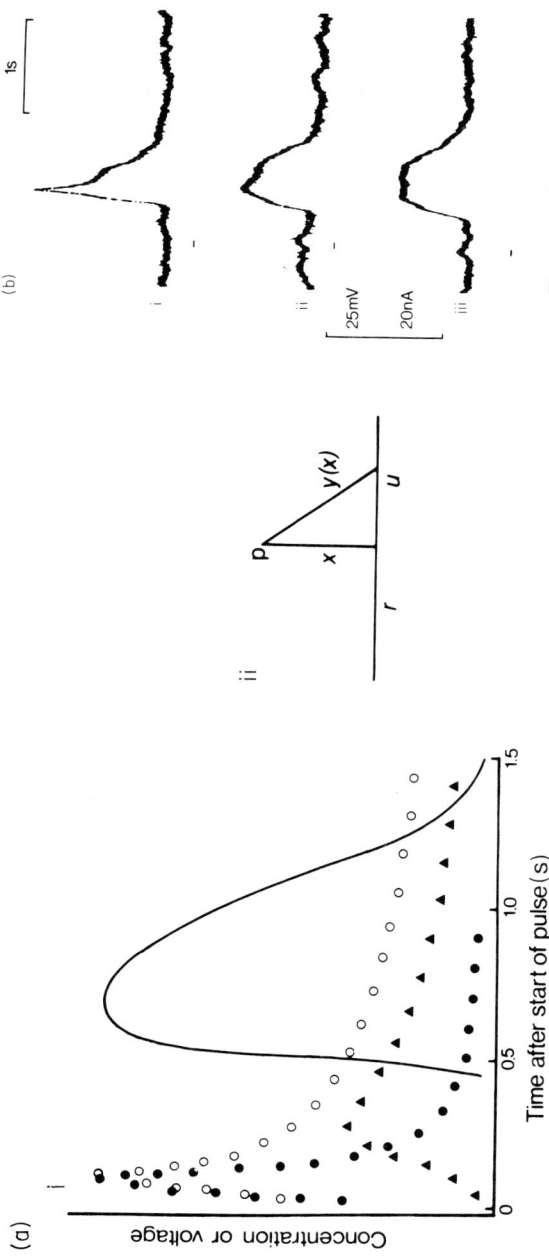

Figure 50 (a)(i) Comparison of a typical voltage response with the calculated time-course of concentration change of acetylcholine 8 μm (circles) and 32 μm (triangles) from a point source. The concentration curves were calculated numerically from diffusion equations for a continuous point source of 100 ms duration, the diffusion constant being taken as 8.10^{-6} cm^2 s^{-1}. The vertical scale is arbitrary, though linear. Concentrations for the 32 μm curve were multiplied by 10 for display purposes. The voltage curve was redrawn from a trace obtained from an 8-day culture when a 100 ms pulse of acetylcholine was applied 4 μm from the surface of the clump. Open circles represent average concentrations at the surface of the whole clump, scaled to the same peak height as the 8 μm curve. (ii) Schematic drawing of geometry assumed for calculation of average concentrations. Acetylcholine is released at point P, distance x above centre of circular clump of radius r. $y(x) = \sqrt{(x^2 + u^2)}$ where u is a dummy radius variable. (b) Responses produced by equal pulses of acetylcholine applied at various distances vertically above the impaled cell. The separations were: (iii) <5 μm, (ii) 8 μm, (i) 15 μm. Note the spike formation and very small increase in latency at the larger separations: 7-day culture. (Reproduced from Purves, 1974, by permission of the British Pharmacological Society.)

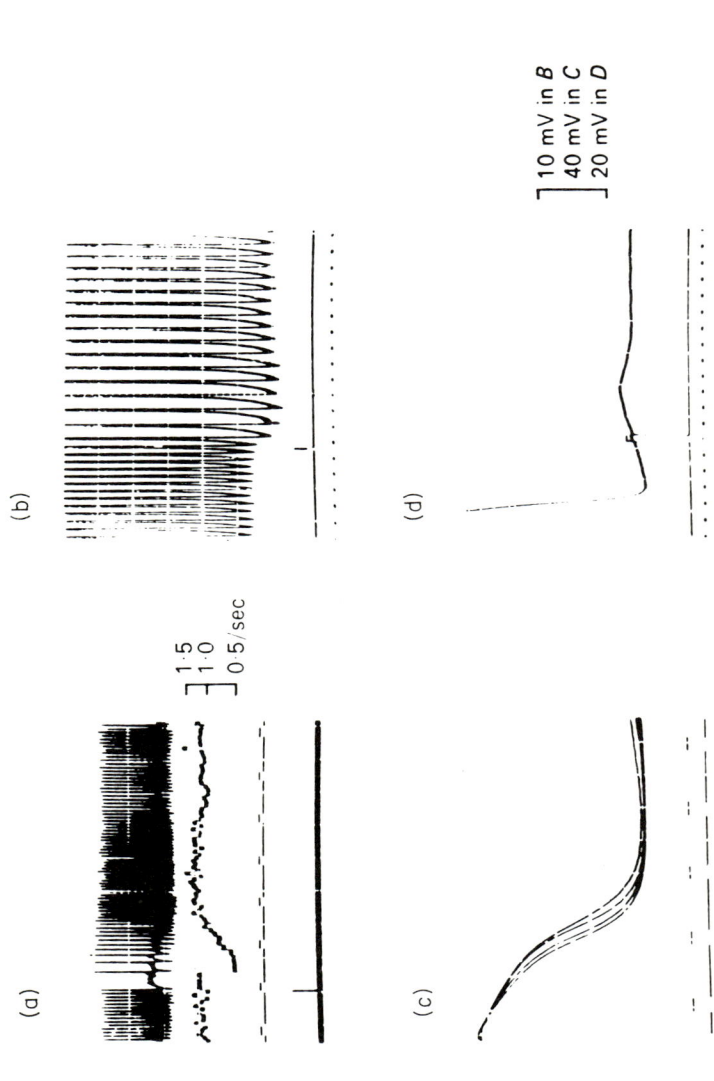

Figure 51 Responses of small clusters of cultured ventricular cells to ionophoretic application of carbachol or acetylcholine. (a) Pulse of carbachol (10 nC in 100 ms) at time indicated by bottom trace. Upper trace shows photoelectric record of contractions of very small cluster (four cells). Second trace: heart rate. Third trace; 10 s time marker. (b) Action potentials recorded intracellularly, showing hyperpolarization in response to a pulse of acetylcholine (40 nC in 170 ms). Time marker: 1 s intervals. (c) Superimposed traces showing shortening of consecutive action potentials following 15 nC pulse of acetylcholine. The action potential whose downstroke is furthest to the right was recorded immediately before the pulse. Time marker: 100 ms intervals. (d) Hyperpolarization in response to a pulse of carbachol (13 nC in 40 ms). Note the long latency. Time marker: 100 ms intervals. (Reproduced from Hill-Smith and Purves, 1978, by permission of the Physiological Society.)

Similarly delayed responses have been shown following the iontophoretic ejection of noradrenaline on to the anococcygeus muscle (Large, 1983) and following the ejection of either acetylcholine or noradrenaline on to cardiac muscle (Hill-Smith and Purves, 1978). In the latter case, using rat ventricular cells in tissue culture acetylcholine was found to produce hyperpolarizations with latencies of around 250 ms and lasting for several seconds (Figure 51). Catecholamines on the other hand showed latencies of several seconds before a chronotropic response became apparent.

PART III MYENTERIC PLEXUS

The activity of neurones in the enteric plexuses has been championed by North (1982) as a useful model of the CNS. Much of the work on this preparation has involved bath perfusion, but the iontophoretic application of compounds has proved invaluable in dissecting different components of response. Acetylcholine, for example, can mimic both a fast cholinergic e.p.s.p. which is nicotinic in nature as well as a slower muscarinic depolarization (North and Tokimasa, 1982; Figure 52). Exactly similar responses have recently been recorded from frog dorsal root ganglion cells (Morita and Katayama, 1984).

Amines have also been tested in this preparation: 5-HT, for example, produced both depolarizing and hyperpolarizing responses of different neurones, probably due to a decrease and increase respectively of potassium conductance (Johnson et al., 1980).

Somatostatin has interesting effects which may have much wider implications for the study of neuronal responses: applied by perfusion the peptide causes a hyperpolarization, but when applied by microiontophoresis it provokes depolarization (Katayama and North, 1980). This may reflect the differential access of somatostatin applied by these methods to dendritic and largely somal receptors.

As a final illustration of the utility of this preparation, it is possible to show a loss of sensitivity to opiate agonists or myenteric neurones after chronic treatment of the tissues or animals with morphine. The opiate antagonist naloxone now causes excitation of neurones (Karras and North, 1981). This effect has also been demonstrated in the CNS (Aghajanian, 1978) and taken to be an electrophysiological manifestation of the opiate withdrawal phenomenon.

PART IV CENTRAL NERVOUS SYSTEM (CNS)

Undoubtedly the largest number of microiontophoretic studies has been concerned with the central nervous system. These studies have yielded information on: (a) the qualitative sensitivity of neurones to putative neurotransmitters and drugs; (b) quantitative estimates of variations of sensitivity in different CNS regions or of different cell types and following lesions or the administration of drugs; (c) the pharmacology of transmitter receptors; (d) the

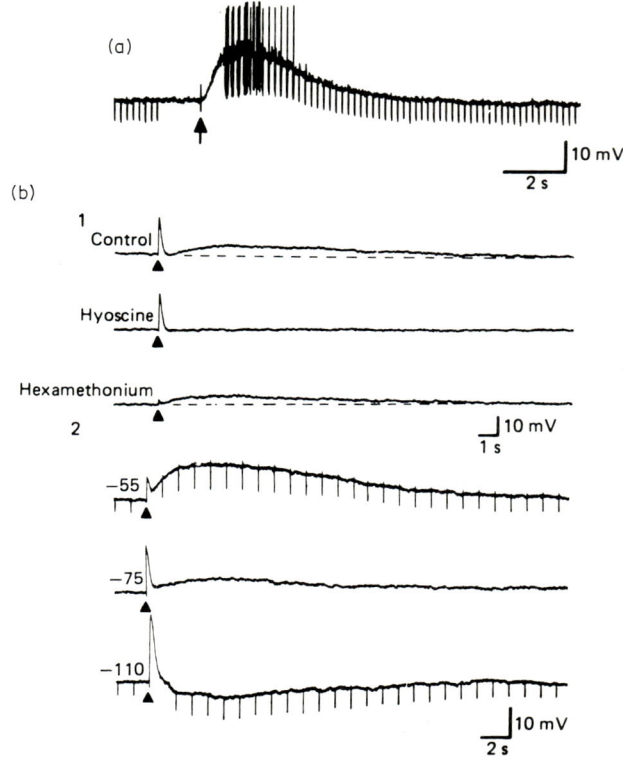

Figure 52 Nicotinic and muscarinic depolarizations in the same cell. (a) Evoked by nerve stimulation. A single pulse stimulus (arrow) evoked a fast e.p.s.p. followed by a much larger and longer lasting slow e.p.s.p. (b) Evoked by ACh ionophoresis (triangles, 20 nA for 1 ms). (1) Hyoscine (1 μM) completely abolished the slow depolarization but did not affect the rapid depolarization. After washing out the hyoscine, hexamethonium (200 μM) was used to abolish the rapid depolarization. (2) At resting potential (-55 mV) ACh ionophoresis caused both a rapid and a slow depolarization. The rapid (nicotine) depolarization became larger with membrane hyperpolarization. The slow (muscarinic) depolarization became smaller and reversed polarity with membrane hyperpolarization. Note the increase in input resistance accompanying the muscarinic effect of ACh. (Reproduced from North and Tokimasa, 1982, by permission of the Physiological Society.)

effects of modifiers of putative transmitter effects (antagonistic or enhancing substances) on synaptic transmission; (e) the localization of receptors on different parts of the neuronal surface; and (f) the mechanisms and ionic conductances underlying transmitter effects, including fluctuation analysis.

In the following pages several classes of neuroactive compounds will be discussed in order to highlight important or instructive results from each of these applications of microiontophoresis.

PART V EXCITATORY AMINO ACIDS

Some of the earliest iontophoretic studies demonstrated marked excitatory activity of several simple dicarboxylic acids, including L-glutamic and L-aspartic acids (Curtis and Watkins, 1960) and these have become recognized as the primary candidates for a neurotransmitter role at a wide variety of synapses (Watkins and Evans, 1981).

Responses to some of these amino acids, especially glutamate and aspartate, terminate rapidly when an ejecting iontophoretic current is switched off. It has never been entirely clear to what extent this is due to the kinetics of iontophoresis (Figure 17) and to what extent it reflects the presence of avid uptake processes but Haldeman and McLennan (1973) and Johnston *et al.* (1980) have shown a potentiation of amino acid responses by inhibitors of uptake mechanisms.

McCabe (1972) on the other hand has described long-lasting changes of cortical neurone firing rate following iontophoresis of glutamate sufficient to at least double the resting firing rate. Little attention seems to have been paid to this observation, which may be of some relevance to a discussion of phenomena such as long-term potentiation in the hippocampus.

V.1 Variations of Sensitivity

One of the arguments most often voiced against the idea that glutamate or aspartate might be neurotransmitters in the CNS is that virtually all neurones seem to respond to these agents. Various approaches have been made to counter this argument by showing that cells, or particular parts of cells such as dendrites, receiving a synaptic input which is suspected on neurochemical grounds of releasing an excitatory amino acid transmitter have a different sensitivity to the amino acid than non-innervated areas or cells. The localized application of compounds by microiontophoresis, of course, is in principle ideally suited to such problems.

The growth of interest in quinolinic acid, for example, stems not only from the fact that it is an endogenous compound able to act selectively on the N-methylaspartate (NMA) receptor (Stone and Perkins, 1981a; Perkins and Stone, 1983a) (Figure 53) but also that there are marked regional differences of neuronal sensitivity (Perkins and Stone, 1983a,b).

The popular hypothesis that the toxic effects of compounds like kainate are linked to their excitant properties has received further circumstantial support from the finding that neurones in the rat mesencephalic trigeminal nucleus, which are not sensitive to kainate's neurotoxic actions, are not excited by kainate (De Montigny and Lund, 1980); neither are they affected by GABA, acetylcholine, glutamate, glycine, catecholamines or histamine (Figure 54).

Morgan *et al.* (1972) reported that in the cat lateral geniculate nucleus a gradient of relative sensitivity to aspartate and glutamate could be detected, correlating with the distance of the cells' receptive fields from the centre of the visual field. Gent and Wolstencroft (1976a) later reported a similar gradient

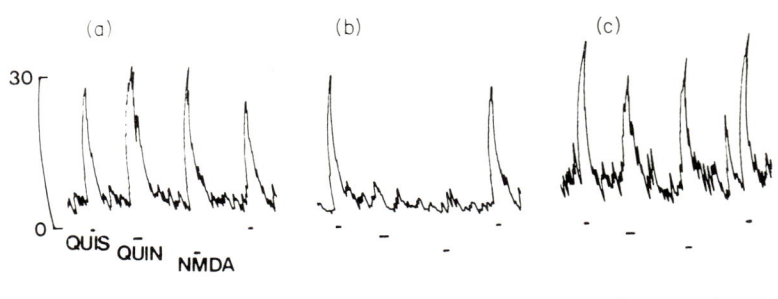

Figure 53 Record of the firing rate of a neurone in the cerebral cortex excited by the iontophoresis of quisqualic acid, 16 nA (QUIS), quinolinic acid, 22 nA (QUIN) and NMDA, 20 nA. panel (a) shows a series of control responses; (b) was taken 2 min after beginning an ejection of 2-amino-5-phosphono-valeric acid, 6 nA. Note the blockade of quinolinic acid and NMDA, but not quisqualic acid. Panel (c) shows recovery, 2 min after (b). Ordinate: firing rate in spikes/second. Time bar: 1 min. (Reproduced from Stone and Perkins, 1981, by permission of Elsevier Biomedical Press B.V.)

on cells in the rat ventrobasal thalamus responding to vibrissal movement. The upper caudal vibrissae projected to the superior caudal thalamus where cells showed a lower glutamate : aspartate ratio than the mean, whereas cells in the inferior rostral thalamus showed much higher ratios. Sensitivity was assessed using plateau responses, and the range of potency ratios ranged from 0.38 to 2.24 across the gradient.

Duggan (1974) claimed that 22 of 23 Renshaw cells in the cat cord were more sensitive to iontophoretic aspartate than glutamate whereas interneurones activated with short latency by nerve stimulation showed the reverse pattern. McCulloch *et al.* (1974) confirmed this finding in principle by showing a potency ratio of kainate (used as a glutamate analogue) to NMA (an aspartate analogue) of less than 10 on Renshaw cells but generally greater than 10 on short latency interneurones. However, with the more recent evidence that glutamate and aspartate receptors are not identical with those for kainate and NMA the relevance of this work remains unclear. Biscoe *et al.* (1976) found that non-Renshaw interneurones in the rat were indeed more sensitive to glutamate than aspartate but Renshaw cells demonstrated no consistent differences between these agonists. Hutchinson *et al.* (1978) later came to the conclusion that both Renshaw cells and other interneurones in the rat are more sensitive to glutamate than aspartate, with no significant differences detectable between the different cell types.

Since the corticofugal pathways were among the first supraspinal pathways suggested to release an excitatory amino acid transmitter (Stone, 1973b) a study was conducted of the relative glutamate : aspartate sensitivity of neurones in the cerebral cortex, cuneate nucleus and caudate nucleus activated monosynaptically by stimulation of the pyramidal tract or the cerebral cortex and cells which could not be so activated (Stone, 1979b).

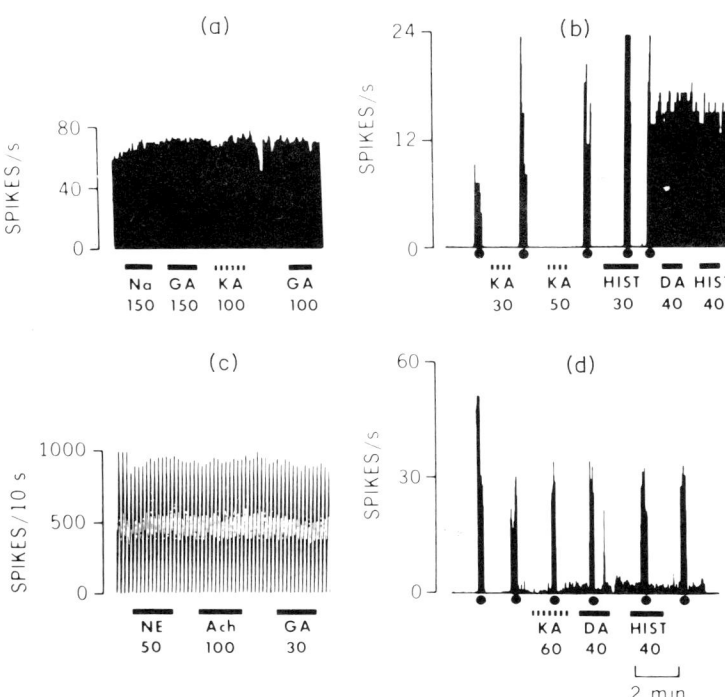

Figure 54 Integrated firing rate histograms of NMT neurones. (a) and (c) Tonic muscle spindle afferent excited by fixing the jaws open. (b) Periodontal afferent; the dot (●) indicates pressure applied to ipsilateral upper incisor tooth. In the latter part of the record, the pressure was maintained. (d): Phasic spindle afferent; the dot (●) indicates stretch of jaw closing muscles. KA: kainate; Na: sodium; GA: GABA; HIST: histamine; DA: dopamine; NE: noradrenaline; ACh: acetylcholine. Iontophoretic currents are indicated in nanoamperes. (Reproduced from Montigny and Lund, 1980, by permission of Pergamon Press Ltd.)

No significant differences could be detected in the glutamate : aspartate potency ratios.

This type of relative potency investigation as a clue to transmitter identity has now become very unpopular. Part of the reason for this is undoubtedly the variation in results from different laboratories, which is in turn a reflection of the difficulty involved in using microiontophoresis for comparative quantitative studies. Potency differences may indeed result from different receptor densities, but they could also be influenced by local uptake and inactivation or simply a different location of amino acid receptors on different parts of the cell surface. Indeed in most non-regularly organized regions of the CNS the different electrode/neurone orientations may account for some of the observed variations of sensitivity. A better recording system in some laboratories, for example, may result in drugs being applied further from the cell soma than in laboratories where a close approach to the spike-generating apparatus is needed. Another closely related biological factor is the existence of extrajunctional receptors. These are well characterized in neuromuscular systems (see this chapter, Pt. I) but their contribution to responses to iontophoretically applied substances in the CNS is largely unknown. If they exist on a large scale they would clearly invalidate any attempts to correlate normal sensitivity and synaptic input.

A final biological factor which cannot be ignored in experiments of this kind is the possibility that subtle variations of receptor pharmacology exist between different cell types independently of synaptic input. The influence of well-recognized variations of iontophoretic ejection between micropipettes or even barrels (see Ch. 4, Pt. III) can be minimized by using a large series of pipettes and testing a random mixture of the cell types of interest with each one (Biscoe *et al.*, 1976; Perkins and Stone, 1983a). Pipette variation will nevertheless always make some contribution to sensitivity studies.

Slightly more weight may be given to studies in which microiontophoresis is used to determine whether the removal of a synaptic input leads to a change of neuronal sensitivity as has been shown for hippocampal CA 1 pyramidal cells after destruction of commissural fibres (Segal, 1977) and cells in the neostriatum after chronic decortication (McLennan, 1980). In the hippocampal study a non-selective increase of amino acid sensitivity was observed, whereas in neostriatum a selective enhancement of glutamate responsiveness was seen. In studies such as these one still cannot differentiate with certainty, using iontophoresis alone, between a compensatory up-regulation of receptor number or affinity and a loss of uptake and inactivation sites as explanations of the changes. Indeed in McLennan's (1980) study binding experiments were also performed which revealed no change of glutamate or kainate binding. The increased sensitivity to glutamate probably resulted from the removal of nerve terminal uptake mechanisms.

V.2 Pharmacology

The development of a series of antagonists together with the discovery of potent amino acid analogues with very high agonist potencies (Biscoe *et al.*, 1975) led to the tentative proposal by McLennan and Lodge (1979) that there may exist three populations of receptor, an aminoadipate-sensitive receptor capable of responding best to NMA and ibotenic acid, a site sensitive to glutamic acid diethyl ester (GDEE) mediating responses to quisqualic acid and glutamate, with a third receptor being reserved primarily for kainic acid, which was not readily blocked by either GDEE or α-aminoadipate (Watkins and Evans, 1981).

With the additional discovery that phosphonate analogues of amino acids, such 2-amino-5-phosphonovaleric acid (Davies *et al.*, 1981; Perkins *et al.*, 1981) are very effective in blocking the actions of compounds like NMA and homocysteic acid but not quisqualic acid or kainic acid, with the converse selectivity being shown by some dipeptides, the concept of these three receptors became fairly well established (Watkins and Evans, 1981).

Among the more interesting or unusual agents with the ability to block excitant amino acid responses are streptomycin (Stone and Perkins, 1983), the anticonvulsant phenytoin (Sastry and Phillis, 1976; Stone, 1981a) and benzodiazepines (Davies and Polc, 1978; Assumpcao *et al.*, 1979). The endogenous tryptophan metabolite kynurenic acid is also an effective antagonist of amino acid excitation (Perkins and Stone, 1982).

The dissociative anaesthetics such as ketamine and phencyclidine will selectively block activation of the NMA receptor (Figure 45) (Anis *et al.*, 1983), an observation which could be very significant for an appreciation of the role of NMA receptors in cerebral function. The effects of other anaesthetics on amino acid responses has been discussed in Chapter 6, Part XI.

V.3 Synaptic Activation

One of the goals of the idealistic iontophoreticist is to use a selective pharmacological antagonist to block selectively one of a series of test agonists in parallel with a synaptic input. This would come close to fulfilling the 'identity of action' criterion for a neurotransmitter, if only from a pharmacological viewpoint. Although this cannot be said to have been achieved as yet, several groups have attempted such work, and a few have come close to success.

In the spinal cord most recent studies seem to be in agreement that the phosphonates, D-glutamyl-glycine (DGG) and 2,3-piperidine dicarboxylate (PDA), can block long latency polysynaptic activation of spinal interneurones, implying the involvement of a transmitter acting on NMA receptors (Peet *et al.*, 1983; Davies and Watkins, 1983). There is still disagreement, however, about the monosynaptic input from primary afferents. Davies and Watkins (1983) claim that this input can be blocked by DGG and PDA, which would imply the physiological activation of a kainate or quisqualate receptor population, whereas Peet *et al.* (1983) have been unable to block the monosynaptic pathway using any of these amino acid antagonists.

In the hippocampus Nature has managed to balance anatomical neatness and experimental accessibility with a pharmacological complexity which seems to defy analysis. Nevertheless the evidence suggests that perforant path synapses on to dentate granule cells involve the activation of a quisqualate- or kainate-like receptor (Hicks and McLennan, 1979; Crunelli *et al.*, 1983). The Schaffer collateral–commissural pathway to CA 1 pyramidal cells has been said to be blocked (Hicks and McLennan, 1979) or not to be blocked (Collingridge *et al.*, 1983) by iontophoretically applied NMA receptor blockers. Long-term potentiation, however, can be prevented in some situations by certain of the amino acid antagonists (Collingridge *et al.*, 1983) (Figure 55).

Stone (1979b) showed that aminoadipate would block both glutamate excitation of Purkinje cells as well as parallel fibre-evoked synaptic activation. However, this was only possible when the safety factor of this input was reduced

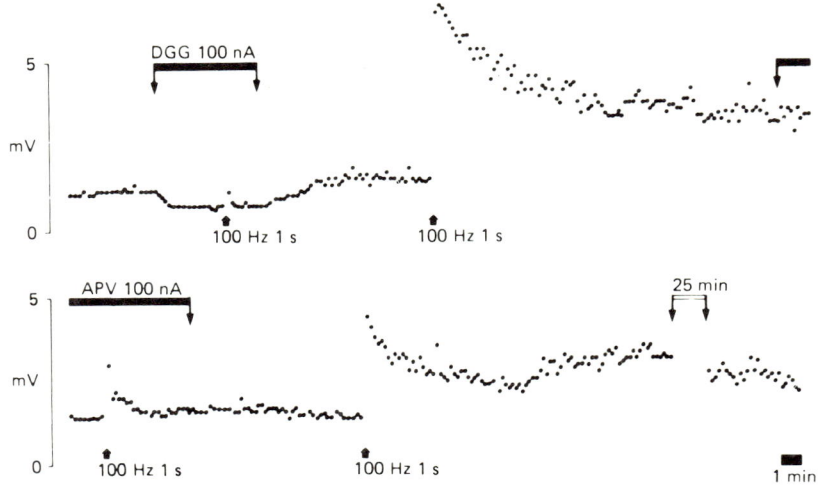

Figure 55 Effects of antagonists on the population spike and on the generation of l.t.p. The amplitude of the population spike was recorded in stratum pyramidale in response to 0.1 Hz stimulation of the Schaffer collateral–commissural projection and antagonists were administered ionphoretically in stratum radiatum for the durations indicated by the bars. The pathway was stimulated at 100 Hz at the times shown by the arrows below the trace. DGG reduced the amplitude of the population spike and prevented l.t.p. in response to high frequency stimulation. Following recovery from the effects of DGG, l.t.p. was produced using a period of identical high frequency stimulation. After 17 min, APV was applied and had no effect on the population spike; 2 min later the stimulus intensity was reduced (lower record) and 3 min later the effects of high frequency stimulation were again tested. Although some short-lasting post-tetanic potentiation resulted, l.t.p. was prevented. After the APV injection had been terminated for 8 min, 100 Hz stimulation for 1 s was again able to produce l.t.p. which did not recover completely over the time that responses were measured (45 min). (Reproduced from Collingridge *et al.*, 1983, by permission of the Physiological Society.)

by depressing Purkinje cell excitability with GABA. Corticofugal activity as well as thalamocortical activity can be blocked by iontophoretic aminoadipate or 2-APV (Stone, 1976, 1979a; Hicks *et al.*, 1981; Hicks and Guedes, 1981). Kemp and Sillito (1982) have reported that aminoadipate would block responses to NMA of neurones in the visual cortex at doses which did not affect glutamate or visually evoked activity. At doses which depressed glutamate responses, however, visually evoked activity was suppressed (Figure 56).

Ikeda and Sheardown (1982) have found that iontophoretic aspartate would excite and enhance the visually evoked activation of the 'sustained' but not 'transient' classes of cells in the cat retina. Furthermore 2-APV would block the visually evoked excitation of the 'sustained' cells only (Figure 57). This would seem to be an extremely promising area in which to approach a definite identification of an aspartate-like compound as a neurotransmitter.

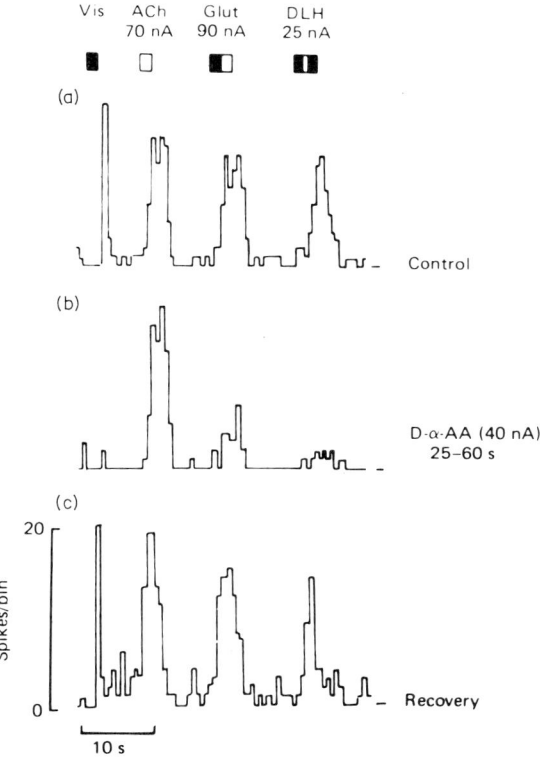

Figure 56 Peristimulus time histograms (PSTHs) illustrating the selective effect of D-α-aminoadipate (D-α-AA) on the responses of a dLGN neurone (LG II, 271) to visual stimulation (vis) and pulsed ionophoretic application of drugs. Visual stimulus is a spot of light flashed within the receptive field centre. Duration of flash and drug pulses is indicated by the symbols above records. Magnitudes of the drug ejection currents are indicated above symbols. Calibration bar on ordinate indicates number of spikes per bin. Calibration of abscissa indicates 10 s. Bin size 400 ms, one trial, cell type, off X. (a) Control run illustrating responses to visual stimulus, acetylcholine (ACh), L-glutamate (Glut) and (DL-homocysteic acid (DLH). (b) Responses to the same sequence as in (a) but during ionophoretic application of D-α-AA in a time period after onset of application as indicated to the right of the records. (c) Recovery run after cessation of D-α-AA application. (Reproduced from Kemp and Sillito, 1982, by permission of the Physiological Society.)

V.4 Localization of Receptors

Dudar (1974) used the hippocampal slice preparation to show that glutamate, applied iontophoretically into a region corresponding approximately to the apical dendrites, caused excitation of CA 1 pyramidal cells. Similar results were obtained by Yamamoto and Sawada (1982) and, during intracellular recordings,

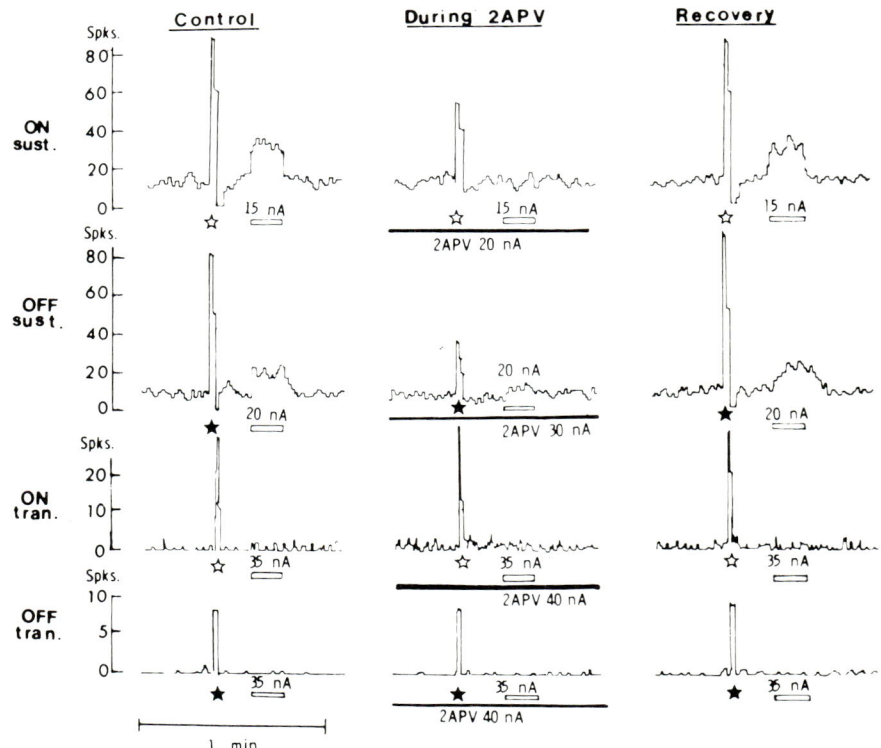

Figure 57 Pen recorder tracings illustrating the effect of 2APV on the visually driven (marked by the stars) and L-aspartate-induced (marked by the open bars) excitations of on-centre and off-centre 'sustained' and on-centre and off-centre 'transient' retinal ganglion cells. The visual stimulus was an optimal spot located at the receptive field centre (spot luminance, 20 cd/m^2; background luminance, 10 cd/m^2; spot size, chosen so that it produced optimal response from the cell, i.e. 0.5° for both 'sustained' and 1° for both 'transient' cells; stimulus duration, 2 s). The control traces were obtained before the application of 2APV, the traces in the middle column 1 min after the beginning of 2APV application and the traces in the right column 1 min after the termination of 2APV application. Note that 2APV reduced both visually and L-aspartate-induced excitations of the 'sustained' cells but had no effect on 'transient' cells. (Reproduced from Ikeda and Sheardown, 1982, by permission of Pergamon Press Ltd.)

by Hablitz and Langmoen (1982) although by using 4 μm steps these latter authors were able to detect several regions of sensitivity as their iontophoretic electrode traversed the dendritic field, presumably due to activation of different branches of the dendritic tree.

Glutamate iontophoresis on to spinal motoneurone dendrites *in vivo* has also been shown to evoke depolarization with a latency less than that seen by iontophoresis at the soma (Zieglgänsberger and Champagnat, 1979).

Chujo *et al.* (1975) and Crepel *et al.* (1982) have studied the sensitivity of Purkinje cell dendrites *in vitro*. The latter group demonstrated that glutamate sensitivity was greater in the dendritic region than at the soma, and that sensitivity to aspartate declined in the more distal dendritic regions whereas glutamate sensitivity did not. Quisqualic acid, but not NMA was also excitatory when applied to the dendrites.

V.5 Mechanism of Action

Intracellular studies have been performed in attempts to understand the mechanism of action of excitatory amino acids at the membrane level. The first studies were performed using glutamate iontophoresed on to spinal neurones *in vivo* (Zieglgänsberger and Puil, 1973) and indicated an increase of membrane conductance, probably to sodium ions. Herrling (1981) and Hablitz and Langmoen (1982) have reached similar conclusions in the hippocampus, although both an increase and decrease of membrane conductance to glutamate were seen by Engberg *et al.* (1979b) *in vivo* and by MacDonald and Wojtowicz (1982) in tissue culture. The increased conductance may be associated with uptake of the glutamate (Engberg *et al.*, 1979b). L-Aspartate appears to produce normally a voltage-dependent decrease of membrane potassium conductance as does homocysteate (Engberg *et al.*, 1979b) while quisqualate produces a voltage-independent increase (MacDonald and Porietis, 1982). In supraspinal regions NMA and homocysteate may activate calcium (Dingledine, 1983) or sodium currents (Flatman *et al.*, 1983).

Intracellular studies combined with iontophoresis are also of great value in comparing qualitatively the type of excitation produced by different agonists. Herrling *et al.* (1983), for example, have shown marked similarities between the effects of NMA and quinolinic acid in the caudate nucleus, both compounds

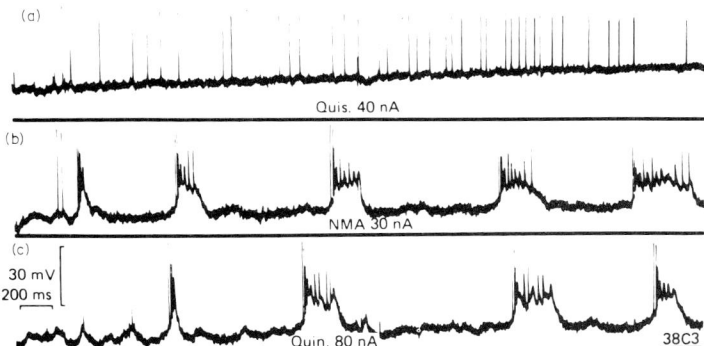

Figure 58 The effects of quisqualate, NMA and quinolinate on the membrane potential and firing pattern of a neurone displaying pronounced plateaux. (a) Quisqualate depolarized the membrane and elicited repetitive firing but no plateaux up to a level where the action potentials were largely inactivated. (b) and (c) Both NMA and quinolinate provoked very distinct plateaux. With quinolinate it was usually necessary to apply more current to reach excitation levels equal to those of NMA on the same cell. (Reproduced from Herrling *et al.*, 1983, by permission of the Physiological Society.)

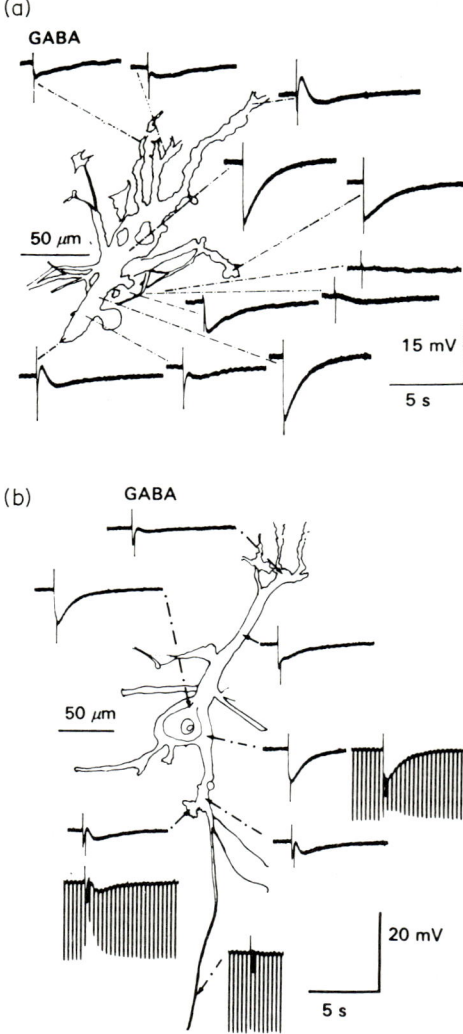

Figure 59 Ionophoresis of identical GABA pulses on to surface of two different spinal cord cells (a) and (b) shows non-uniform topography of sensitivity and response complexity. Monophasic, hyperpolarizing responses associated with conductance increase present at cell body, while multiphasic responses coupled to conductance increase observed on processes. Withdrawing the ionophoretic pipette from the surface in 10 μm steps (at lower right-hand part of cell in (a)) shows progressive depression in response amplitude and slowing of kinetics. Responses illustrated are representative of three evoked at each site on each cell. Resting potential: −53 mV (a), −55 mV (b). Downward deflexions in (b) are voltage responses to constant current (−1 nA) pulses. GABA ionophoretic pulses: 22 nA, 100 ms (a); 24 nA, 100 ms (b). (Reproduced from Barker and Ransom, 1978, by permission of the Physiological Society.)

producing rhythmic bursts of depolarization, whereas quisqualate induces only a sustained and progressive tonic depolarization (Figure 58). This is consistent with an action of quinolinate on the NMA type of receptor.

PART VI INHIBITORY AMINO ACIDS

Both glycine and 4-aminobutyric acid (GABA) are now widely recognized as potent inhibitors of neuronal activity in the CNS, usually causing hyperpolarization associated with an increased membrane conductance to chloride. GABA can, however, cause depolarization of ganglion cells (Obata, 1974) and recent studies have shown that this amino acid can also have depolarizing actions if applied to certain parts of the neuronal surface. Barker

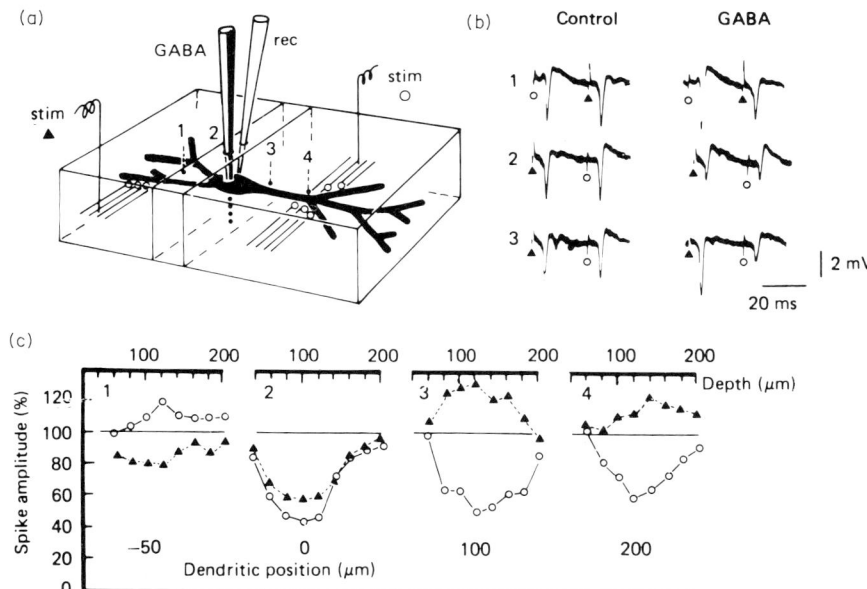

Figure 60 Reciprocal effect of GABA on two separate synaptic inputs to CA 1 pyramidal cells. (a) Diagram to show the two orthodromic inputs in stratum radiatum (open circle) and stratum oriens (filled triangle). GABA was delivered by an iontophoretic electrode in a series of tracks, lying in a plane parallel to the main dendritic axis. Four of the tracks are labelled 1-4. (b) Population spikes to orthodromic activation of the two inputs shown in (a), labelled with the same symbols. The left-hand traces were taken before, the right-hand traces were taken during GABA application (40 nA, 4 s). Lines 1-3 indicate that GABA was delivered in tracks called 1-3 in (a). Upward deflexions are positive (c) The four panels 1-4 refer to GABA application in tracks 1-4 of 6a). The ordinate gives the size of the radiatum- (open circles) and oriens- (filled triangles) induced population spikes in per cent control values. The abscissa gives the depth of GABA ejection. When applied in track 2, there was a similar effect on the response from the two inputs, while GABA applied in tracks 1, 3 and 4 gave reciprocal effects. (Reproduced from Andersen *et al.*, 1980, by permission of the Physiological Society.)

and Ransom (1978a), for example, used cultured mouse cord and brain neurones to reveal the variation of response size and polarity which resulted from GABA iontophoresis (Figure 59). Application directly on to the soma elicited chloride-dependent hyperpolarizations similar to those described *in vivo*; application on the cell processes resulted in a component of depolarization which appeared to involve an increase of sodium conductance. Exactly analogous findings have now been made on hippocampal pyramidal cells using the slice preparation (Djorup *et al.*, 1981; Alger and Nicholl, 1982) and Andersen *et al.* (1980) have extended this work to show that locally applied GABA can differentially affect synaptic input (which is suppressed) and distant synapses (which are facilitated) (Figure 60).

It has been suggested that some of the depolarizing effects of GABA could be due to an electrogenic sodium influx coupled to the GABA uptake carrier mechanism (Krnjević *et al.*, 1977). Consistent with this is the observation that intracellular iontophoretic ejections of GABA cause hyperpolarization, assumed to reflect a net reversal of the GABA transport system (Constanti *et al.*, 1980) (Figure 61). However, it would seem unlikely that a carrier-mediated process contributes significantly to GABA-induced depolarization of hippocampal dendrites, as the response is not affected by the presence of nipecotic acid, a potent inhibitor of GABA transport (Djorup *et al.*, 1981). Both the depolarizing and hyperpolarizing effect of GABA can be blocked by bicuculline (Wong and Watkins, 1982).

VI.1 Pharmacology

Whereas glycine is selectively antagonized by strychnine (Curtis *et al.*, 1971a), picrotoxin and bicuculline have become firmly established as the GABA antagonists of choice, although the latter must be used as a quaternary methylated salt to avoid the rapid degradation of the neat alkaloid (Curtis *et al.*, 1971b; Johnston *et al.*, 1972). Doubts about the value of bicuculline (Straughan *et al.*, 1971; Hill *et al.*, 1973) do not seem to have been borne out (Dray, 1975), even though the selectivity of the alkaloid has been questioned again more recently (Mayer and Straughan, 1981; Okamoto and Sakai, 1981). Interestingly, intravenous bicuculline does not appear to block GABA inhibitions (Kelly and Renaud, 1973). The suggested use of tubocurarine as a GABA antagonist (Hill *et al.*, 1973) has not received wide acceptance (Curtis *et al.*, 1974).

There are reports of benzodiazepine potentiation of neurally evoked inhibitory phenomena, usually assumed to be GABA mediated and studied in parallel with responses to iontophoretic GABA (Gallagher, 1978; Geller *et al.*, 1978; Sinclair *et al.*, 1982). Such potentiation has not been observed by other groups (Felix and Steiner, 1976; Wolf and Haas, 1977; Assumpcao *et al.*, 1979; Jiang, 1981) and may depend on the dose of benzodiazepine (MacDonald and Barker, 1978). One possible explanation is that both hyperpolarizing (somatic) and depolarizing (dendritic) responses can be recorded to iontophoretic GABA and both of these

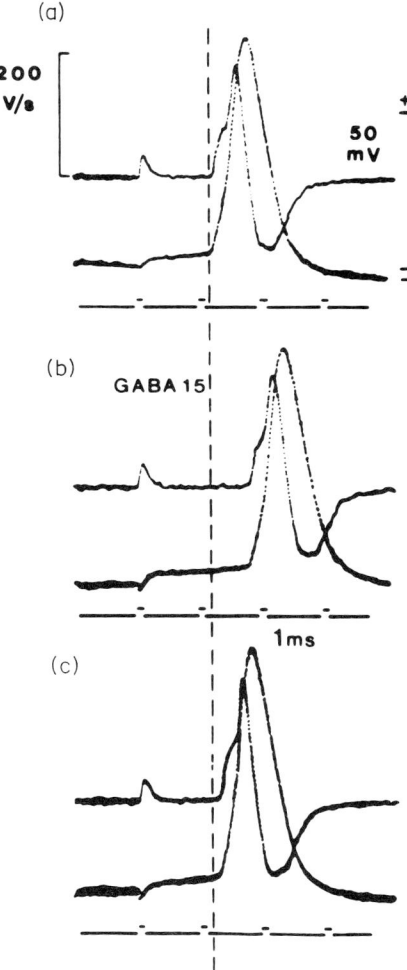

Figure 61 Reduction in excitability caused by intraneuronal injection of GABA. Spikes were evoked by identical intracellular depolarizing current pulses (2.5 nA, 10 ms throughout). In each case, lower trace is record of membrane potential and upper trace (partly superimposed) is first time derivative of action potential. (a) Initial control. (b) During injection of GABA (15 nA), membrane potential shifts downward indicating hyperpolarization, and both latency and amplitude of spike are increased (c) Very substantial recovery 90 s after end of injection. Initial resting potential was −66 mV. Time-scale trace provides a constant level of reference for changes in potential. (Reproduced from Constanti et al., 1980, by permission of the Canadian Journal of Physiological Pharmacology.)

may be enhanced by benzodiazepines (Jahnsen and Laursen, 1981). The net observable interaction with GABA would depend on the area of brain, electrode and cell orientation, and the concentration and diffusional spread of GABA and the drug.

Other anticonvulsant drugs such as valproic acid may act partly by enhancing GABA-related processes (MacDonald and Bergey, 1979; Gent and Phillips, 1980; Kerwin *et al.*, 1980).

VI.2 Synaptic Blockade

Less frequently than one might imagine, synaptic inhibition is encountered which cannot be blocked by strychnine or bicuculline (Duggan *et al.*, 1981) or which can be reduced only partially by these compounds as in the case of the subthalamic–pallidal pathway (Perkins and Stone, 1980b). Unfortunately negative results are far less conclusive than positive when using microiontophoresis because the relationship between electrode and innervation is unknown. A differentiation between agonists may be produced readily by an antagonist because the concentrations around the pipette tip are of the same order. The antagonist concentration at synapses 1 mm distant, however, may be only a few per cent of that at the tip. In spite of difficulties such as these some very elegant studies have been performed, particularly in the visual system. Sillito (1975, 1977) has demonstrated that bicuculline can markedly modify the visual response characteristics of neurones in the visual cortex. This is most strikingly seen as a loss of directional sensitivity of simple cells and of some complex cells (Sillito, 1977). The possibility raised by this work of dissecting pharmacologically the relative contribution of excitatory and inhibitory influences on sensory response properties awaits extension to other sensory receiving areas. In the cat retina *in vivo*, Ikeda and Sheardown (1983) have been able to distinguish beautifully between synaptic inhibitory mechanisms probably mediated by GABA and glycine. Thus GABA enhanced, while bicuculline blocked post-excitatory inhibition at the receptive field centre, and surround inhibition, of on-centre but not off-centre ganglion cells. Conversely glycine augmented and strychnine blocked the equivalent inhibitory phenomena at off-centre, but not on-centre cells.

Some of the iontophoretic studies on the type and cell surface localization of responses to GABA have been mentioned above, but it has also been shown that the dendrites of Purkinje cells show different regions of maximal sensitivity to glycine and GABA (Okamoto and Sakai, 1980) (Figure 62).

PART VII   ACETYLCHOLINE

Studies of acetylcholine sensitivity in the CNS have proved popular with practitioners of microiontophoresis because the parent compound as well as the various receptor-specific synthetic analogues can all be applied easily by this method, and because of the ready availability of potent and selective

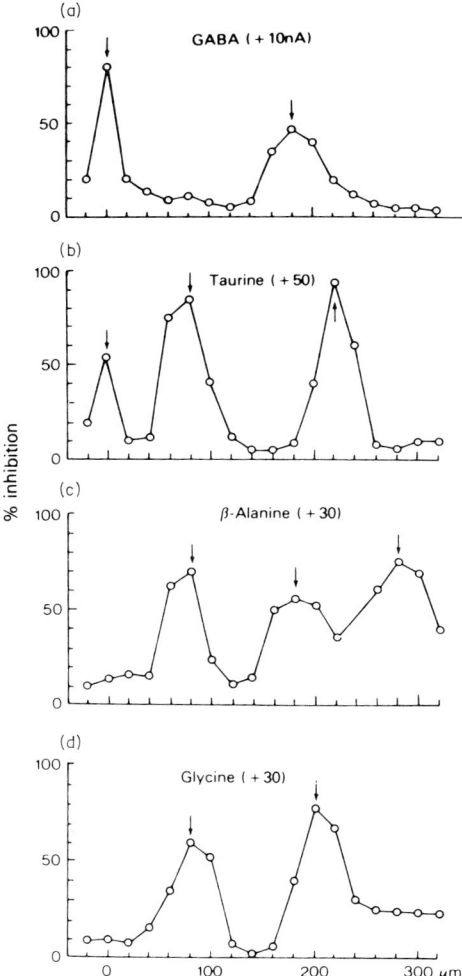

Figure 62 Typical distributions of sensitive spots to γ-aminobutyric acid (GABA (a), taurine (b), β-alanine (c) and glycine (d)) on individual cells. Ordinate scales: per cent inhibition of discharge frequency induced by the amino acid. Abscissa scales: distance (μm) from the Purkinje cell body along a line passing through the Purkinje cell body and perpendicular to the pial surface, 0 μm being the position of the cell body and 300 μm being near the pial surface. Each of the amino acids was ejected by the current given in parentheses at all the spots tested. The most sensitive spots are indicated by the arrow. (Reproduced from Okamoto and Sakai, 1980, by permission of the British Pharmacological Society.)

antagonists at those receptors. Nevertheless an exemplary degree of caution is required even here, because the high local concentrations of atropine, for example, which can be achieved by iontophoresis may be sufficient to cause a depression of action potential height with an increase of width (Curtis and Phillis, 1960). Equally, it was realized long ago that iontophoretically applied d-tubocurarine is not a very effective antagonist of acetylcholine at apparently nicotinic receptors (Curtis and Eccles, 1958b) and that it can have marked excitatory effects which are unrelated to acetylcholine sensitivity. Part of this latter problem probably results from the ability of tubocurarine to block the inhibitory actions of compounds like GABA (Hill et al., 1973) and 5-hydroxytryptamine (Mayer and Straughan, 1981) and to potentiate acetylcholine as a result of anticholinesterase properties (Miller and McLennan, 1974). For this reason dihydro-β-erythroidine has often been used as the central nicotinic antagonist of choice in iontophoretic studies.

Apparently, even α-bungarotoxin can be pushed out of micropipettes by iontophoresis or pressure sufficiently to block acetylcholine excitation (but not ventral-root-evoked responses) (Duggan et al., 1976). Spinal interneurones have not received as much attention as Renshaw cells but many are clearly sensitive to acetylcholine and related compounds. The paper by Myslinski and Randić (1977) summarizes and discusses much of the preceding work. That study also revealed a primarily nicotinic excitatory action of acetylcholine on Clarke's column and dorsal horn interneurones while a muscarinic inhibitory action was seen on dorsal spinocerebellar tract neurones.

Almost every region of brain has been examined for its sensitivity to iontophoretically applied cholinergic agents. Most of the earlier work *in vivo* (discussed in Tebecis, 1974 and Krnjević, 1974) was concerned primarily with establishing the direction of responses to cholinomimetics and whether the effects involved muscarinic, nicotinic or 'mixed' receptors. (The term 'mixed' does not distinguish between a mixed population of independent muscarinic and nicotinic receptors and a single population of receptors with properties intermediate between the two classical extremes.)

Many of these studies examined only cells encountered randomly in a particular region of brain, but others have often succeeded in relating the direction of responses to cholinomimetics with some specific function. Beckman and Eisenman (1970), for example, were able to distinguish between warm-sensitive interneurones which were excited by acetylcholine but inhibited by noradrenaline and cold-sensitive cells which were not affected by acetylcholine but were excited by noradrenaline.

Supraoptic neurones were found by Dreifuss and Kelly (1972) to be excited by a nicotinic action of acetylcholine, whereas Barker *et al.* (1971) reported that most supraoptic neurones experienced a muscarinic inhibition in response to cholinomimetics. Although the reasons for this difference are not clear, a more recent study by Bioulac *et al.* (1978) was able to show an interesting distinction between tonically firing supraoptic neurones, which probable release oxytocin, and phasically firing cells which are thought to release vasopressin. On the latter cells acetylcholine had a predominantly excitatory action, though only when the ejection was made during the silent periods. If applied during the discharge of the cell, however, acetylcholine had no effect. In contrast 99 out of 124 tonically active cells were inhibited by acetylcholine. In the cochlear nuclei Caspary *et al.* (1983) have noted that acetylcholine had opposite effects in the dorsal and ventral groups: there was activation of many neurones in the ventral nucleus whereas a reduction of tone-induced responses was seen in the dorsal nucleus.

In the cerebral cortex deep pyramidal tract cells are excited by acetylcholine (Krnjević, 1964; Stone, 1972a). Several authors have also described an inhibitory action of acetylcholine, also largely muscarinic in nature, in more superficial levels of the cortex and an excitatory action which appears to have a primarily nicotinic pharmacology, in the same superficial layers (Stone, 1972a; Krnjević, 1974).

Many of these observations have recently been substantiated in the careful study of Lamour *et al.* (1982) (Figure 63) although the nicotinic component of excitation was more evenly distributed throughout the cortex (see also McLennan and Hicks, 1978). As the sensitivity of cortical neurones to iontophoretically applied cholinesterase-resistant cholinomimetics is not changed after chronic undercutting of the cortex, any cholinergic neurones are assumed to be wholly intracortical (Reiffenstein and Triggle, 1972). As in the case of smooth muscle, responses to acetylcholine of central neurones often show a rather slow onset and prolonged time-course and the question arises of whether these represent a problem of access of cholinomimetic substances to the receptive surface, or whether they reflect a real biological delay. Several studies using *in vitro* preparations indicate the latter. Firstly, close apposition of the micro-iontophoretic electrode to the surface of Purkinje cells in an *in vitro* cerebellar slice (Crepel and Dhanjal, 1982) or of pyramidal cells in the hippocampal slice (Dodd *et al.*, 1981) still leads to slow acetylcholine responses. In the latter study the acetylcholine depolarizations were found to have a latency to onset about four times greater than an approximately equipotent application of glutamate, and outlasted an ejection about ten times longer than glutamate. Using cultures of neuroblastoma cells, Kato *et al.* (1983) have been able to distinguish a transient nicotinic depolarizing response and a later muscarinic phase exactly analogous to the components described by North and Tokimasa (1982) in myenteric plexus. Cultures of hippocampal slices have also been useful to confirm the muscarinic depolarization seen by Dodd *et al.* (1981) and Gähwiler and Dreifuss (1982). Evidence for cholinergic synapses in neocortex has been reported usually as a result of blocking a synaptic pathway with iontophoretically applied atropine. In this way excitation produced by reticular formation stimulation has been blocked (Spehlman and Daniels, 1973) as has inhibition from the same site (Phillis and York, 1968) and excitation from certain specific thalamic nuclei (Stone, 1972a; Hicks *et al.*, 1981).

One of the more exciting of recent studies of acetylcholine effects is by Sillito and Kemp (1983). They have found that acetylcholine will enhance the stimulus-evoked responses of visually driven cortical units, without affecting the overall

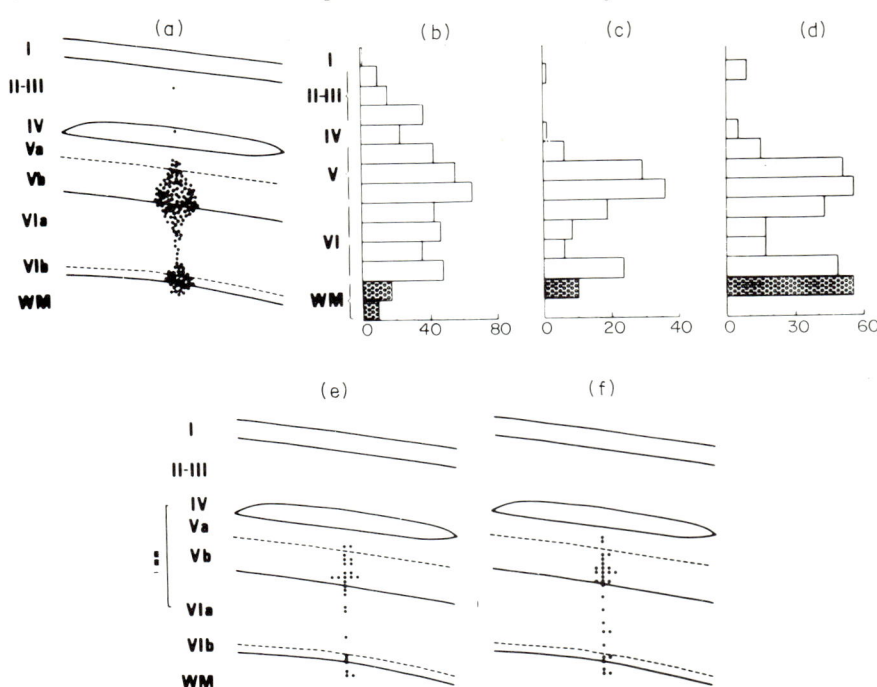

Figure 63 Laminar distribution of the excitatory responses to acetylcholine in rat first somatosensory cortex, under urethane (a) to (d), pentobarbital (e) and holothane (f)

(a) Positions in the cortical layers of 137 neurones which were excited by ACh at currents less than 120 nA. Each dot represents one cell. Cortical layers are numbered from I to VI, and layers V and VI have been subdivided according to previous authors. Dashed line indicates the limit between Va and Vb and VIa and VIb. A neuronal aggregate, chracteristic of SI cortex has been represented in layer IV. During the experiments, neurones were sampled within SI in the forelimb or hindlimb representation but they have been pooled in the figure. The position in depth of each neurone corresponds to the accurate position of the unit as determined by the reconstruction of the electrode tracks based on the dye deposit made at the final recording site. All the units represented in this figure (as well as in (b), (c) and (d) were recorded during penetrations which reached the white matter (WM) below the anatomical limit of the cortex.

(b) In (b), (c) and (d), the cortex has been subdivided in 12 bins of 180 μm each, and the part of the white matter underlying the cortex in two bins of 180 μm (dotted area). The correspondence between these bins and the cortical layers was established using mean layer dimensions calculated on sections taken from 10 different brains. According to these calculations, layer V corresponds, for example, to three bins of 180 μm, i.e. 540 μm, and layer VI to four bins. The number of units recorded per bin is given in (b).

(c) Absolute number of units excited by ACh per bin. Notice that no unit was excited by ACh in the second (deepest) bin of the white matter.

(d) Percentage of ACh-excited units per bin. Notice the clear distribution of bins with a high percentage of ACh-excited units in two peaks: one corresponding to the lower part of layer V (i.e. Vb) and upper part of VI, the other to the lowest part of layer VI (i.e. VIb) and the white matter immediately underlying it.

(e),(f) Distribution of the excitatory responses under pentobarbital (e) and holothane (f). Same conventions as in (a) (Reproduced from Lamour et al., 1982, by permission of Pergamon Press Ltd.)

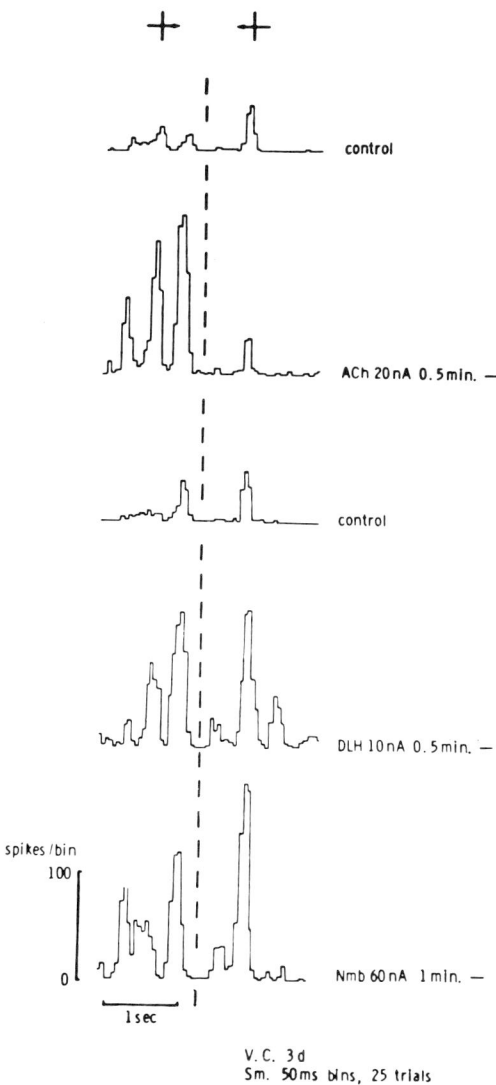

Figure 64 Comparison of the action of ACh. N-Methylbicuculline and DL-homocysteic acid (DLH) on the response of a multimodal 'S' cell to the two directions of motion of an optimally oriented bar of light. Records in sequence from top to bottom show: control run, effect of ACh applied with 20 nA ejecting current starting 0.5 min before record taken, control for recovery from ACh effect, effect of DLH applied with a 10 nA ejecting current starting 0.5 min before records taken, effect of N-methylbicuculline applied with 60 nA ejecting current starting 1.0 min before trials taken. Bin size 50 ms, 3.0 s cycle, 25 trials. Vertical calibration shows range corresponding to 0–100 counts/bin. (Reproduced from Sillito and Kemp, 1983, by permission of Elsevier Biomedical Press B.V.)

excitability of the cell. Thus orientation and direction specificity of neurones is preserved and increased relative to non-preferred stimulus responses. The contrast with a compound such as homocysteate which increases excitability and responsiveness to all inputs is striking (Figure 64). The phenomenon is reminiscent of the effects of some amines which can also increase signal-to-noise ratio by potentiating evoked activity and suppressing background (see this chapter, Pt. VIII). Perhaps this is a general principle of transmitter action in the CNS.

VII.1 Mechanisms

The mechanism of action of the excitatory effects of acetylcholine has been investigated by Krnjević et al. (1971a). Acetylcholine produced an increase of membrane resistance with a reversal potential of about -87 mV and with no evidence of anomalous rectification. Intracellular injection of Cl^- shifted the chloride equilibrium potential but not the acetylcholine reversal potential. The authors proposed that a decrease of potassium permeability was probably involved. Barium ions, which can block potassium channels also cause excitation (Krnjević et al., 1971b). From the same laboratory it was also reported that hypoxia or metabolic inhibitors such as dinitrophenol could selectively reduce excitatory responses to acetylcholine on cortical neurones (Godfraind et al., 1971) but Curtis and Felix (1971) subsequently pointed out that dinitrophenol would block not only muscarinic excitation but also excitation by excitatory amino acids. However, these latter studies were performed on Renshaw cells in the spinal cord.

VII.2 Field Potentials

An excellent illustration of the combination of localized iontophoretic administration with the recording of evoked potentials can be found in work by Ropert and Krnjević (1982), Rovira et al. (1983) and Cherubini et al. (1982) who have examined the effects of iontophoretically applied acetylcholine on field potentials in the hippocampus *in vivo*. When applied near the pyramidal somata, a range of muscarinic and nicotinic agonists were found to enhance the CA 1 population spike in response to commissural stimulation, but when applied into the dendritic region muscarinic and nicotinic agonists had opposite effects, muscarinics depressing and nicotinics enhancing the field e.p.s.p. and population spike (Figures 64 and 66).

PART VIII NORADRENALINE (NOREPINEPHRINE)

Early iontophoretic studies showed that noradrenaline would cause a depression of neuronal firing in the cat cerebral cortex (Krnjević and Phillis, 1963a) and a huge number of experiments have revealed similar responses in most areas of the CNS (Tebecis, 1974; Krnjević, 1974). This inhibition often

Practical Applications 163

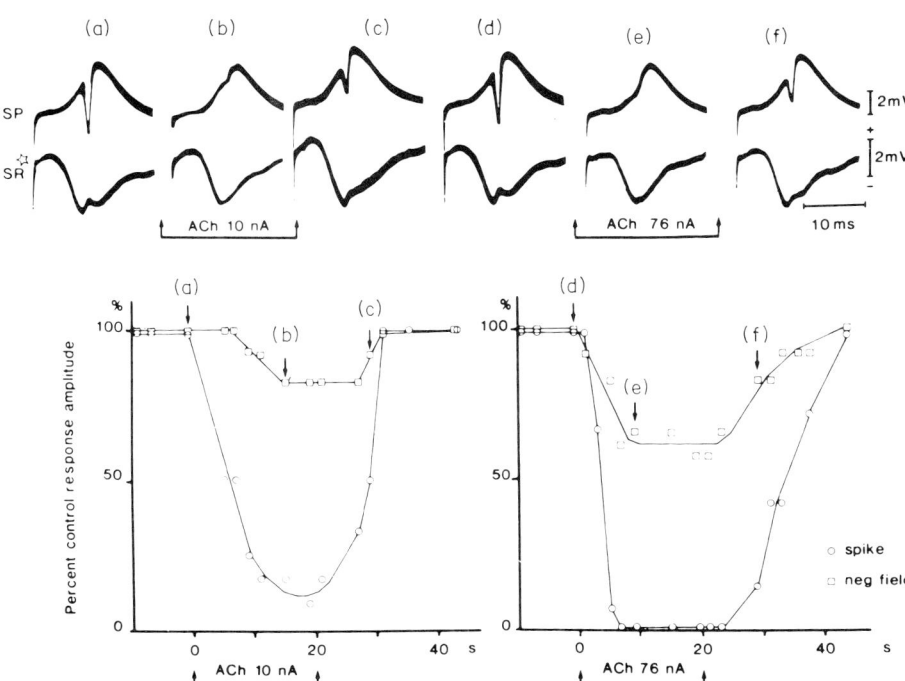

Figure 65 Effects of dendritic applications of acetylcholine on the negative dendritic field and the somatic population spike double recording system. In (a), traces obtained simultaneously from stratum pyramidale (SP) and stratum radiatum (SR). ACh was applied in stratum radiatum (asterisk) for 20 s. The dendritic negative wave (SR) is only slightly reduced but the somatic population spike is practically abolished. The results from this experiment are represented graphically in the lower part of the figure. (Reproduced from Rovira et al., 1983, by permission of Pergamon Press Ltd.)

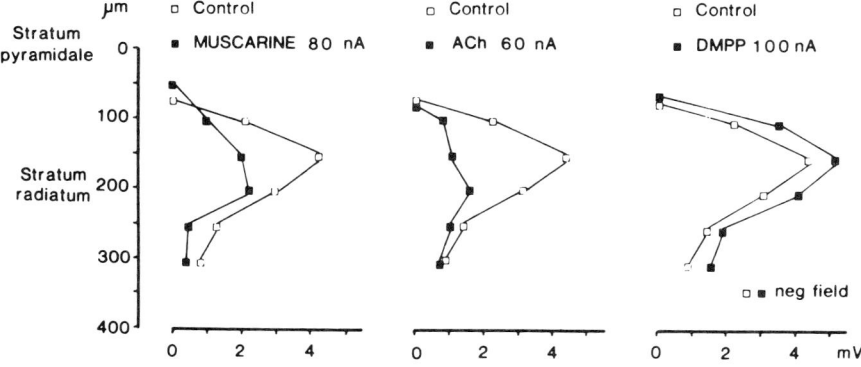

Figure 66 Depth profiles of dendritic actions of cholinomimetics. The agents were applied successively (for 20 s once per minute) at intervals of 50 μm. (Reproduced from Rovira et al., 1983, by permission of Pergamon Press Ltd.)

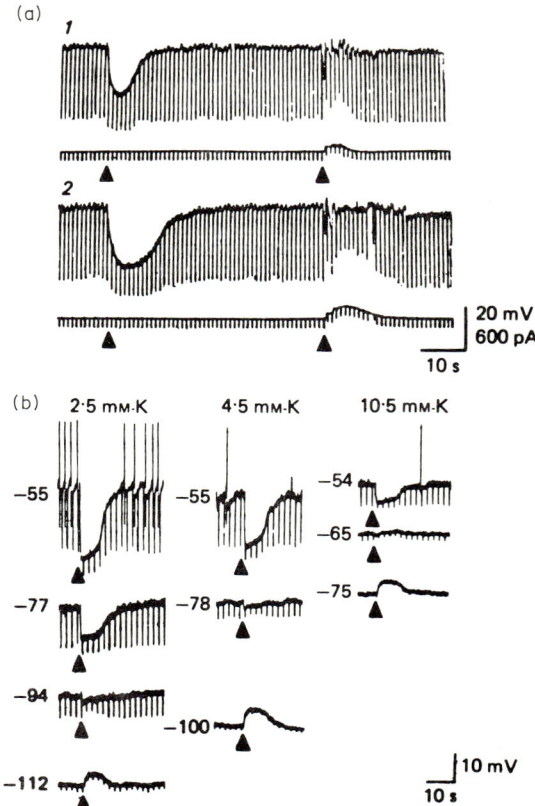

Figure 67 Noradrenaline activates potassium conductance. (a) Pressure application of noradrenaline (50 ms, 10 p.s.i. (68 kPa); ▲) produced a hyperpolarization and an increase of membrane conductance. Top traces are membrane potential and bottom traces are membrane current. (1) and (2) are from the same neurone. Noradrenaline was applied twice in each trace. The full amplitude of the noradrenaline-induced hyperpolarization is seen after the first application. Following the second application the membrane potential was maintained at rest by the manual-clamp technique. Twice as much noradrenaline was applied in (2) as in (1). (b) Determination of the noradrenaline reversal potential in solutions of varying potassium content. A single pressure ejection pulse (50 ms, 10 p.s.i. (68 kPa) was applied at each triangle. Left panel, in normal (2.5 mM) potassium; as the membrane was hyperpolarized, the noradrenaline potential became smaller and reversed at −100 mV. Middle panel, in 4.5 mM potassium; the reversal potential was decreased to −85 mV. Right panel, in 10.5 mM potassium; the reversal potential was −65 mV.
(Reproduced from Egan et al., 1983, by permission of the Physiological Society.)

seems to involve a voltage-dependent hyperpolarization accompanied by an increased membrane resistance (Marshall and Engberg, 1979; Siggins et al., 1971a) although Egan et al. (1983) have demonstrated a hyperpolarizing action of noradrenaline associated with a decreased membrane resistance, on neurones of the locus coeruleus in a slice preparation in vitro (Figure 67).

The biochemical basis of these hyperpolarizations has been the subject of much argument. The suggestion that they may be mediated by an increase in the intracellular concentration of cyclic AMP (Bloom, 1975) was mentioned in an earlier section. The failure of other groups to repeat some of the original cyclase-related observations prompted new hypotheses, most notably that the noradrenaline-induced hyperpolarizations were due to a calcium-dependent activation of Na^+-K^+-ATPase (Phillis, 1976). The main contribution of iontophoresis to this idea was the demonstration that a range of ATPase inhibitors including several glycosides and ethacrynic acid could block depressant responses to noradrenaline (Sastry and Phillis, 1977b). The involvement of calcium arose form experiments of Phillis and Limacher (1974) who observed that some metallic cations such as manganese and lanthanum, thought to act as calcium antagonists, would block depressant responses to amines. Freedman et al. (1975) later used a computer summing technique to circumvent the pronounced direct depressant effects of these ions. They were able to conclude that despite this background depression there was no blockade of noradrenaline responses (Figure 40).

Freedman et al. (1977) later showed that in spite of the depression of spontaneous Purkinje cell firing by noradrenaline, there was little change, or some augmentation of responses evoked by stimulation of climbing or mossy fibres. The same preservation of chemically induced responses (excitatory or inhibitory) (Moises et al., 1979) and synaptically evoked activity has now been shown also in the cerebral cortex (Waterhouse and Woodward, 1980; Waterhouse et al., 1980) and hippocampus (Segal, 1982b). However, noradrenaline reduced orthodromic activation of cells in the spinal trigeminal nucleus (Sasa et al., 1979). The enhancement of evoked activity in hippocampus may be due to a blockade by noradrenaline (and cyclic AMP) of a calcium-activated potassium conductance which contributes to repolarization or accommodation to depolarization (Madison and Nicoll, 1982).

Overt excitatory effects of noradrenaline have also been seen in many areas of CNS (Szabadi, 1979). In some regions these excitatory effects have become a source of argument, most particularly in the cerebral cortex. Johnson et al. (1969a) reported a much higher proportion of excitatory responses to noradrenaline in halothane anaesthetized or *encéphale isolé* cats compared with barbiturate anaesthetized animals (a similar change was seen for isoprenaline and 5-hydroxytryptamine). As there was also a significant difference in the depth distribution of spontaneously active cells under these conditions the authors favoured the concept that different cell populations, with different noradrenaline responses, were being sampled. Szabadi et al. (1977) have recently attempted to correlate the direction of responses to noradrenaline with background firing rate: the lower the rate the more likely is a cell to be excited by noradrenaline.

However, many other groups have observed noradrenaline responses which are almost always depressant, whether in unanaesthetized, *cerveau isolé* or methoxyflurane anaesthetized animals (Frederickson et al., 1973), urethane anaesthesia (Stone, 1973a; Ewart and Logan, 1978; Reader et al., 1979) or halothane (Freedman *et al.*, 1975) and in a number of species (Jordan *et al.*, 1972; Stone and Taylor, 1977). Stone (1971) suggested that, since iontophoretically applied noradrenaline would cause vasoconstriction with a time-course comparable with neuronal excitatory responses (Stone, 1972b) these two phenomena might be related. This idea was predictably challenged (Boakes *et al.*, 1971; Szabadi and Bradshaw, 1972) and defended (Stone, 1972d) (see Ch. 5, Pt. IV).

Another proposal was that excitant effects of noradrenaline depended on the pH of the solution in the iontophoretic pipette (Frederickson *et al.*, 1971) (see also Ch. 6, Pt. VI). Ejection from solutions at pH 4 or less were said to result in significantly more excitatory responses than when using pH 5. This was in conflict with Johnson *et al.* (1969b) and could not be confirmed by Stone (1972c) or Bevan *et al.* (1973a,b), although the latter authors failed even to observe effects of H^+ ejection, widely acknowledged as affecting neuronal excitability (Hewes and Frederickson, 1974).

This discrepancy (proportion of excitatory responses) persists between laboratories even today, although there are fresh attempts to resolve the problem. Armstrong-James and Fox (1983) have combined the iontophoretic ejection of noradrenaline in the urethane-anaesthetized rat cerebral cortex with their electrochemical assay for noradrenaline around the pipette tip. The two main findings of interest were, firstly, that neurones would respond to local concentrations of noradrenaline of between 10 nM and 10 μM and, secondly, that the lower concentrations were often associated with excitatory responses, particularly of the more deeply located cells (Figure 68). As excitatory responses to noradrenaline appear to show tachyphylaxis far more readily than inhibitory responses (Boakes *et al.*, 1971; Stone, 1973a), it is possible to propose on the basis of the Armstrong-James and Fox study (1983) that the higher the local noradrenaline concentration the more rapidly will any excitatory effect desensitize, leaving only a depressant response observable. Armstrong-James and Fox (1983) also reported that some cells exhibited a change of firing rate for up to an hour after an application of 100 nM noradrenaline.

It must be emphasized at this point that excitatory effects of noradrenaline are obtained so consistently in some regions that the question of their origin, artefactual or otherwise has not arisen. Particularly satisfying are those studies which have revealed a physiological or anatomical correlate of noradrenaline responses. For example, cells in the cat dorsal raphe nucleus are frequently depressed by noradrenaline, although the more ventrally located cells in the same nucleus are excited (Key *et al.*, 1980). Still in the hindbrain, cells of the lateral vestibular nucleus can be excited by noradrenaline while medial nucleus neurones are depressed (Kirsten and Sharma, 1976b). In the hypothalamic paraventricular nucleus correlations have been observed for cells which have a neurosecretory function, and which are depressed by noradrenaline, and cells which are not neurosecretory and which are usually excited by the amine (Moss *et al.*, 1972). Similarly cells identified antidromically in the medial preoptic nucleus are inhibited by noradrenaline and dopamine whereas neurones in the

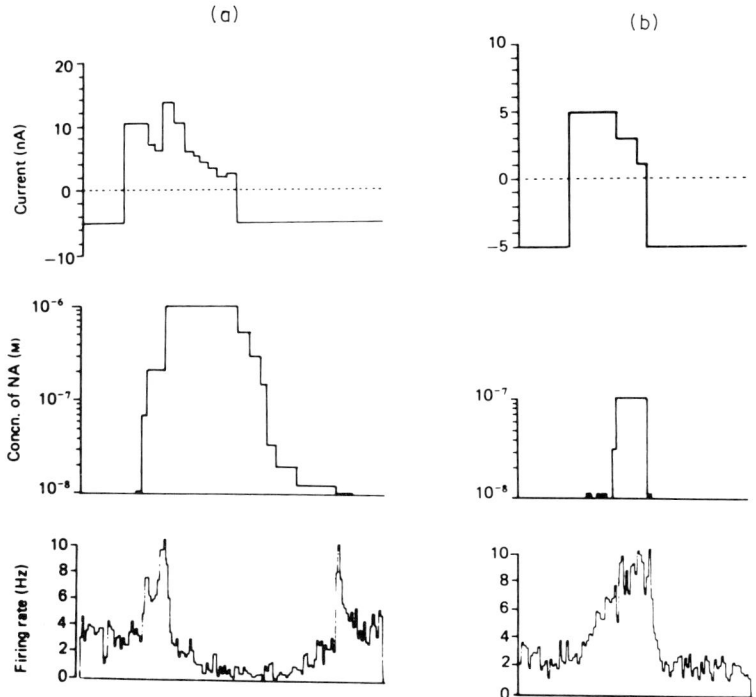

Figure 68 (a) Changes in firing rate (lowermost trace) of a cell located at 1200 μm in the deep cortical zone, in reply to changing concentrations of NA from less than 10^{-8} to 10^{-6} M. Receptive field was on distal hind foot pad. (b) Response of the same cell to maintaining extracellular concentration of NA at 10^{-7} M. Upper trace: iontophoretic current. Middle trace: extracellular concentration of noradrenaline measured electrochemically (see Ch. 4, Pt. III.1.a). (Reproduced from Armstrong-James and Fox, 1983, by permission of the Physiological Society.)

arcuate–ventromedial region are activated (Moss *et al.*, 1978). Warm-sensitive neurones in the preoptic and anterior hypothalamic nuclei are often inhibited by noradrenaline, whereas cold-sensitive cells are frequently excited (Beckman and Eisenman, 1970; Jell, 1973; Murakami, 1973; Hori and Nakayama, 1973).

Attempts to demonstrate a development of postsynaptic supersensitivity to noradrenaline have met with varying success, but an increase in the size or duration of excitatory (Menkes *et al.*, 1983) and inhibitory responses (Segal and Bloom, 1974; de Montigny *et al.*, 1980) has been recorded. In the cerebral cortex the proportion of excitatory responses to noradrenaline decreases dramatically after degeneration of the medial forebrain bundle (Jones and Roberts, 1979a).

Neuronal responses to iontophoretic noradrenaline, apparently excitatory as well as inhibitory, can be enhanced by antidepressant drugs (Bevan *et al.*, 1975; Jones and Roberts, 1979b; Menkes and Aghajanian, 1981; Egan *et al.*, 1983). However, this potentiation can occur even after the loss of most amine-containing terminals (Jones and Roberts, 1979a) and it may be restricted to certain layers of the cortex (Bunney and Aghajanian, 1976). Higher doses of antidepressants may cause blockade of noradrenaline (Ewart and Logan, 1978; Jones and Roberts, 1979b).

The pharmacology of responses to iontophoretically applied noradrenaline has been studied by several groups. Only excitatory responses could be readily blocked by α or β blocking drugs in the study of Johnson *et al.* (1969b) whereas depressant responses were subsequently blocked by β antagonists (Stone, 1973a; Freedman *et al.*, 1975; Hoffer *et al.*, 1971b). Bevan *et al.* (1977) have postulated excitatory α responses and depressant β responses in the neocortex, and some reports have appeared which are consistent with this concept in other areas (Menkes *et al.*, 1983; Vandermaelen and Aghajanian, 1983) and in cultured glia (Hirata *et al.*, 1983). Receptors of the α_2 subtype can be inhibitory (Cahusac and Hill, 1983).

Since amines are taken up into neurones by high and low affinity processes, Krnjević *et al.* (1978) and Nistri *et al.* (1978) reasoned that at times of high aminergic activity or when extracellular concentrations of amines are elevated, for example as a result of antidepressant therapy, the amine levels inside cells might rise to an extent which would have effects on the membrane biophysics. Accordingly this group showed that intracellular iontophoretic administration of catecholamines produced a depolarization with increased input resistance, with a corresponding diminution of spike height and after-hyperpolarization. It would be most interesting to know how the intracellular concentrations achieved by iontophoresis compare with those which could be achieved naturally.

PART IX DOPAMINE

Dopamine was first tested iontophoretically in the cerebral cortex (Krnjević and Phillis, 1963a) where profound suppression of spontaneous cell firing was observed. This action has been confirmed since by several authors (Bunney and Aghajanian, 1976; Stone, 1976) although, as for noradrenaline, excitatory effects have been reported by Bevan *et al.* (1978). Naturally most attention has centred on the effects of dopamine in the neostriatum where its action is usually inhibitory in the caudate nucleus (Connor, 1970; Feltz and de Champlain, 1972). Excitatory effects were noted by York (1972) in the putamen, but this was not confirmed by Ben-Ari and Kelly (1976).

Herrling and Hull (1980) have recently performed an intracellular analysis of dopamine's actions on cat caudate neurones. They recorded a depression of spontaneous firing, consistent with the above studies, but associated with a depolarization. In order to explain this the authors proposed that dopamine might hyperpolarize near the axon hillock, thus suppressing action potential production, but depolarize elsewhere in the cell, possibly the dendrites. The question then arises of whether the production of excitatory or inhibitory responses may depend largely on the relative orientation of cells and electrode.

The effects of dopamine injected into motoneurones were similar to the effects of noradrenaline (Nistri *et al.*, 1978).

Bunney and Aghajanian (1976) have performed a laminar analysis of amine responses in the rat cerebral cortex. They found that neurones in layers II and III, which receive a dense noradrenergic projection, were more sensitive to noradrenaline than dopamine, whereas the reverse pattern was noted in layers V and VI which receive a greater dopamine-containing projection. These authors also reported that desipramine would enhance noradrenaline responses in II and III but not deeper layers while benztropine enhanced dopamine responses only in V and VI.

Dopamine receptors are present not only on innervated cells but also on the dopaminergic cell bodies themselves—the so-called autoreceptors. Activation of such receptors by dopamine or apomorphine causes marked inhibition of cell firing and these effects can be blocked by neuroleptic drugs (Aghajanian and Bunney, 1977; Sedvall, 1975).

Generally iontophoretic studies of dopamine response pharmacology have proved consistent with behavioural and neurochemical work. Phenothiazines, for example, will block dopamine but not noradrenaline responses in the cortex (Bunney and Aghajanian, 1976; Stone, 1976) and striatum (York, 1972). Iontophoretically applied α-flupenthixol can also block the effects of dopamine (Ben-Ari and Kelly, 1976) although the same authors observed that intravenously administered α-flupenthixol or pimozide did not modify neuronal responses to iontophoretic dopamine. Gonzales-Vegas (1974) has summarized his own work on the concept that compounds such as bulbocapnine may produce their catatonic effects by blocking dopamine responses in the striatum.

In one of the few iontophoretic studies designed to detect presynaptic effects of drugs, Brown and Arbuthnott (1983) have shown that whereas fluphenazine blocks the direct depressant actions of dopamine in the striatum, sulpiride does not. Sulpiride does, however, enhance the excitatory effects of stimulating corticostriatal fibres while not affecting glutamate excitation directly. These findings are consistent with the idea that sulpiride can block dopamine receptors on corticostriatal terminals, those receptors normally functioning to inhibit the corticostriate transmitter (probably glutamate) release.

Only a limited success has been achieved using microiontophoresis to correlate neuronal responses to dopamine with responses to synaptic input. York (1972) did correlate the excitation of cells in the putamen to iontophoretic dopamine activation by nigral stimulation and Connor (1970) reported that caudate neurones depressed by nigral stimulation were also depressed by dopamine. Both these responses could be blocked by α-methyldopamine. Conversely, after destruction of the ascending aminergic pathways by 6-hydroxydopamine, Feltz and de Champlain (1972) were able to show a large increase in the number of caudate neurones responding to iontophoretic dopamine.

PART X 5-HYDROXYTRYPTAMINE (5-HT)

In most areas of the CNS the anatomical or physiological identification of units has revealed clear correlations with the type of 5-HT response obtained making it seem very likely that response variations reflect a real, biological difference between the target cells. Thus cat sympathetic preganglionic neurones are usually excited by 5-HT (De Groat and Ryall, 1967) whereas parasympathetic preganglionic cells are frequently depressed (Ryall and De Groat, 1972). Jordan *et al.* (1979) have described excitant effects of 5-HT on all the spinothalamic neurones tested which were associated with deep receptive fields, while a separate population of cells, mainly showing responses to high threshold input from very wide areas of body surface, were depressed.

Perkins and Stone (1983c) have described a differential sensitivity to 5-HT of neurones in the rat globus pallidus. Neurones which showed high spontaneous firing rates were not affected by either 5-HT or stimulation of the dorsal raphe nucleus, but cells with very low spontaneous activity, or which were silent until activated by an amino acid, were clearly inhibited both by 5-HT and raphe stimulation. It is not known whether there are other anatomical or physiological differences between these two cell populations.

There have been relatively few intracellular studies of the mechanism underlying 5-HT responses. In hippocampal slices Segal (1980) showed that 5-HT hyperpolarized CA 1 pyramidal cells with a decrease of membrane resistance, possibly due to an increase of potassium conductance. These effects were maximal with somatic and minimal with dendritic applications of 5-HT. Using cultured spinal neurones Cottrell and Green (1982) detected depolarizing responses to pressure-ejected 5-HT, which could be associated with either an increase or a decrease of membrane resistance in different cells.

Iontophoresed intracellularly into motoneurones, 5-HT produced little change of membrane potential or conductance, but reduced spike latency and augmented depolarizing and hyperpolarizing after-potentials (Nistri *et al.*, 1978).

Varying degrees of success have been reported in manipulating responses to iontophoretic 5-HT with appropriate drugs. The depressant responses in particular have proved almost invariably resistant to blockade by compounds known to block 5-HT in peripheral tissues although Segal (1976) and Segal and Bloom (1974) described some reduction of these responses in the hippocampus by cyproheptadine and methysergide, and Sastry and Phillis (1977a) have reported a blockade of neocortical depressant responses by metergoline. This latter blockade was achieved in parallel with a diminution of raphe-evoked inhibition of neurones.

In the early study by Roberts and Straughan (1967) it was noted that lysergic acid diethylamide (LSD) and its brominated derivative would reduce some excitatory responses to 5-HT in the cortex. This interaction was subsequently confirmed in the reticular formation (Boakes *et al.*, 1970). Briggs (1977) also confirmed this blockade of 5-HT and showed that it occurred in parallel with the blockade of excitation of reticular formation units elicited by raphe stimulation. Bradley and Briggs (1974) demonstrated that psychotomimetic tryptamine derivatives shared this action of LSD, while non-psychotomimetic analogues did not.

PART XI PURINES

Among the first purine compounds to be applied by microiontophoresis were the cyclic nucleotides which were found to mimic closely the depressant effects of noradrenaline on cerebellar Purkinje cells. A series of papers reported on the pharmacological manipulations of noradrenaline-induced depressions of Purkinje cell firing by agents known to interfere with adenylate cyclase activation (Bloom, 1975). Similar work has since been carried out in other areas including the hippocampus (Segal and Bloom, 1974) and cerebral cortex (Stone and Taylor, 1977; Jones and Roberts, 1979b). Some of this work has been the subject of considerable controversy, some groups being unable to confirm the observations made using cyclic AMP on Purkinje cells (Godfraind and Pumain, 1971; Jordan et al., 1972; Lake and Jordan, 1974) and these reports and the replies to them (Siggins et al., 1971b; Bloom et al., 1974) are most instructive for anyone contemplating microiontophoresis.

Cyclic GMP has also been applied iontophoretically. Consistent with the hypothesis that this nucleotide mediates cellular responses to acetylcholine, it was found to excite cortical neurones which were excited by acetylcholine (Stone et al., 1975; Hoffer et al., 1977; Stone and Taylor, 1977).

Intracellular work by Swartz and Woody (1979) showed a decrease of membrane conductance in response to extracellular acetylcholine and a similar change in response to intracellularly iontophoresed cyclic GMP, supporting the findings of Stone et al., (1975). In the spinal cord too Krnjević et al. (1976) recorded changes of membrane potential which were usually depolarizing for both acetylcholine and cyclic GMP intracellularly, and larger doses of cyclic GMP outside the cell had the same effect. Apart from the similar changes of membrane potential, however, most of the effects of cyclic GMP and acetylcholine were found to be dissimilar, acetylcholine producing for example an increase of membrane resistance, a slowing of spike repolarization and no effect on post-spike hyperpolarization. The authors, therefore, concluded that cyclic GMP could not be viewed as a second messenger for cholinergic actions. However, compounds applied intracellularly are being injected into an exceedingly complex system in which substances would normally be restricted to specific metabolic compartments. Responses to injected materials may never be observed physiologically.

In a separate study from the same laboratory (Krnjević and Van Meter, 1976) it was noted that intracellularly applied cyclic AMP tended to hyperpolarize cells, a finding consistent with many of the studies described above and supporting the view that cyclic AMP and cyclic GMP may have opposite effects on membrane potential (Stone et al., 1975). In addition it was reported that the cyclic AMP hyperpolarization was associated with an increased membrane resistance as noted by Siggins *et al.* (1971a).

Apart from cyclic nucleotides there has arisen much interest in the possible transmitter or modulator role of purines such as adenosine and adenosine triphosphate (ATP) (Stone, 1981b). Phillis *et al.* (1974) were among the earliest workers to investigate systematically the effects of a large number of purines and pyrimidines applied iontophoretically to cortical neurones.

Using iontophoretic applications of adenosine restricted to either the dendrites or the soma of pyramidal cells in the hippocampal slice, Segal (1982a) has shown that both presynaptic inhibition of transmitter release (reflected in a reduction of p.s.p. size) and a direct postsynaptic hyperpolarizing action associated with a conductance increase can be demonstrated (Figure 69).

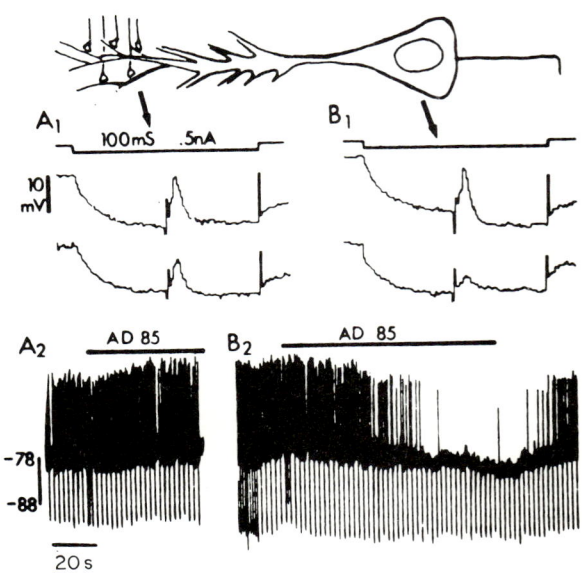

Figure 69 Comparison of dendritic (A) and somatic (B) application of adenosine in the same cell. (A_1, B_1) Computer averages of responses to hyperpolarizing current pulses and to stimulation of the stratum radiatum. (A_2, B_2) Chart recording of resting potentials and responses to hyperpolarizing current pulses. Dendritic application caused a decrease in e.p.s.p. without a change in resting potential whereas somatic application affected both. (Reproduced with permission from Segal, 1982.)

In spite of the interest being shown in adenosine receptors only two papers have specifically addressed the question of which purine receptor might be involved in the depression of neuronal firing. Stone (1982) showed that $(-)N^6$-phenylisopropyladenosine (PIA) and 5' N-ethylcarboxamide adenosine (NECA) were both able to mimic adenosine or AMP in causing a depression of spontaneous neuronal firing in the cerebral cortex (Figure 70). The PIA responses tended to outlast by many minutes the ejecting pulse and this was

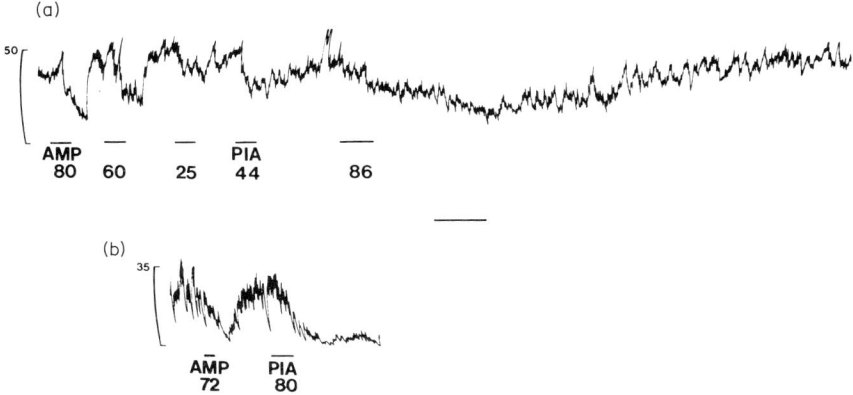

Figure 70 Records of the firing rates of two cortical neurones. Cell (a) dose-dependent suppression of firing rate in response to the iontophoretic application of AMP with currents of 80, 60 and 25 nA. The application of N^6-phenylisopropyladenosine (PIA) with currents of 44 and 86 nA produced responses which were comparable to those of AMP with respect to peak inhibition, but which were much longer lasting. Cell (b) illustrative of four cells encountered where AMP (here 72 nA) produced typical depressions of firing, but PIA produced a profound depression of firing which did not recover over the next 15–20 min. Ordinate: firing rate in spikes per second. Time scale: 1 min. (Reproduced from Stone, 1982, by permission of Elsevier Biomedical Press B.V.)

interpreted to imply the slow metabolism or removal of PIA, perhaps giving an exaggerated impression of its potency (Figure 70). As this kind of slow, prolonged action can also be seen on isolated perfused tissues this interpretation may not be correct. However, coupled with the observation that fewer cells responded to (−)PIA than to NECA, whether applied by iontophoresis or pressure ejection, Stone (1982) concluded that the depression of most cells involved an Ra/A_2 receptor. The blockade of purine responses by iontophoretically applied xanthines (Perkins and Stone, 1980a; Stone and Perkins, 1981b) is consistent with this conclusion.

In the study by Phillis (1982) NECA was shown to be a better depressant of cell firing than PIA and the prolonged time-course of the PIA effects was also confirmed. This author thus came to the same conclusion, that an A_2 receptor was involved in the neuronal inhibition.

As a neurotransmitter candidate ATP has received much more attention than adenosine, probably because the latter exhibits such a wide spectrum of effects. However, the effects of ATP on single CNS neurones is less clear than for adenosine. In the study of Phillis *et al.* (1974) ATP was found to have a depressant action on all the neurones tested in the cerebral cortex, although the authors noticed a transient initial excitation of a small number of more superficial units.

In order to clarify the role of an ATP receptor in neuronal firing Stone and Perkins (1981b) used a series of non-hydrolysable analogues of ATP

(β-, γ-methylene ATP; P_1P_5-diadenosine pentaphosphate) applied iontophoretically to cortical neurones. All these compounds caused depression of firing, usually weak, with no evidence of excitation. The occasional excitatory responses seen by Phillis *et al.* (1974) may, therefore, reflect only a non-specific effect, such as metal chelation.

At the same time Stone and Perkins (1981b) reported a strong depressant response to nicotinamide adenine dinucleotide (NAD) a finding of some potential importance in view of the almost millimolar concentrations of this compound in brain.

Interest in ATP has recently been rekindled in areas other than cerebral cortex. Salt and Hill (1983), for example, have described frequent excitant responses to ATP of neurones in the caudal trigeminal nucleus, although the authors are careful to point out that similar excitations were seen with iontophoretic pyrophosphate. Jahr and Jessell (1983) have also seen clear excitatory responses to iontophoretic ATP of most (91%) of a sample of dorsal root ganglion cells in tissue culture and of a smaller population (27%) of dorsal horn neurones in culture. The effect was shared by stable ATP analogues but not by chelating agents and appeared to be due to an increase of sodium conductance.

PART XII PEPTIDES

Microiontophoresis or pressure ejection has been used to apply a wide range of endogenous and synthetic peptides to neurones *in vivo* and *in vitro*. Partly because of the lack of selective antagonists, however, there has been little progress in relating the observed responses to a physiological role, and as a result attention has been concentrated on the mechanism of the observed responses, and potential interactions with neurotransmitters. Substance P, for example, appears to interact selectively with acetylcholine (Henry *et al.*, 1975; Belcher and Ryall, 1977; Krnjević and Lekić, 1977; Lamour *et al.*, 1983). The latter group has shown that the depressant effect of substance P is directed towards the nicotinic but not muscarinic excitatory receptor on Renshaw cells.

Iontophoretic substance P will also enhance the response of spinal cord neurones to noxious stimuli but not innocuous ones, in some cases leading to the occurrence of responses in initially unresponsive units (Henry, 1976; Randić and Miletić, 1977). Some excitatory effects of substance P can be mimicked by capsaicin, also applied iontophoretically, at least in the trigeminal nucleus (Salt and Hill, 1980).

There is no evidence for an increase of sensitivity of spinal neurones to the substance P analogue, eledoisin related peptide, after chronic dorsal rhizotomy (Roberts and Wright, 1981) but interest has arisen in the possible role of substance P in the therapeutic effects of drugs such as antidepressants. Jones and Olpe (1984) for instance have shown that chronic treatment of rats with desipramine leads to an apparent selective increase in the sensitivity of cingulate neurones to iontophoretic substance P but not glutamate. Acute injections of desipramine have no such action.

With regard to the development of substance P antagonists G. Engberg et al. (1981) have reported that the excitation by substance P of neurones in locus coeruleus could be blocked by [D-Pro^2, D-Trp^{7,9}] substance P, at a time when acetylcholine and glutamate responses were unchanged, but in the trigeminal nucleus, Salt et al. (1982) have failed to block susbtance P excitation by the same putative antagonist.

Yarbrough (1976) reported that thyrotropin releasing hormone (TRH) would selectively enhance the excitatory effects of acetylcholine on cortical neurones, with no effect on resting firing rates, but this could not be confirmed by Renaud et al. (1979). The latter group, on the other hand, reported that TRH would depress the responses of cortical neurones to excitatory amino acids, with a degree of selectivity being shown for blocking glutamate rather than aspartate (or acetylcholine). Braitman et al. (1980) then tactfully published results which implied that both previous groups were partially correct: acetylcholine responses were indeed potentiated by TRH on 5 of 14 neurons, at least 12 of which were pyramidal tract cells. Responses to glutamate, however, were not enhanced on most of this population and acetylcholine responses were not potentiated on 9 non-pyramidal tract cells. Equally Braitman et al. (1980) stated that glutamate responses were *reduced* by TRH on 5 of 12 cells tested.

The most recent contribution to this topic is from Stone (1983a) who again observed an enhancement of acetylcholine responses (9 of 15 cells in the neocortex) but obtained no evidence for a reduction of sensitivity to amino acids in spite of using NMA and quisqualic acid as agonists selective for different amino acid receptors. Interestingly a major metabolite of TRH, histidylproline diketopiperazine, which shares some of the behavioural actions of TRH, was able to mimic most of the electrophysiological actions of the parent peptide.

In contrast to most peptides the potent excitatory action of somatostatin in hippocampal slices is relatively rapid in onset and termination, though the significance of this remains obscure (Dodd and Kelly, 1978). Cholecystokinin is also frequently excitatory (Dodd and Kelly, 1981) while angiotensin has excitant properties which appear to be restricted to the subfornical organ and related structures (Felix and Akert, 1974; Felix and Phillips, 1978). Neurotensin is also frequently excitatory (Stanzione and Zieglgänsberger, 1983) while the tripeptide Met–Tyr–Lys is inhibitory to spinal neurones (Logan et al., 1982). Normanton and Gent (1983) have shown that two sleep-inducing peptides, delta sleep-inducing peptide and arginine vasotocin, can both cause depression of rat brainstem neurones though with very different response characteristics, suggesting that they may not work in the same way, at least at this level.

Finally it should be re-emphasized that peptides do present special problems for microiontophoresis. Larger molecules in particular tend to be adsorbed on to charged surfaces which include the internal wall of a micropipette tip. Some peptides may also undergo denaturation or degradation during iontophoretic experiments, as reported by Gozlan et al. (1977) for substance P. This problem may be exacerbated if very high ejecting currents are applied for long periods of time through high resistance tips: any change of local temperature may have a major impact on the stablity of a peptide. It may be an advisable precaution to use assay methods, or pharmacological means (Belcher and Ryall, 1977) to rule out any contribution to the observed responses of possible breakdown products.

PART XIII OPIATES AND OPIOIDS

Microiontophoresis has proved exceedingly valuable for opiate studies since it allows the testing of discrete units activated respectively by noxious or non-noxious stimuli in the same preparation. In most such studies the applied opiates have depressed noxious stimulus-evoked activity (Davies and Dray, 1978; Henry, 1978; Duggan *et al.*, 1979) though usually in parallel with effects on spontaneous or chemically induced firing (Calvillo *et al.*, 1974; Andersen *et al.*, 1978; Hill and Pepper, 1978). Duggan *et al.* (1979) reported that iontophoresis of morphine near the cell bodies of lamina V neurones in the cat cord had little effect on evoked activity, though when applied from a separate pipette on to the dendrites in layer II (substantia gelatinosa) of layer V cells, morphine selectively depressed responses evoked by noxious but not non-noxious stimuli.

Napier *et al.* (1983) have shown that iontophoretically applied naloxone can block striatally induced inhibition of pallidal neurones, consistent with the idea of an enkephalinergic link between the two structures. The study did not, however, exclude a contribution from the non-opiate actions of naloxone (such as GABA blockade) mentioned below.

Microiontophoresis has also proved a popular means for comparing qualitatively opiate responses in normal and in opiate-tolerant animals. Thus inhibitory responses to morphine were encountered less frequently in the neocortex of morphine-tolerant rats than in controls (Satoh *et al.*, 1976). Aghajanian (1978) and Fry *et al.* (1980) showed that iontophoretically applied naloxone would elicit a large increase of firing of locus coeruleus neurones in morphine-tolerant rats, presumably a correlate of the withdrawal phenomenon in such animals. Also using iontophoresis Zieglgänsberger *et al.* (1982) have shown that tolerance may develop to opiate alkaloids but not opioid peptides on some neurones.

As for morphine itself the opioid peptides have been tested iontophoretically in many regions of CNS (Bradley *et al.*, 1976; Gent and Wolstencroft, 1976b; Nicoll *et al.*, 1977; Young *et al.*, 1977; Palmer *et al.*, 1978; North, 1979; Klemm, 1980) but some of the excitatory effects seen in the hippocampus appear to be mediated indirectly due to effects on transmitter release (Haas and Ryall, 1980) or a naloxone-sensitive depression of local inhibitory interneurones (Zieglgänsberger *et al.*, 1979; Lee *et al.*, 1980; Nicoll *et al.*, 1980).

Some of the longer length opioid-related peptides such as endorphins and C-fragment have also been tested iontophoretically (Gent *et al.*, 1977; Nicoll *et al.*, 1977; Henry, 1978). Most recently attempts have been made to test iontophoretically peptides such as kyotorphin (Satoh *et al.*, 1980; Stone, 1983b) Correlations have been made between the occurrence and direction of responses to kyotorphin and met-enkephalin, or kyotorphin and D-phenylalanine though only enkephalin responses (inhibitory in globus pallidus, mixed in cortex) were blocked by iontophoretic naloxone (Stone, 1983b).

No one yet seems to have pursued a report that indirect effects of some kind are involved in modulating opiate sensitivity in the cerebral neocortex, since D-Ala^2-metenkephalinamide no longer inhibits neocortical neurones after destruction of catecholaminergic pathways ascending to this area (Palmer and Hoffer, 1980).

A large number of studies have dealt only with effects of morphine or other opiates on neuronal firing rate in various regions of CNS together with the sensitivity of those effects to blockade by naloxone. Many of those studies have been summarized in reviews by North (1979) and Klemm (1980) and will not be discussed here except to caution that iontophoretic naloxone can also antagonize GABA (Dingledine et al., 1978) and substance P (Davies and Dray, 1977) and may not block opiate responses which can be prevented by systemic naloxone (Hill and Pepper, 1978). Naloxone and tests of agonist stereospecificity may, therefore, be misleading (Fry et al., 1979).

PART XIV NON-MAMMALIAN CNS

The CNS of sub-mammalian species has provided a wealth of experimental material for iontophoreticists, since many such organisms possess large neurones which can be readily identified visually and are highly consistent in their localization from specimen to specimen. Among vertebrates the lamprey has been studied occasionally (Beranek et al., 1970; Gold and Martin, 1981) but the goldfish has probably been more popular. In a classic series of papers Diamond and his colleagues detailed the responses to iontophoretically applied amino acids of the large Mauthner neurones of this species (Diamond, 1968; Diamond and Roper, 1973; Diamond et al., 1973). The dependence on conductance changes and neuronal localization of the effects of GABA and glutamate and the interaction of their responses with synaptic potentials has remained an exemplary model of transmitter function. The relatively large and easily accessible retina of the goldfish has also been popular for iontophoretic studies (Ishida et al., 1984).

In many cases the transmitter released by identified neurones is reasonably well established and studies have begun to concentrate on pharmacological interactions and the distribution of receptor subtypes. The giant synapse of the squid for example, thought to use glutamate as its transmitter, has been subjected to fluctuation analysis (Bevan et al., 1975) while the giant dopamine-containing neurone of *Planorbis* has been studied for responsiveness to other compounds as well as the ionic basis of its own synaptic actions (Logan and Cottrell, 1975; Berry and Cottrell, 1979) (Figure 71).

The snail, *Helix*, has also provided much useful information and most recently has been used to examine the effects of excitatory amino acids and related compounds (Roberts and Walker, 1982) and the modulatory interactions

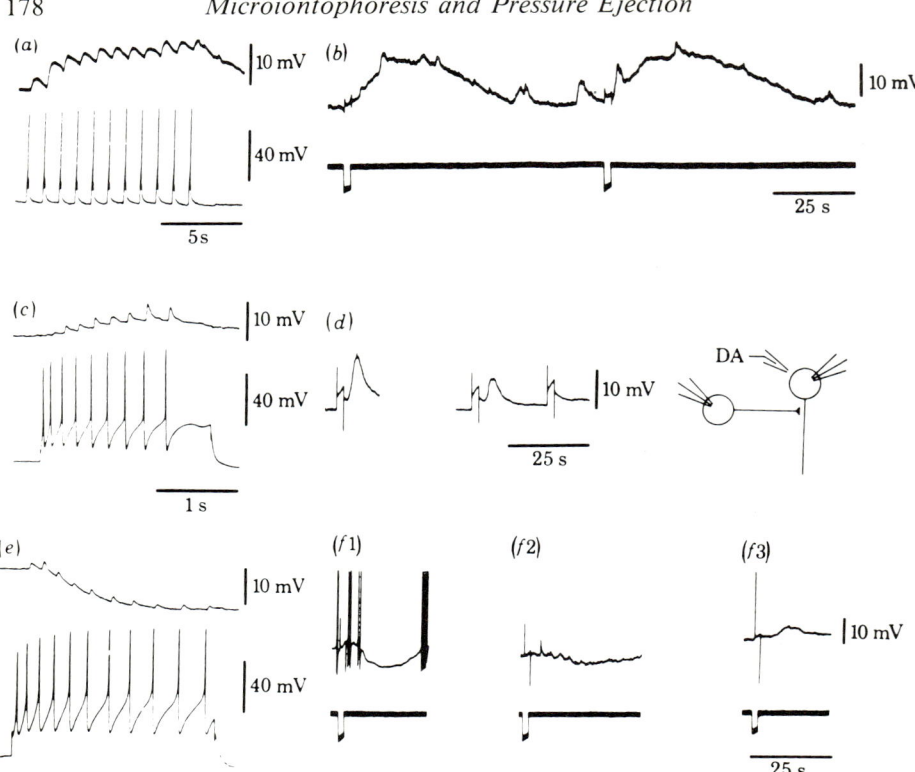

Figure 71 Excitatory responses (upper traces) to stimulation of the dopamine neurone (lower traces), and to iontophoresis of dopamine (DA). (a) Each presynaptic action potential produced an e.p.s.p. which reached its peak in about 300 ms and lasted about 1 s. (b) Iontophoretic application of dopamine on to a neurone, receiving the type of e.p.s.p. shown in (a) produced a long-lasting depolarization showing little desensitization. The iontophoretic current (400 nA) is monitored on the lower trace. (c) In some postsynaptic neurones the e.p.s.p.s produced by the dopamine neurone were much more rapid (150 ms) and peaked in about 20 ms. Note the difference in time-scale from (a). (d) Iontophoresis of dopamine on to a neurone receiving e.p.s.p.s of the type shown in (c) produced a short-lasting depolarization showing intense desensitization. The second application of dopamine (note artefacts) was made about 2 min after the first and produced a response which was greatly reduced. The third application produced a negligible response. Current intensity (not shown) was about 500 nA in each case. (e) Example of a biphasic input (depolarizing–hyperpolarizing) from the dopamine neurone. The depolarizing phase was rapid. (f1) Neurones receiving biphasic input from the dopamine neurone showed only a hyperpolarizing response to dopamine when recorded at the resting potential (iontophoretic current 400 nA). (f2) When hyperpolarized to −95 mV the response was occasionally biphasic but usually purely hyperpolarizing. (f3) Cooling abolished the hyperpolarization and revealed a rapid depolarization. The delay in response is presumably largely caused by the distance of the iontophoretic pipette from the receptors. (Reproduced from Berry and Cottrell, 1979, by permission of the Royal Society.)

between transmitters, such as the effect of 5-HT on acetylcholine sensitivity (Yurchenko and Rozsa 1984). Serotonin is of great interest in this species since at least one specific neurone appears to utilize the compound as its transmitter, although the mechanism of action of serotonin postjunctionally is unknown (Cottrell, 1981). The existence of several different types of responses to 5-HT involving different pharmacological receptors and conductance mechanisms has been reported in detail by Gerschenfeld and Paupardin-Tritsch (1974). It is interesting to note that compounds, such as glutamate, which seem to be universally excitant in higher animals, are not necessarily excitant in invertebrates (Cottrell et al., 1972; Sawada et al., 1984).

The large Retzius cells of the leech, *Hirudo*, have also received attention from microelectropharmacologists, both with respect to their responsiveness to exogenous agents (James and Walker, 1979) and with respect to the possible transmitter released by some Retzius cells themselves, possibly 5-HT (Henderson, 1983). Investigators have come closer to distinguishing between synaptic and extrasynaptic receptors on leech neurones than on neurones in almost any other CNS, since the cell bodies which are the areas most easily studied are generally devoid of synapses. Sargent *et al.* (1977) described the responses of cells to a variety of iontophoretically applied putative transmitters, and showed that cells with different functions (mechanoreceptive, nociceptive, motoneurones, etc.) had different complements of transmitter responses, defined either in terms of their qualitative characteristics or their pharmacology.

The greatest volume of invertebrate research though has undoubtedly been performed on *Aplysia* and related *Navanax* species. Ever since the first iontophoretic applications of acetylcholine to ganglion cells of *Aplysia* (Tauc and Gerschenfeld, 1962), *Aplysia* have provided some of the most fascinating answers to the question of whether multiple receptor types can exist on the same neurone. Levitan and Tauc (1972) thus reported on the separation of two distinct responses to acetylcholine showing different pharmacology and distributed differently over the axo-somatic region. Kehoe (1972a) investigated further the underlying ionic mechanisms of these responses as well as commenting on their possible physiological role (Kehoe, 1972b).

The effects of amines on *Aplysia* neurones have been examined (Woodruff and Walker, 1969; Ascher, 1972) and more recently the mechanisms of some of these responses such as to histamine have been studied in more detail (Gruol and Weinreich, 1979; McCaman and Weinreich, 1982). Ascher and Chesnoy-Marchais (1982) have begun to examine the interactions of different classes of agonist including cholinomimetics and amines at the level of desensitization processes and conductance mechanisms. The possibility that cyclic AMP might be involved in some transmitter responses has been strengthened by the demonstration that when pressure-injected into *Aplysia* neurones the nucleotide will cause a voltage-dependent inward current similar to that seen with 5-HT application extracellularly (Pellmar and Carpenter, 1981).

Most of the studies on transmitter sensitivity and pharmacology in invertebrates, however, have involved bath application, hence the fragmentary

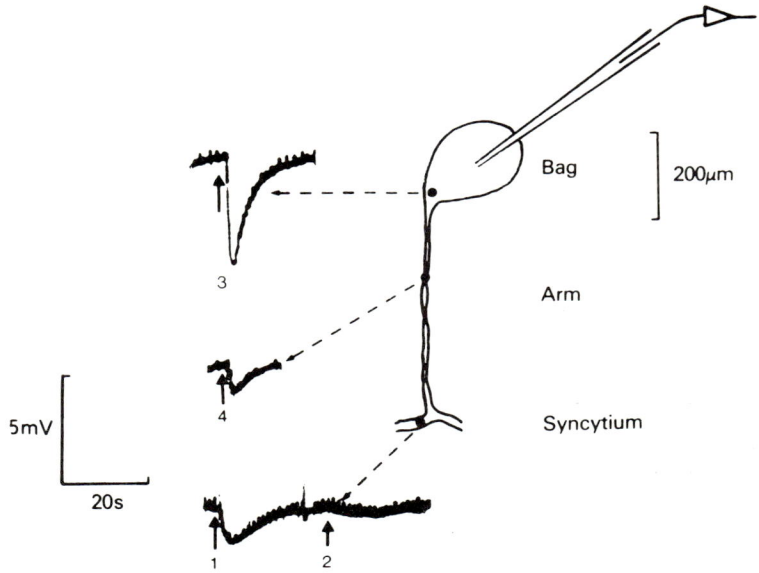

Figure 72 Effect of γ-aminobutyric acid (GABA) iontophoresis on the bag membrane potential when GABA is applied to different regions of the muscle cell. This preparation was made from a caudal section of *Ascaris*. A standard current pulse of 0.4 μC (at the vertical arrow) was used to deliver GABA to the different regions marked (●). Even though this preparation was at 22 °C, small depolarizing potentials were still observed. The effect of GABA release over the syncytium was tested first (1). The GABA pipette was raised 50 μm but then only caused a small response (2). Application of GABA to the bag produced the largest response (3). No response to GABA iontophoresis was observed when the GABA pipette was placed 100 μm from the edge of the bag, except for small responses observed over the arm (4). (Reproduced from Martin, 1980, by permission of the British Pharmacological Society.)

nature of the present discussion of the contribution made by microiontophoresis. The same often applies to sensory neurones such as the crayfish stretch receptor (Deisz and Lux, 1977) although Martin (1980) has successfully used microiontophoresis to resolve a long-standing debate concerning the localization of GABA sensitivity on *Ascaris* muscle. The restricted application of GABA clearly indicates that maximal sensitivity resides in the bag region (Figure 72).

CHAPTER 8

The Ejection of Dyes and other Markers

I	Which Marker to Use	181
II	Checking Ejection	183

PART I WHICH MARKER TO USE

Various marker substances have been ejected by microiontophoresis or pressure for the following purposes:

1. To mark the position of an iontophoretic barrel tip in a tissue so that the anatomical placement of the tip can be later verified histologically. Such direct confirmation of the location of cells studied is essential if differences of neuronal sensitivity or pharmacology are to be correlated with the position of cells in adjacent or nearly adjacent areas of brain, such as layers of the cerebral cortex or the pars compacta and reticulata of the substantia nigra. In most of these cases, however, the extracellular ejection of a dye from one barrel of a multibarrel assembly will be adequate.
2. If an intracellular study is conducted into the membrane properties of a neurone it would be preferable to mark that particular neurone, in order to identify it individually and in order to comment, perhaps, on the relationship between membrane properties or chemical sensitivity and neuronal geometry.
3. If the prime objective of a study is to examine the geometry and synaptic connections of a specific cell or type of cell, it will be necessary to eject into the cell a compound which will reach by diffusion or axonal transport as many branches of the cell as possible.

A number of factors may need to be considered in determining which marker to use. For extracellular use these include permanence of the spot, since some compounds such as Fast Green and Methyl Blue fade in colour or diffuse away readily from the site of deposition. The subsequent treatment of tissue may also be important; Prussian Blue for example is not visible after

Table 2
Dyes and markers

Compound	Solution used	Ejection parameters	Comment and use (Extracellular E; Intracellular I)	Reference
Potassium ferrocyanide	0.5 M	(−) 3–10 μA; 10–15 min	E/I; stain with 1.1 M $FeCl_3$ to produce Prussian Blue	Kerkut and Walker (1962) Talbot et al. (1967)
Methyl Blue	Saturated	(−) 1–3 μA; 1–3 min	E/I	Thomas and Wilson (1966) Holubar et al. (1967)
Fast Green	Saturated	(−) 10–12 μA; 5–10 min	E	Thomas and Wilson (1965)
Alcian Blue	3–8%	(+) 0.5–1 μA; 0.5–1 min	E; produces clear, permanent spot	Lee et al. (1969)
Neutral Red	Final conc. approx. 14 mg/l see ref.	(+) 100–150 nA	E	Maillis (1974)
Procion Yellow	5%	(−) 10 nA; about 5–10 min (−) 10–50 nA 0.5 s, 1 Hz, 30 min	E/I fluorescent	Zieglgansberger and Reiter (1974) Stretton and Kravitz (1968)
Procion Brilliant Red	4%	(−) 40 nA; 1 min	E/I fluorescent	Harris and Ribchester (1975)
Lucifer Yellow (Lithium)	5%	(−) 1–2 nA; 0.2 s pulses at 3 Hz; 5–10 min	E/I fluorescent	Gutnick et al. (1983)
Pontamine Sky Blue	2.5%	(−) 2–5 μA; 3–10 min	E very popular	Lodge et al. (1974) Boakes et al. (1974)
Horseradish peroxidase	Typically 2.5% in KCl/Tris pH 7	(−) 10 nA; 0.2 s pulses at 5 Hz; 10–20 s	I	Ono et al. (1982) Sakai et al. (1978)
Cobalt	1–50 mM	(+) 50 nA, 0.5 s, 1 Hz, 1 h	E/I allows excellent resolution of branches	Pitman et al. (1971)
Arsenazo III	80 mg/ml	200 nA; 0.8 s pulses at 1 Hz Pressure	I; monitoring calcium	Brown et al. (1977) Ahmed and Connor (1979) Gormon and Thomas (1980)

Golgi–Cox preparation. Generally speaking it is also preferable to use markers which can be ejected using relatively low iontophoretic currents since this probably reduces the likelihood of the electrode blocking, and precludes the tissue coagulation that can result from currents in the microampere range (see Ch. 6, Pt. VIII) (Holubar *et al.*, 1967). However, the substances ejected with the lowest currents tend to be fluorescent and access must, therefore, be available to suitable fluorescence microscopy facilities. If only one or a few spots are deposited in an experiment and the required tissue sections are thin it may additionally be important to use a dye which is clearly visible during the cutting process. Prussian Blue, for example, only becomes visible after treatment with ferric chloride.

Similarly cobalt chloride only becomes visible as cobalt sulphide is formed during treatment with ammonium sulphide. The pictures which can be obtained using cobalt, however, are excellent: even fine branches of axons and dendrites down to about $1 \mu m$ diameter are usually resolvable after intracellular iontophoresis and, since cobalt sulphide is electron opaque, the method can even be used to examine synaptic contacts using electron microscopy (Pitman *et al.*, 1971).

In Table 2 are listed a few examples of dyes and markers used in the past, with the parameters used for their deposition by microiontophoresis. The last compound listed in Table 2, however, is typical of substances used for highly specific purposes. Arsenazo III is iontophoresed intracellularly in order to study calcium movements; the calcium–dye complex exhibits a different absorbance spectrum from the parent dye and the change of absorbance at around 600 nm can be used to monitor free calcium levels (Brown *et al.*, 1977; Ahmed and Connor, 1979; Gorman and Thomas, 1980). The fluorescent compound aequorin has been used to similar purpose (Eckert *et al.*, 1977; Lux and Heyer, 1977).

In order to study the detailed projections of a neurone or pathway many groups have now tended to move away from the dyes indicated in Table 2 and to use instead radiolabelled neurotransmitters (Pentreath and Cottrell, 1974) or similar substances which can be iontophoresed intracellularly and distributed throughout the neurone by axoplasmic transport without having any toxic effects on that process or on the neurone: tritiated adenosine could be another example.

Finally Kettenmann *et al.* (1983) have devised a unique means of identifying cells of neuronal (as distinct from glial) origin in cultures by ejecting a neurone-specific antibody from micropipettes. The antibody binds to the neuronal surface, permitting subsequent identification by immunofluorescent methods, but does not affect the electrical properties of the cell.

PART II CHECKING EJECTION

Histological procedures can be tedious and, in the case of studies where axonal transport of materials is involved, can require waiting several hours or even days before the result of a dye injection is known. This problem is worst for autoradiographic studies where several weeks of anticipation may be involved.

It is clearly highly desirable to be reasonably certain that at the end of the waiting period a dye mark of some kind will be awaiting the enquiring eye of the experimenter. A 50% failure in such studies is an unacceptable waste of time and effort. It is always wise to check before and after an ejection of dye into a tissue that the electrode is indeed passing dye. The ability to pass current, it will be recalled, is not an adequate test.

A simple spectrophotometric method may well suffice for the coloured or fluorescent dyes, and ejection into a small volume of fluid followed by scintillation counting will confirm the ejection of radiolabelled materials. A method has also been described for rapidly detecting horseradish peroxidase ejected in pre-experimental checks of this kind (Alheid *et al.*, 1981).

References

Adams, P. R. (1976). 'A comparison of the time course of excitation and inhibition by iontophoretic decamethonium in frog endplate', *Br. J. Pharmacol.*, **57**, 59–66.

Aghajanian, G. K. (1978). 'Tolerance of locus coeruleus neurones to morphine and suppression of withdrawal response by clonidine', *Nature*, **276**, 186–188.

Aghajanian, G. K., and Bunney, B. S. (1977). 'Pharmacological characterisation of dopamine autoreceptors by microiontophoretic single cell studies', *Adv. Biochem. Psychopharm.*, **16**, 433–438.

Ahmed, Z., and Connor, J. A. (1979). 'Measurement of calcium influx under voltage clamp in molluscan neurones using the metallochromic dye Arsenazo III', *J. Physiol.*, **286**, 61–82.

Aleksanyan, Z. A., Skvaril, J. and Bures, J. (1972). 'Stability of firing patterns of hypothalamic neurones subjected to direct electrical or chemical stimulation affected by current', *Exp. Brain Res.*, **15**, 29–38.

Alger, B. E., and Nicoll, R. A. (1982). 'Pharmacological evidence for two kinds of GABA receptors on rat hippocampal pyramidal cells studied *in vitro*', *J. Physiol.*, **328**, 125–142.

Alheid, G. F., Edwards, S. B., Kitai, S. T., Park, M. R., and Switzer, R. C. (1981). 'Methods for delivering tracers'. In *Neuroanatomical Tract Tracing Methods*. Eds. L. Heimer and M. J. Roberts. Plenum, New York, pp. 91–116.

Andersen, P., Dingledine, R., Gjerstad, L., Langmoen, I. A., and Laursen, A. M. (1980). 'Two different responses of hippocampal pyramidal cells to application of GABA', *J. Physiol.*, **305**, 279–296.

Andersen, R. K., Lund, J. P., and Puil, E. (1978). 'Enkephalin and substance P effects related to trigeminal pain', *Can. J. Physiol. Pharmacol.*, **56**, 216–222.

Anis, N. A., Clark, R. B., Gration, K. A. F., and Usherwood, R. N. R. (1981). 'Influence of agonists on desensitisation of glutamate receptors on locust muscle', *J. Physiol.*, **312**, 345–364.

Anis, N. A., Berry, S. C., Burton, N. R., and Lodge, D. (1983). 'The dissociative anaesthetics, ketamine and phencyclidine, selectively reduce excitation of central mammalian neurones by N-methylaspartate', *Br. J. Pharmacol.*, **79**, 565–576.

Anwyl, R. (1977). 'Permeability of the postsynaptic membrane of an excitatory glutamate synapse to sodium and potassium', *J. Physiol.* **273**, 367–388.

Anwyl, R., and Narahashi, T. (1980a). 'Desensitisation of the acetylcholine receptor of denervated rat soleus muscle and the effect of calcium', *Br. J. Pharmacol.*, **69**, 91–98.

Anwyl, R., and Narahashi, T. (1980b). 'Comparison of desensitisation and time dependent block of the acetylcholine receptor responses by chlorpromazine, cytochalasin B, triton X-100 and other agents', *Br. J. Pharmacol.*, **69**, 99–106.

Armstrong-James, M., and Fox, K. (1983). 'Effects of iontophoresed noradrenaline on the spontaneous activity of neurones in rat primary cortex', *J. Physiol.*, **335**, 427–448.

Armstrong-James, M., Fox, K., Kruk, Z. L., and Millar, J. (1981). 'Quantitative iontophoresis of catecholamines using multibarrel carbon fibre microelectrodes', *J. Neurosci. Meth.* **4**, 385–406.

Ascher, P. (1972). 'Inhibitory and excitatory effects of dopamine on *Aplysia* neurones', *J. Physiol.*, **225**, 173–209.

Ascher, P., and Chesnoy-Marchais, D. (1982). 'Interactions between three slow potassium responses controlled by three distinct receptors in *Aplysia* neurones', *J. Physiol.*, **324**, 67–92.

Assumpcao, J. A., Bernardi, N., Brown, J., and Stone, T. W. (1979). 'Selective antagonism by benzodiazepines of neuronal responses to excitatory aminoacids in the cerebral cortex', *Br. J. Pharmacol.*, **67**, 563–568.

Bagust, J., and Kerkut, G. A. (1981). 'Observations on the use of anaesthetics in the preparation of *in vitro* CNS material', *Neuropharm.*, **20**, 73–78.

Baldwin, D. J. (1980). 'Dry bevelling of micropipette electrodes', *J. Neurosci. Meth.*, **2**, 153–161.

Barasi, S., and Roberts, M. H. T. (1974). 'The modification of lumbar motoneurone excitability by stimulation of a putative 5-hydroxytryptamine pathway', *Br. J. Pharmacol.*, **52**, 339–348.

Barasi, S., and Roberts, M. H. T. (1977). 'Responses of motoneurones to electrophoretically applied dopamine', *Br. J. Pharmacol.*, **60**, 29–35.

Barcroft, H., Bonnar, W. McK., Edholm, O. G., and Effray, A. S. (1943). 'On sympathetic vasoconstrictor tone in human skeletal muscle', *J. Physiol.*, **102**, 21–31.

Barker, J.L., and Ransom, B. R. (1978a). 'Amino acid pharmacology of mammalian central neurones grown in tissue culture', *J. Physiol.*, **280**, 331–354.

Barker, J. L., and Ransom, B. R. (1978b). 'Pentobarbitone pharmacology of mammalian central neurones grown in tissue culture', *J. Physiol.*, **280**, 355–372.

Barker, J. L., Crayton, J. W., and Nicoll, R. A. (1971). 'Supraoptic neurosecretory cells: adrenergic and cholinergic sensitivity', *Science*, **171**, 208–210.

Beckman, A. L., and Eisenman, J. S. (1970). 'Microelectrophoresis of biogenic amines on hypothalamic thermosensitive cells', *Science*, **170**, 334–336.

Begent, N., and Born, G. V. R. (1970). 'Determination of the iontophoretic release of adenosine diphosphate from micropipettes', *Br. J. Pharmacol.*, **40**, 592–593.

Belcher, G., and Ryall, R. W. (1977). 'Substance P and Renshaw cells: a new concept of inhibitory synaptic interactions', *J. Physiol.*, **272**, 105–119.

Ben-Ari, Y., and Kelly, J. S. (1976). 'Dopamine evoked inhibition of single cells in the feline putamen and basolateral amygdala', *J. Physiol.*, **256**, 1–21.

Benitez, H. H., Murray, M. R., and Woolley, D. W. (1955). 'Effects of serotonin and its antagonists upon oligodendroglia *in vitro*,' *Anat. Rec.*, **121**, 466.

Beranek, R., Martin, A. R., and Wickelgren, W. O. (1970). 'Effects of iontophoretically applied drugs on spinal interneurones of the lamprey', *J. Physiol.*, **207**, 653–665.

Berry, M. S., and Cottrell, G. A. (1979). 'Ionic basis of different synaptic potentials mediated by an identified dopamine containing neurone in *Planorbis*', *Proc. Roy. Soc.*, **B203**, 427–444.

Bevan, P., Bradshaw, C. M., Roberts, M. H. T., and Szabadi, E. (1973a). 'Effect of pH on the release of noradrenaline from micropipettes', *J. Pharm. Pharmacol.*, **25**, 1007–1008.

Bevan, P., Bradshaw, C. M., Roberts, M. H. T., and Szabadi, E. (1973b). 'The excitation of neurones by noradrenaline', *J. Pharm. Pharmacol.*, **25**, 309–314.

Bevan, P., Bradshaw, C. M., and Szabadi, E. (1975). 'Effects of iprindole on responses of single cortical and caudate neurones to monoamines and acetylcholine', *Br. J. Pharmacol.*, **55**, 17–26.

Bevan, P., Bradshaw, C. M., and Szabadi, E. (1977). 'The pharmacology of adrenergic neuronal responses in the cerebral cortex: evidence for excitatory α and inhibitory β receptors', *Br. J. Pharmacol.*, **59**, 635–642.

Bevan, P., Bradshaw, C. M., Pun, R. Y. K., Slater, N. T., and Szabadi, E. (1978). 'Responses of single cortical neurones to noradrenaline and dopamine', *Neuropharmacol.*, **17**, 611-617.

Bevan, P., Bradshaw, C. M., Pun, R. Y. K., Slater, N. T., and Szabadi, E. (1979). 'The relative contribution of iontophoresis and electro-osmosis to the electrophoretic release of noradrenaline from multibarrelled micropipettes', *Br. J. Pharmacol.*, **67**, 478-479.

Bevan, S. J. Katz, B., and Miledi, R. (1975). 'Membrane potential fluctuations produced by glutamate in nerve cells of the squid', *Proc. Roy. Soc.*, **191**, 561-565.

Bioulac, B., Gaffori, O., Harris, M., and Vincent, J. D. (1978). 'Effects of acetylcholine, sodium glutamate and GABA on the discharge of supraoptic neurones in the rat', *Brain Res.*, **154**, 159-162.

Biscoe, T. J., Evans, R. H., Headley, P. M., Martin, M., and Watkins, J. C. (1975). 'Domoic and quisqualic acids as potent aminoacid excitants of frog and rat spinal neurones', *Nature*, **255**, 166-167.

Biscoe, T. J., Headley, P. M., Lodge, D., Martin, M. R., and Watkins, J. C. (1976). 'The sensitivity of rat spinal interneurones and Renshaw cells to L-glutamate and L-aspartate', *Exp. Brain Res.*, **26**, 547-551.

Biscoe, T. J., Martin, M. R., and Rickets, C. (1978). 'A concentric multibarrelled microelectrode for use in microiontophoresis', *J. Physiol.*, **277**, 25-26.

Blatt, M. R., and Slayman, C. L. (1983). 'Potassium chloride leakage from microelectrodes and its impact on the membrane parameters of a nonexcitable cell', *J. Memb. Biol.*, **772**, 223-234.

Bloom, F. E. (1974). 'To spritz or not to spritz: the doubtful value of aimless iontophoresis', *Life Sci.*, **14**, 1819-1834.

Bloom, F. E. (1975). 'The role of cyclic nucleotides in central synaptic function', *Revs. Physiol. Biochem. Pharmacol.*, **74**, 1-104.

Bloom, F. E., Siggins, G. R., and Hoffer, B. J. (1974). 'Interpreting the failures to confirm the depression of cerebellar Purkinje cells by cyclic AMP', *Science*, **185**, 627.

Bloom, F. E., Siggins, G. R., and Henriksen, S. J. (1981). 'Electrophysiologic assessment of receptor changes following chronic drug treatment', *Fed. Proc.*, **40**, 166-172.

Boakes, R. J., Bradley, P. B., Briggs, I., and Dray, A. (1970). 'Antagonism of 5HT by LSD-25 in the CNS: a possible neuronal basis for the actions of LSD-25', *Br. J. Pharmacol.*, **40**, 202-218.

Boakes, R. J., Bradley, P. B., Candy, J. M., and Wolstencroft, J. H. (1971). 'Actions of noradrenaline, other sympathomimetic amines and antagonists on neurones in the brain stem of the cat', *Br. J. Pharmacol.*, **41**, 462-479.

Boakes, R. J., Bradley, P. B., Candy, J. M., and Dray, A. (1972). 'Noradrenaline artefacts', *Nature New Biol.*, **239**, 151-152.

Boakes, R. J., Bramwell, G. J., Briggs, I., Candy, J. M., and Tempesta, E. (1974). 'Localisation with Pontamine sky blue of neurones in the brainstem responding to microiontophoretically applied compounds', *Neuropharmacol.*, **13**, 475-479.

Bolton, T. B. (1976). 'On the latency and form of the membrane responses of smooth muscle to the iontophoretic application of acetylcholine or carbachol, *Proc. Roy. Soc.*, **B194**, 99-119.

Bradley, P.B., and Briggs, I. (1974). 'Further studies on the mode of action of psychotomimetic drugs: antagonism of the excitatory action of 5HT by methylated derivatives of tryptamine', *Br. J. Pharmacol.*, **50**, 345-354.

Bradley, P.B., and Candy, J. M. (1970). 'Iontophoretic release of acetylcholine, noradrenaline, 5HT and D-LSD from micropipettes', *Br. J. Pharmacol.*, **40**, 194-201.

Bradley, P. B., and Dray, A. (1973). 'Modification of the responses of brain stem neurones to transmitter substances by anaesthetic agents', *Br. J. Pharmacol.*, **48**, 212-224.

Bradley, P. B., and Dray, A. (1974). 'Morphine and neurotransmitter substances: microionophoretic study in the rat brain stem', *Br. J. Pharmacol.*, **50**, 47-56.

Bradley, P. B., Briggs, I., Gayton, R. J., and Lambert, L.A. (1976). 'Effects of iontophoretically applied methionine enkephalin on single neurones in rat brainstem', *Nature*, **261**, 425–426.

Bradshaw, C. M., and Szabadi, E. (1974). 'The measurement of dose in microelectrophoretic experiments', *Neuropharmacol.*, **13**, 407–416.

Bradshaw, C. M. Roberts, M. H. T., and Szabadi, E. (1973). 'Kinetics of the release of noradrenaline from micropipettes: interaction between ejecting and retaining currents', *Br. J. Pharmacol.*, **49**, 667–677.

Bradshaw, C. M., Pun, R. Y. K., Slater, N. T., and Szabadi, E. (1981). 'A procedure for comparing the mobilities of unlabelled drugs used in microelectrophoresis experiments', *J. Pharmacol. Meth.*, **5**, 67–74.

Braitman, D. J., Auker, C. R., and Carpenter, D. O. (1980). 'TRH has multiple actions in cortex', *Brain Res.*, **194**, 244–248.

Briano, R. A. (1983). 'A reproducible technique for breaking glass micropipettes over a wide range of tip diameters', *J. Neurosci. Meth.*, **9**, 31–34.

Briggs, I. (1977). 'Excitatory responses of neurones in rat bulbar reticular formation to bulbar raphe stimulation and to iontophoretically applied 5HT, and their blockade by LSD-25', *J. Physiol.*, **265**, 327–340.

Briggs, I. (1979). 'Excitatory effects of TRH on medullary reticular neurones', *Neurosci, Lett.*, **15**, 33–36.

Brown, J. E., Brown, P. K., and Pinto, L. H. (1977). 'Detection of light induced changes of intracellular calcium concentrations in *Limulus* ventral photoreceptors using arsenazo III', *J. Physiol.*, **267**, 299–320.

Brown, J. R., and Arbuthnott, G. W. (1983). 'The electrophysiology of dopamine D2 receptors: a study of the actions of dopamine on corticostriatal transmission', *Neuroscience*, **10**, 349–355.

Brown, K. T., and Flaming, D. G. (1975). 'Instrumentation and technique for beveling fine micropipette electrodes', *Brain Res.*, **86**, 172–180.

Brown, K. T., and Flaming, D. G. (1979). 'Technique for precision beveling of relatively large micropipettes', *J. Neurosci. Meth.*, **1**, 25–35.

Bunney, B. S., and Aghajanian, G. K. (1976). 'Dopamine and norepinephrine innervated cells in rat prefrontal cortex: pharmacological differentiation using microiontophoretic techniques', *Life Sci.*, **19**, 1783–1792.

Bureš, J., Petrán, M., and Zachar, J. (1967). *Electrophysiological Methods in Biological Research*. Academic Press, London.

Cahusac, P. M. B., and Hill, R. G. (1983). 'α_2 Adrenergic receptors on neurones in the region of the lateral reticular nucleus of the rat', *Neurosci. Lett.*, **42**, 279–284.

Calvillo, O., Henry, J. L., and Neuman, R. S. (1974). 'Effects of morphine and naloxone on dorsal horn neurones in the cat', *Can. J. Physiol. Pharmacol.*, **52**, 1207–1211.

Candy, J. M., Boakes, R. J., Key, B. J., and Worton, E. (1974). 'Correlation of the release of amines and antagonists with their effects', *Neuropharmacol.*, **13**, 423–430.

Carette, B. I. (1978). 'A new method of manufacturing multibarrelled micropipettes with projecting recording barrel', *Electroenceph. Clin. Neurophysiol.*, **44**, 248–250.

Carslaw, H. S., and Jaeger, J. C. (1959). *Conduction of Heat in Solids*. Oxford University Press, London.

Caspary, D. M., Harvey, D. C., and Faingold, C. L. (1983). 'Effects of acetylcholine on cochlear nucleus neurones', *Exp. Neurol.*, **82**, 491–498.

Catchlove, R. F. H., Krnjević, K., and Maretic, H. (1972). 'Similarity between effects of general anaesthetics and dinitrophenol on cortical neurones', *Can. J. Physiol. Pharmacol.*, **50**, 1111–1114.

Cherubini, E., Rovira, C., Ben-Ari, Y., and Padjen, A. (1982). 'Simultaneous recording of somatic and dendritic field potentials and combined microiontophoresis in the rat Ammon's horn *in situ*: effects of GABA and acetylcholine', *Neurosci. Lett.*, **31**, 19–24.

References

Chesnut, T. J. (1983). 'Two component desensitisation at the neuromuscular junction of the frog', *J. Physiol.*, **336**, 229–241.

Chujo, T., Yamada, Y., and Yamamoto, C. (1975). 'Sensitivity of Purkinje cell dendrites to glutamic acid', *Exp. Brain Res.*, **23**, 293–300.

Clark, R. B., Gration, K. A. F., and Usherwood, P. N. R. (1982). 'Influence of sodium and calcium ions and membrane potential on receptor desensitisation', *Comp. Biochem. Physiol.*, **72**, 1–8.

Clarke, G., Forrester, P. A., and Straughan, D. W. (1974). 'A quantitative analysis of the excitation of single cortical neurones by acetylcholine and L-glutamic acid applied microiontophoretically', *Neuropharmacol.*, **13**, 1047–1056.

Clarke, G., Hill, R. G., and Simmonds, M. A. (1973). 'Microintophoretic release of drugs from micropipettes: use of ^{24}Na as a model', *Br. J. Pharmacol.*, **48**, 156–161.

Cleugh, J., and Gaddum, J. H. (1963). 'The stability of purified preparations of substance P', *Experientia*, **19**, 72–73.

Coceani, F., and Viti, A. (1972). 'The release of prostaglandin E_1 from micropipettes *in vitro*', *Brain Res.*, **45**, 469–477.

Cohen, S. A., and Fishbach, G. D. (1977). 'Clusters of acetylcholine receptors located at identified nerve muscle synapses *in vitro*', *Dev. Biol.*, **59**, 24–38.

Collingridge, G. L., Kehl, S. J., and McLennan, H. (1983). 'Excitatory aminoacids in synaptic transmission in the Schaffer collateral-commissural pathway of the rat hippocampus', *J. Physiol.*, **334**, 33–46.

Comis, S. D., Hayward, T. L., Hodges, D. C., and Hollins G. (1972). 'An improved electrically operated microtap', *Br. J. Pharmacol.*, **45**, 190–191.

Connor, J. D. (1970). 'Caudate nucleus neurones: correlation of the effects of substantia nigra stimulation with iontophoretic dopamine', *J. Physiol.*, **208**, 691–703.

Constanti, A., Krnjević, K., and Nistri, A. (1980). 'Intraneuronal effects of inhibitory aminoacids', *Can. J. Physiol. Pharmacol.*, **58**, 193–204.

Cottrell, G. A. (1981). 'An unusual synaptic response mediated by a serotonin neurone', *Quart. J. Exp. Physiol.*, **66**, 475–485.

Cottrell, G. A., and Green, K. A. (1982). 'Responses of mouse spinal neurones in culture to locally applied serotonin', *J. Physiol.*, **325**, 25–26.

Cottrell, G. A., Macon, J., and Szczepaniak, A. C. (1972). 'Glutamic acid mimicking of synaptic inhibition on the giant serotonin neurone of the snail', *Br. J. Pharmacol.*, **45**, 684–688.

Courtice, C. J. (1976). 'A current pump monitor for microiontophoresis circuits', *J. Physiol.*, **258**, 42–43.

Crawford, J. M. (1970). 'Anaesthetic agents and the chemical sensitivity of cortical neurones', *Neuropharmacol.*, **9**, 31–46.

Crepel, F., and Dhanjal, S. S. (1982). 'Cholinergic mechanisms and neurotransmission in the cerebellum of the rat: an *in vitro* study', *Brain Res.*, **244**, 59–68.

Crepel, F., Dhanjal, S. S., and Sears, T. A. (1982). 'Effects of glutamate, aspartate and related derivatives on cerebellar Purkinje cell dendrites in the rat: an *in vitro* study', *J. Physiol.*, **329**, 297–318.

Cross, B. A., and Dyer, R. G. (1971). 'Unit activity in rat diencephalic islands—the effects of anaesthetics', *J. Physiol.*, **212**, 467–482.

Crossman, A. R., Walker, R. J., and Woodruff, G. N. (1974). 'Problems associated with iontophoretic studies in the caudate nucleus and substantia nigra', *Neuropharmacol.*, **13**, 547–552.

Crunelli, V., Forda, S., and Kelly, J. S. (1983). 'Blockade of aminoacid induced depolarisations and inhibition of epsps in rat dentate gyrus', *J. Physiol.*, **341**, 627–640.

Cull-Candy, S. G. (1978). 'Glutamate sensitivity and distribution of receptors along normal and denervated locust muscle fibres', *J. Physiol.*, **276**, 165–181.

Cull-Candy, S. G., Miledi, R., and Uchitel, D. D. (1982). 'Properties of junctional and extrajunctional acetylcholine receptor channels in organ cultured human muscle fibres', *J. Physiol.*, **333**, 251–267.
Curtis, D. R. (1964). 'Microelectrophoresis', In *Physical Techniques in Biological Research*, vol. 5A. Ed. W. L. Nastuk. Academic Press, New York, pp. 144–190.
Curtis, D. R. (1968). 'A method for assembly of "parallel" micropipettes', *Electroenceph. Clin. Neurophysiol.*, **24**, 587–589.
Curtis, D. R. (1976). 'The use of transmitter antagonists in microelectrophoretic investigations of central synaptic transmission.' In *Drugs and Central Synaptic Transmission*. Eds. P. B. Bradley and B. N. Dhawan. Macmillan, London. pp. 7–36.
Curtis, D. R., and Eccles, R. M. (1958a). 'The excitation of Renshaw cells by pharmacological agents applied electrophoretically', *J. Physiol.*, **141**, 435–445.
Curtis, D. R., and Eccles, R. M. (1958b). 'The effect of diffusional barriers upon the pharmacology of cells within the CNS', *J. Physiol.*, **141**, 446–463.
Curtis, D. R., and Felix, D. (1971). 'Muscarinic action of acetylcholine', *Nature*, **234**, 355.
Curtis, D. R., and Phillis, J. W. (1960). 'The action of procaine and atropine on spinal neurones', *J. Physiol.*, **153**, 17–34.
Curtis, D. R., and Watkins, J. C. (1960). 'The excitation and depression of spinal neurones by structurally related amino acids', *J. Neurochem.*, **6**, 117–141.
Curtis, D. R., Phillis, J. W., and Watkins, J. C. (1959). 'The depression of spinal neurones by GABA and beta-alanine', *J. Physiol.*, **146**, 185–203.
Curtis, D. R., Perrin, D., and Watkins, J. C. (1960). 'The excitation of spinal neurones by the iontophoretic application of agents which chelate calcium', *J. Neurochem.*, **6**, 1–20.
Curtis, D. R., Duggan, A. W., and Johnston, G. A. R. (1971a). 'The specificity of strychnine as a glycine antagonist', *Exp. Brain Res.*, **12**, 547–565.
Curtis, D. R., Duggan, A. W., Felix, D., and Johnston, G. A. R. (1971b). 'Bicuculline, an antagonist of GABA and synaptic inhibition in the spinal cord of the cat', *Brain Res.*, **32**, 69–96.
Curtis, D. R., Game, J. A., and McCulloch, R. M. (1974). 'Antagonism of inhibitory aminoacid action by tubocurarine', *Br. J. Pharmacol.*, **52**, 101–103.
Davies, J., and Dray, A. (1977). 'Substance P and opiate receptors', *Nature*, **268**, 351–352.
Davies, J., and Dray, A. (1978). 'Pharmacological and electrophysiological studies of morphine and enkephalins on rat supraspinal neurones', *Br. J. Pharmacol.*, **63**, 87–96.
Davies, J., Francis, A. A., Jones, A. W., and Watkins, J. C. (1981). '2-Amino-5-phosphono-valerate (2APV), a potent and selective antagonist of aminoacid induced and synaptic excitation', *Neurosci. Lett.*, **21**, 77–82.
Davies, J., and Polc, P. (1978). 'Effect of a water-soluble benzodiazepine on the responses of spinal neurones to acetylcholine and excitatory aminoacid analogues', *Neuropharmacol.*, **17**, 217–220.
Davies, J., and Watkins, J. C. (1983). 'Role of excitatory aminoacid receptors in mono and polysynaptic excitation in the cat spinal cord', *Exp. Brain Res.*, **49**, 280–290.
De Groat, W. C., and Ryall, R. W. (1967). 'An excitatory action of 5HT on sympathetic preganglionic neurones', *Exp. Brain Res.*, **3**, 299–305.
Deisz, R. A., and Lux, H. D. (1977). 'Diphenylhydantoin prolongs postsynaptic inhibition and iontophoretic GABA action on the crayfish stretch receptor', *Neurosci. Lett.*, **5**, 199–204.
del Castillo, J., and Katz, B. (1955). 'On the localisation of acetylcholine receptors', *J. Physiol.*, **128**, 157–181.
del Castillo, J., and Katz, B. (1957). 'A study of curare action with an electrical micromethod', *Proc. Roy. Soc.*, **B146**, 339–356.

de Montigny, C., and Lund, J. P. (1980). 'A microiontophoretic study of the action of kainic acid and putative neurotransmitters in the rat mesencephalic trigeminal nucleus', *Neuroscience*, **5**, 1621–1628.
de Montigny, C., Wang, R. Y., Reader, T. A., and Aghajanian, G. K. (1980). 'Monoaminergic denervation of the rat hippocampus: microiontophoretic studies on pre- and postsynaptic supersensitivity to norepinephrine and serotonin', *Brain Res.*, **200**, 363–376.
Diamond, J. (1968). 'The activation and distribution of GABA and L-glutamate receptors on goldfish Mauthner neurones: an analysis of dendritic remote inhibition', *J. Physiol.*, **194**, 669–723.
Diamond, J., and Roper, S. (1973). 'Analysis of Mauthner cell responses to iontophoretically delivered pulses of GABA, glycine and L-glutamate', *J. Physiol.*, **232**, 113–128.
Diamond, J., Roper, S., and Yasargil, G. M. (1973). 'The membrane effects and sensitivity to strychnine of neural inhibition of the Mauthner cell, and its inhibition by glycine and GABA', *J. Physiol.*, **232**, 87–112.
Dingledine, R. (1983). 'N-methylaspartate activates a voltage dependent calcium conductance in rat hippocampal pyramidal cells', *J. Physiol.*, **343**, 385–405.
Dingledine, R., Iversen, L. L., and Breuker, E. (1978). 'Naloxone as a GABA antagonist: evidence from iontophoretic, receptor binding and convulsant studies' *Eur. J. Pharmacol.*, **47**, 19–27.
Dionne, V. E. (1976). 'Characterisation of drug iontophoresis with a fast microassay technique', *Biophys. J.*, **16**, 705–717.
Djorup, A., Jahnsen, H., and Laursen, A. M. (1981). 'The dendritic response to GABA in CA1 of the hippocampal slice', *Brain Res.*, **219**, 196–201.
Dodd, J., and Kelly, J. S. (1978). 'Is somatostatin an excitatory transmitter in the hippocampus? *Nature*, **273**, 674–675.
Dodd, J., and Kelly, J. S. (1981). 'The actions of cholecystokinin and related peptides on pyramidal neurones of the mammalian hippocampus', *Brain Res.*, **205**, 337–350.
Dodd, J., Dingledine, R., and Kelly, J. S. (1981). 'The excitatory action of acetylcholine on hippocampal neurones of the guinea-pig and rat maintained *in vitro*', *Brain Res.*, **207**, 109–128.
Dray, A. (1975). 'Comparison of bicuculline methochloride with bicuculline and picrotoxin as antagonists of aminoacid and monoamine depression of neurones in the rat brainstem', *Neuropharmacol.*, **14**, 887–891.
Dray, A., Hanley, M. R., Pinnock, R. D., and Sandberg, B. E. B. (1983). 'A comparison of the release of substance P and some synthetic analogues from micropipettes by microiontophoresis or pressure', *Neuropharmacol.*, **22**, 859–864.
Dreifuss, J. J., and Kelly, J. S. (1972). 'The activity of identified supraoptic neurones and their responses to acetylcholine applied by microiontophoresis', *J. Physiol.*, **220**, 105–118.
Dreyer, F., and Peper, K. (1974). 'Iontophoretic application of acetylcholine: advantages of high resistance micropipettes in connection with an electric current pump', *Pflug. Arch. Ges. Physiol.*, **348**, 263–272.
Dudar, J. D. (1974). '*In vitro* excitation of hippocampal pyramidal cell dendrites by glutamic acid', *Neuropharmacol.*, **13**, 1083–1089.
Dudel, J. (1975). 'Kinetics of postsynaptic action of glutamate pulses applied iontophoretically through high resistance micropipettes', *Pflug. Arch. Ges. Physiol.*, **356**, 329–346.
Duggan, A. (1974). 'The differential sensitivity to L-glutamate and L-aspartate of spinal interneurones and Renshaw cells', *Exp. Brain Res.*, **19**, 522–528.
Duggan, A., Hall, J. G., and Lee, C. Y. (1976). 'Alpha-bungarotoxin, cobra neurotoxin and excitation of Renshaw cells by acetylcholine', *Brain Res.*, **107**, 166–170.

Duggan, A., Griersmith, B. T., Headley, P. M., and Hall, J. G. (1979). 'Lack of effect by substance P at sites in the substantia gelatinosa where metenkephalin reduces the transmission of nociceptive imnpulses', *Neurosci. Lett.*, **12**, 313–318.

Duggan, A., Griersmith, B. T., and Johnson, S. M. (1981). 'Supraspinal inhibition of the excitation of dorsal horn neurones by impulses in unmyelinated primary afferents: lack of effect by strychnine and bicuculline', *Brain Res.*, **210**, 231–242.

Dunlap, K, and Fishbach, G. D. (1981). 'Neurotransmitters decrease the calcium conductance activated by depolarisation of embryonic chick sensory neurones', *J. Physiol.*, **317**, 519–535.

Dyball, R. E. J., and McPhail, C. I. (1974). 'Unit activity in the supraoptic and paraventricular nuclei—the effects of anaesthetics', *Brain Res.*, **67**, 43–50.

Eckert, R., Tillotson, D., and Ridgway, E. B. (1977). 'Voltage-dependent facilitation of calcium entry in voltage clamped aequorin injected molluscan neurones', *Proc. Nat. Acad. Sci. USA*, **74**, 1748–1752.

Edwall, L., and Scott, D. (1971). 'Influence of changes in microcirculation on the excitability of the sensory unit in the tooth of the cat', *Acta Physiol. Scand.*, **82**, 555–566.

Egan, T. M., Henderson, G., North, R. A., and Williams, J. T. (1983). 'Noradrenaline mediated synaptic inhibition in rat locus coeruleus neurones', *J. Physiol.*, **345**, 477–488.

Engberg, G., Svensson, T. H., Rosell, S., and Folkers, K. (1981). 'A synthetic peptide as an antagonist of substance P', *Nature*, **293**, 222–223.

Engberg, I., Kallstrom, Y., and Marshall, K. C. (1972). 'Double micromanipulator for independent impalements of one neurone with two electrodes', *Acta Physiol. Scand.*, **84**, 4A–5A.

Engberg, I., Flatman, J. A., and Lambert, J. D. C. (1975). 'A simple and cheap method of screening glass microelectrodes', *Br. J. Pharmacol.*, **55**, 312–313.

Engberg, I., Flatman, J. A., and Lambert, J. D. C. (1979a). 'A comparison of extracellular and intracellular recording during extracellular microiontophoresis', *J. Neurosci. Meth.*, **1**, 219–233.

Engberg, I., Flatman, J. A., and Lambert, J. D. C. (1979b). 'The actions of excitatory aminoacids on motoneurones in the feline spinal cord', *J. Physiol.*, **288**, 227–260.

Erhardt, M., and Junier, N. (1982). 'A method for manufacturing long-shanked glass microelectrodes', *J. Neurosci. Meth.*, **6**, 85–90.

Ewart, W. R., and Logan, J. G. (1978). 'The effects of desipramine on the noradrenaline mediated responses in rat cortical cell firing rate', *J. Physiol.*, **276**, 77–78.

Felix, D., and Akert, K. (1974). 'The effects of angiotensin II on neurones of the cat subfornical organ', *Brain Res.*, **76**, 350–353.

Felix, D., and Phillips, M. I. (1978). 'Effects of angiotensin II on central neurones', pp. 104–106 in Ryall and Kelly (1978).

Felix, D., and Steiner, F. A. (1976). 'Antagonistic effects of GABA and benzodiazepines on vestibular and cerebellar neurones', *Nature*, **260**, 346–347.

Feltz, P., and de Champlain, J. (1972). 'Enhanced sensitivity of caudate neurones to microiontophoretic injections of dopamine in 6-hydroxydopamine treated cats', *Brain Res.*, **43**, 601–605.

Feltz, A., and Trautmann, A. (1982). 'Desensitization at the frog neuromuscular junction: a biphasic process', *J. Physiol.*, **322**, 257–272.

Feltz, A., Large, W. A., and Trautmann, A. (1977). 'Analysis of atropine action at the frog neuromuscular junction', *J. Physiol.*, **269**, 109–130.

Fischbach, G. D., and Lass, Y. (1978). 'Acetylcholine noise in cultured chick myoballs: a voltage clamp analysis', *J. Physiol.*, **280**, 515–526.

Flaming, D. G., and Brown, K. T. (1982). 'Micropipette puller design. Form of the heating filament and effects of filament width on tip length and diameter', *J. Neurosci. Meth.*, **6**, 91–102.

Flatman, J. A., Schwindt, P. C., Crill, W. E., and Stafstrom, C. E. (1983). 'Multiple actions of NMDA on cat neocortical neurones *in vitro*', *Brain Res.*, **266**, 169–173.
Frank, E., and Fischbach, G. D. (1979). 'Early events in neuromuscular junction formation *in vitro*: induction of acetylcholine receptor clusters in the postsynaptic membrane of newly formed synapses', *J. Cell. Biol.*, **83**, 143–158.
Frederickson, R. C. A., Jordan, L. M., and Phillis, J. W. (1971). 'The action of noradrenaline on cortical neurones: effects of pH', *Brain Res.*, **35**, 556–560.
Frederickson, R. C. A., Jordan, L. M., and Phillis, J. W. (1973). 'A technique for microelectrophoretic study of single neurones in the awake non-paralysed cat', *Neuropharmacol.*, **12**, 77–82.
Freedman, R., Hoffer, B. J., and Woodward, D. J. (1975). 'A quantitative microiontophoretic analysis of the response of central neurones to noradrenaline: interactions with cobalt, manganese, verapamil and dichloroisoprenaline', *Br. J. Pharmacol.*, **54**, 529–540.
Freedman, R., Hoffer, B. J., Woodward, D. J., and Puro, D. (1977). 'Interaction of norepinephrine with cerebellar activity evoked by mossy and climbing fibres', *Exp. Neurol.*, **55**, 269–288.
Freeman, J. A. (1971). 'A simple multichannel spike height discriminator', *J. Appl. Physiol.*, **31**, 939–941.
Fries, W., and Zieglgänsberger, W. (1974). 'A method to discriminate axonal from cell body activity and to analyse "silent" cells', *Exp. Brain Res.*, **21**, 567–574.
Fry, J. P., Herz, A., and Zieglgänsberger, W. (1980). 'A demonstration of naloxone precipitated opiate withdrawal on single neurones in the morphine tolerant dependent rat brain', *Br. J. Pharmacol.*, **68**, 585–592.
Fry, J. P., Zieglgänsberger, W., and Herz, A. (1979). 'Specific versus nonspecific actions of opioids on hippocampal neurones in the rat brain', *Brain Res.*, **163**, 295–306.
Gage, P. W., and Hamill, O. P. (1980). 'Lifetime and conductance of acetylcholine activated channels in normal and denervated toad sartorius muscle', *J. Physiol.*, **298**, 525–538.
Gähwiler, B. H., and Dreifuss, J. J. (1982). 'Multiple actions of acetylcholine on hippocampal pyramidal cells in organotypic explant cultures', *Neuroscience*, **7**, 1234–1256.
Gallagher, D. W. (1978). 'Benzodiazepines: potentiation of a GABA inhibitory response in the dorsal raphe nucleus', *Eur. J. Pharmacol.*, **49**, 133–143.
Gardner, C. R., and Walker, R. J. (1982). 'The roles of putative neurotransmitters and neuromodulators in annelids and related invertebrates', *Progr. Neurobiol.*, **18**, 81–120.
Geller, H. M., and Woodward, D. J. (1972). 'An improved constant current source for microiontophoretic drug application studies', *Electroenceph. Clin. Neurophysiol.*, **33**, 430–432.
Geller, H. M., Taylor, D. A., and Hoffer, B. J. (1978). 'Benzodiazepines and central inhibitory mechanisms', *Arch. Pharmacol.*, **304**, 81–88.
Gent, J. P., and Phillips, N. I. (1980). 'Sodium di-n-propylacetate (valproate) potentiates responses to GABA and muscimol on single central neurones', *Brain Res.*, **197**, 275–278.
Gent, J. P., Morgan, R., and Wolstencroft, J. H. (1974). 'Determination of the relative potency of 2 excitant aminoacids', *Neuropharmacol.*, **13**, 441–447.
Gent, J. P., Smyth, D. G., Snell, C. R. and Wolstencroft, J. H. (1977). 'Effects of C fragment on brain stem neurones in the cat', *Br. J. Pharmacol.*, **60**, 272.
Gent, J. P., and Wolstencroft, J. H. (1976a). 'The relative sensitivity to glutamate and aspartate of cells in the ventrobasal thalamus of the rat which respond to movement of the vibrissae', *J. Physiol.*, **256**, 39–40.
Gent, J. P., and Wolstencroft, J. H. (1976b). 'Effects of methionine enkephalin and leucine enkephalin compared with those of morphine on brainstem neurones in cat', *Nature*, **261**, 426–427.

Gerschenfeld, H. M. (1973). 'Chemical transmission in invertebrate central nervous system and neuromuscular junctions', *Physiol. Revs.*, **53**, 1–119.

Gerschenfeld, H. M., and Paupardin-Tritsch, D. (1974). 'Ionic mechanisms and receptor properties underlying the responses of molluscan neurones to 5HT', *J. Physiol.*, **243**, 427–456.

Godfraind, J. M. (1979). 'Differences in the pharmacology of the excitatory and inhibitory responses evoked by acetylcholine on thalamic neurones in the cat', *Arch. Int. Pharmacodyn.*, **242**, 303–306.

Godfraind, J. M., and Pumain, R. (1971). 'Cyclic AMP and norepinephrine: effects on Purkinje cells in rat cerebellar cortex', *Science*, **174**, 1257–1258.

Gold, M. R., and Martin, A. R. (1983). 'Analysis of glycine activated inhibitory postsynaptic channels in brain stem neurones of the lamprey', *J. Physiol.*, **342**, 99–118.

Gonzalez-Vegas, J. A. (1974). 'Antagonism of dopamine mediated inhibition in the nigrostriatal pathway: a mode of action of some catatonia inducing drugs', *Brain Res.*, **80**, 219–228.

Gorman, A. L. F., and Thomas, M. V. (1980). 'Intracellular calcium accumulation during depolarisation in a molluscan neurone', *J. Physiol.*, **308**, 259–286.

Gozlan, H., Le Gal La Salle, G., Michelot, R., and Ben-Ari, Y. (1977). 'Rapid degradation of substance P and related peptides during microiontophoretic experiments', *Neurosci. Lett.*, **6**, 27–33.

Gration, K. A., Clark, R. B., and Usherwood, P. N. R. (1979). 'Three types of L-glutamate receptor on junctional membrane of locust muscle fibres', *Brain Res.*, **171**, 360–364.

Gruol, D. L., and Weinreich, D. (1979). 'Two pharmacologically distinct histamine receptors mediating membrane hyperpolarisation on identified neurones of *Aplysia californica*', *Brain Res.*, **162**, 281–301.

Gutnick, M. J., and Lobel-Yaakov, R. (1983). 'Carbon dioxide uncouples dye-coupled neuronal aggregates in neocortical slices', *Neurosci. Lett.*, **42**, 197–200.

Guyenet, P. G., Mroz, E. A., Aghajanian, G. K., and Leeman, S. E. (1979). 'Delayed iontophoretic ejection of substance P from glass micropipettes: correlation with time course of neuronal excitation', *Neuropharmacol.*, **18**, 553–558.

Haas, H. L., and Ryall, R. W. (1980). 'Is excitation by enkephalins of hippocampal neurones in the rat due to presynaptic facilitation or to disinhibition?' *J. Physiol.*, **308**, 315–330.

Haas, H. L., Wolf, P., Palacios, J. M., Garbang, M., Barbin, G., and Schwartz, J. C. (1978). 'Hypersensitivity to histamine in the guinea pig brain: microiontophoretic and biochemical studies', *Brain Res.*, **156**, 275–291.

Hablitz, J. J., and Langmoen, I. A. (1982). 'Excitation of hippocampal pyramidal cells by glutamate in the guinea-pig and rat', *J. Physiol.*, **325**, 317–331.

Haigler, H. J., and Aghajanian, G. K. (1974). 'LSD and serotonin: a comparison of effects on serotoninergic neurons and neurons receiving a serotoninergic input', *J. Pharm. Exp. Ther.*, **188**, 688–699.

Haldeman, S., and McLennan, H. (1973). 'The action of two inhibitors of glutamic acid uptake upon aminoacid induced and synaptic excitations of thalamic neurones', *Brain Res.*, **63**, 123–130.

Halgren, E., Babb, T. L., and Crandall, P. H. (1977). 'Responses of human limbic neurones to induced changes in blood gases', *Brain Res.*, **132**, 43–68.

Hall, J. G., Hicks, T. P., McLennan, H., Richardson, T. L., and Wheal, H. V. (1979). 'The excitation of mammalian central neurones by amino acids', *J. Physiol.*, **286**, 29–39.

Harris, J. B., and Ribchester, R. R. (1975). 'A method for the microinjection into mammalian muscle fibres of Procion brilliant red H3BN', *Br. J. Pharmacol.*, **55**, 306–307.

Heikkila, R. E., Manzino, L., Cabbat, F. S., and Hanly, J. G. (1983). 'Ascorbic acid and the binding of dopamine agonists to neostriatal membrane preparations', *Neuropharmacol.*, **22**, 135–137.
Henderson, L. P. (1983). 'The role of 5-HT as a transmitter between identified leech neurones in culture', *J. Physiol.*, **339**, 309–324.
Henn, F. A., and Henn, S. W. (1980). 'The psychopharmacology of astroglial cells', *Progr. Neurobiol.*, **15**, 1–17.
Henry, J. L. (1976). 'Effect of substance P on functionally identified units in cat spinal cord', *Brain Res.*, **114**, 439–452.
Henry, J. L. (1978). 'Peptides and transmission in central nociceptive pathways', pp. 110–112 in Ryall and Kelly (1978).
Henry, J. L., Krnjević, K., and Morris, M. E. (1975). 'Substance P and spinal neurones', *Can. J. Physiol. Pharmacol.*, **53**, 423–432.
Herrling, P. L. (1981). 'The membrane potential of cat hippocampal neurons recorded *in vivo* displays four different reaction mechanisms to iontophoretically applied transmitter agonists', *Brain Res.*, **212**, 331–344.
Herrling, P. L., and Hull, C. D. (1980). 'Iontophoretically applied dopamine depolarises and hyperpolarises the membrane of cat caudate neurones', *Brain Res.*, **192**, 441–462.
Herrling, P. L., Morris, R., and Salt, T. E. (1983). 'Effects of excitatory aminoacids and their antagonists on membrane and action potentials of cat caudate neurones', *J. Physiol.*, **339**, 207–222.
Herz, A., Zieglgänsberger, W., and Farber, G. (1969). 'Microiontophoretic studies concerning the spread of glutamic acid and GABA in brain tissue', *Exp. Brain Res.*, **9**, 221–235.
Herz, A., Zieglgänsberger, W., and von Freytag-Lorighoven, Hj. (1970). 'Development of fields of focal potentials in the caudate nucleus following microelectrophoretic application of glutamic acid and GABA', *Electroenceph. Clin. Neurophys.*, **28**, 247–258.
Hewes, C. R., and Frederickson, R. C. A. (1974). 'Responses of cortical neurones in rat to microelectrophoretically applied hydrogen ion', *Neuropharmacol.*, **13**, 1077–1081.
Hicks, T. P., and Guedes, R. C. A. (1983). 'Neuropharmacological properties of electrophysiologically identified, visually responsive neurones of the posterior lateral suprasylvian area. A microiontophoretic study', *Exp. Brain Res.*, **49**, 157–173.
Hicks, T. P., and McLennan, H. (1979). 'Aminoacids and the synaptic pharmacology of granule cells in the dentate gyrus of the rat', *Can. J. Physiol. Pharmacol.*, **57**, 973–978.
Hicks, T. P., Guedes, R. C. A., and Creutzfeldt, O. D. (1981). 'Selective synaptic antagonism by atropine and aminoadipate of pulvinar and cortical afferents to the suprasylvian visual area', *Brain Res.*, **208**, 456–462.
Hill, R. G., and Pepper, C. M. (1978). 'Selective effects of morphine on the nociceptive responses of thalamic neurones in the rat', *Br. J. Pharmacol.*, **64**, 137–144.
Hill, R. G., and Simmonds, M. A. (1973). 'A method for comparing the potencies of GABA antagonists on single cortical neurones using microiontophoretic techniques', *Br. J. Pharmacol.*, **48**, 1–11.
Hill, R. G., Simmonds, M. A., and Straughan, D. W. (1973). 'A comparative study of some convulsant substances as GABA antagonists in the feline cerebral cortex', *Br. J. Pharmacol.*, **49**, 37–51.
Hill-Smith, I., and Purves, R. D. (1978). 'Synaptic delay in the heart: an ionophoretic study', *J. Physiol.*, **279**, 31–54.
Hirata, H., Slater, N. T., and Kimelberg, H. K. (1983). 'Adrenergic mediated depolarisation of rat neocortical astrocytes in primary culture', *Brain Res.*, **270**, 358–362.

Hoffer, B. J., Neff, N. H., and Siggins, G. R. (1971a). 'Microiontophoretic release of norepinephrine from micropipettes', *Neuropharmacol.*, **10**, 175–180.

Hoffer, B. J., Siggins, G. R., and Bloom, F. E. (1971b). 'Studies of the norepinephrine containing afferents to Purkinje cells of rat cerebellum. II Sensitivity of Purkinje cells to norepinephrine and related substances administered by microiontophoresis', *Brain Res.*, **25**, 523–534.

Hoffer, B. J., Seiger, A., Freedman, R., Olson, L., and Taylor, D. (1977). 'Electrophysiology and cytology of hippocampal formation transplants in the anterior chamber of the eye. II Cholinergic mechanisms', *Brain Res.*, **119**, 107–132.

Holmes, O., and Houchin, J. (1966). 'Units in the cerebral cortex of the anaesthetized rat and the correlations between their discharges', *J. Physiol.*, **187**, 651–671.

Holubar, J., Hanke, B., and Malik, V. (1967). 'Intracellular recording from cortical pyramids and small interneurones as identified by subsequent staining with the recording microelectrode', *Exp. Neurol.*, **19**, 257–265.

Hori, T., and Nakayama, T. (1973). 'Effects of biogenic amines on central thermoresponsive neurones in the rabbit', *J. Physiol.*, **232**, 71–86.

Hosford, D. A., Haigler, H. J., and Turner, R. S. (1981). 'Methionine-enkephalin and morphine: amount ejected micriontophoretically', *J. Neurosci. Meth.*, **4**, 135–140.

Hösli, L., and Hösli, E. (1978). 'Action and uptake of neurotransmitters in CNS tissue culture', *Revs. Physiol. Biochem. Pharm.*, **81**, 135–188

Hughes, I. E. and Smith, J. A. (1978). 'The stability of noradrenaline in physiological saline solutions', *J. Pharm. Pharmacol.*, **30**, 124–126.

Hutchinson, G. B., McLennan, H., and Wheal, H. V. (1978). 'The responses of Renshaw cells and spinal interneurones of the rat to L-glutamate and L-aspartate', *Brain Res.*, **141**, 129–136.

Ikeda, H., and Sheardown, M. J. (1982). 'Aspartate may be an excitatory transmitter mediating visual excitation of "sustained" but not "transient" cells in the cat retina: iontophoretic studies *in vivo*', *Neuroscience*, **7**, 25–36.

Ikeda, H., and Sheardown, M. J. (1983). 'Transmitters mediating inhibition of ganglion cells in the cat retina: iontophoretic studies *in vivo*', *Neuroscience*, **8**, 837–853.

Ishida, A. T., Kaneko, A., and Tachibana, M. (1984). 'Responses of solitary retinal horizontal cells from *Carassius auratus* to L-glutamate and related aminoacids', *J. Physiol.*, **348**, 255–270.

Ito, M., Kostyuk, P. G., and Oshima, T. (1962). 'Further study on anion permeability of inhibitory postsynaptic membrane of cat motoneurones', *J. Physiol.*, **164**, 150–156.

Jahnsen, H., and Laursen, A. M. (1981). 'The effect of a benzodiazepine on the hyperpolarising and depolarising responses of hippocampal cells to GABA', *Brain Res.*, **207**, 214–217.

Jahr, C. E., and Jessell, T. M. (1983). 'ATP excites a subpopulation of rat dorsal horn neurones', *Nature*, **304**, 730–732.

James, V. A., and Walker, R. J. (1979). 'The ionic mechanism responsible for L-glutamate excitation of leech Retzius cells', *Comp. Biochem. Physiol.*, **C64**, 261–266.

Jell, R. M. (1973). 'Responses of hypothalamic neurones to local temperature and to acetylcholine, noradrenaline and 5HT', *Brain Res.*, **55**, 123–134.

Jiang, Z. (1981). 'A comparison of the effects of flurazepam on GABA mediated depression of cerebellar and cerebral cortical neurones', *Can. J. Physiol. Pharmacol.*, **59**, 595–597.

Johnson, E. S., Roberts, M. H. T., Sobieszek, A., and Straughan, D. W. (1969a). 'Noradrenaline sensitive cells in cat cerebral cortex', *Int. J. Neuropharmacol.*, **8**, 549–566.

Johnson, E. S., Roberts, M. H. T., and Straughan, D. W. (1969b). 'Responses of cortical neurones to monoamines under different anaesthetic conditions', *J. Physiol.*, **203**, 261–280.

Johnson, S. M., Katayama, Y., and North, R. A. (1980). 'Multiple action of 5HT on myenteric neurones of the guinea pig ileum', *J. Physiol.*, **304**, 459–470.

Johnston, G. A. R., Beart, P. M., Curtis, D. R., Game, C. J. A., McCulloch, R. M., and Maclachlan, R. M. (1972). 'Bicuculline methochloride as a GABA antagonist', *Nature*, **240**, 219–220.

Johnston, G. A. R., Lodge, D., Bornstein, J. C., and Curtis, D. R. (1980). 'Potentiation of glutamate and aspartate excitation of cat spinal neurones by the stereoisomers of threo-3-hydroxyaspartate', *J. Neurochem.*, **34**, 241–243.

Jones, R. S. G., and Olpe, H. R. (1984). 'An increase in sensitivity of rat cingulate cortical neurones to substance P occurs following withdrawal of chronic administration of antidepressant drugs', *Br. J. Pharmacol.*, **81**, 659–664.

Jones, R. S. G., and Roberts, M. H. T. (1979a). 'Potentiation of responses to monoamines by antidepressants after destruction of monoamine afferents', *Br. J. Pharmacol.*, **65**, 501–510.

Jones, R. S. G., and Roberts, M. H. T. (1979b). 'Potentiation of responses of cortical neurones to cyclic AMP by desipramine', *Neuropharmacol.*, **18**, 701–704.

Jordan, L. M., Lake, N., and Phillis, J. W. (1972). 'Mechanism of noradrenaline depression of cortical neurones: a species comparison', *Eur. J. Pharmacol.*, **20**, 381–384.

Jordan, L. M., Frederickson, R. C. A., Phillis, J. W., and Lake, N. (1973). 'Microelectrophoresis of 5-HT: a clarification of its action on cerebral cortical neurones', *Brain Res.*, **40**, 552–558.

Jordan, L. M., Kenshalo, D. R., Martin, R. F., Haber, L. H., and Willis, W. D. (1979). 'Two populations of spinothalamic tract neurones with opposite responses to 5HT', *Brain Res.*, **164**, 342–346.

Karras, P. J., and North, R. A. (1981). 'Acute and chronic effects of opiates on single neurons of the myenteric plexus', *J. Pharmacol. Exp. Ther.*, **217**, 70–80.

Kasser, R. J., and Cheney, P. D. (1983). 'Double-barreled electrode for simultaneous iontophoresis and single unit recording during movement in awake monkeys', *J. Neurosci. Meth.*, **7**, 235–242.

Katayama, Y., and North, R. A. (1980). 'The action of somatostatin on neurones of the myenteric plexus of the guinea-pig ileum', *J. Physiol.*, **303**, 315–323.

Kato, E., and Narahashi, T. (1982). 'Characteristics of the electrical response to dopamine in neuroblastoma cells', *J. Physiol.*, **333**, 213–226.

Kato, E., Anwyl, R., Quandt, F. N., and Narahashi, T. (1983). 'Acetylcholine induced electrical responses in neuroblastoma cells', *Neuroscience*, **8**, 643–651.

Katz, B., and Miledi, R. (1972). 'The statistical nature of the acetylcholine potential and its molecular components, *J. Physiol.*, **224**, 665–700.

Katz, G. M., and Steinberg, S. (1976). 'Microelectrophoresis and constant current sources'. In *Electrobiology of Nerve, Synapse and Muscle*. Eds J. P. Reuben *et al.* Raven Press, New York, pp. 367–377.

Kehoe, J. (1972a). 'Three acetylcholine receptors in *Aplysia* neurones', *J. Physiol.*, **225**, 115–146.

Kehoe, J. (1972b). 'The physiological role of three acetylcholine receptors in synaptic transmission in *Aplysia*', *J. Physiol.*, **225**, 147–172.

Kelly, J. S. (1975). 'Microiontophoretic application of drugs onto single neurones', In *Handbook of Psychopharmacology*, Vol 2. Eds. L. L. Iversen, S. D. Iversen, and S. H. Snyder. Plenum Press, New York. pp. 29–67.

Kelly, J. S., and Renaud, L. P. (1973). 'On the pharmacology of the GABA receptors on the cuneo-thalamic relay cells of the cat', *Br. J. Pharmacol.*, **48**, 369–386.

Kelly, J. S., Simmonds, M. A., and Straughan, D. W. (1975). 'Microelectrode techniques.' In *Methods in Brain Research*. Ed. P. B. Bradley. Wiley, London. pp. 332–377.

Kelly, M. J., Moss, R. L., and Dudley, C. A. (1977). 'The effects of microionotphoretically applied estrogen, cortisol and acetylcholine on medial preoptic/septal unit activity throughout the estrous cycle of the female rat', *Exp. Brain Res.*, **30**, 53–64.

Kemp, J. A., and Sillito, A. M. (1982). 'The nature of the excitatory transmitter mediating X and Y cell inputs to the cat lateral geniculate nucleus', *J. Physiol.*, **323**, 377–392.

Kerkut, G. A., and Walker, R. J. (1962). 'Marking individual nerve cells through electrophoresis of ferrocyanide from a microelectrode', *Stain Technol.*, **37**, 217–219.

Kerwin, R. W., Olpe, H. R., and Schmutz, M. (1980). 'The effect of dipropylacetate on GABA dependent inhibition in the rat cortex and substantia nigra in relation to its anticonvulsant activity', *Br. J. Pharmacol.*, **71**, 545–551.

Kettenmann, H., Wienrich, M., and Schachner, M. (1983). 'Antibody Ll ejected from a micropipette identifies neurons without altering electrical activity', *Neurosci. Lett.*, **41**, 85–90.

Key, B. J., Boakes, R. J., and Candy, J. M. (1980). 'Responses of cat dorsal raphe neurones to iontophoretically applied noradrenaline', *Neuropharmacol.*, **19**, 139–142.

Kirsten, E. B., and Sharma, J. N. (1976a). 'Microiontophoresis of acetylcholine, histamine and their antagonists on neurones in the medial and lateral vestibular nuclei of the cat', *Neuropharmacol.*, **15**, 743–754.

Kirsten, E. B., and Sharma, J. N. (1976b). 'Characteristics and response differences to iontophoretically applied norepinephrine, D-amphetamine and acetylcholine on neurones in the medial and lateral vestibular nuclei of the cat', *Brain Res.*, **112**, 77–90.

Klemm, W. R. (1980). 'Opiate mechanisms: evaluation of research involving neuronal action potentials', *Progr. Neuropsychopharmacol.*, **5**, 1–34.

Krnjević, K. (1964). 'Microiontophoretic studies on cortical neurones', *Int. Rev. Neurobiol.*, **7**, 41–98.

Krnjević, K. (1974). 'Chemical nature of synaptic transmission in vertebrates', *Physiol. Revs.*, **51**, 418–540.

Krnjević, K., and Lekić, D. (1977). 'Substance P selectively blocks excitation of Renshaw cells by acetylcholine', *Can. J. Physiol. Pharmacol.*, **55**, 958–961.

Krnjević, K., and Morris, M. E. (1974). 'An excitatory action of substance P on cuneate neurones', *Can. J. Physiol. Pharmacol.*, **52**, 736–744.

Krnjević, K., and Phillis, J. W. (1963a). 'Iontophoretic studies of neurones in the mammalian cerebral cortex', *J. Physiol.*, **165**, 274–304.

Krnjević, K., and Phillis, J. W. (1963b). 'Acetylcholine sensitive cells in the cerebral cortex', *J. Physiol.*, **166**, 296–327.

Krnjević, K., and Van Meter, W. G. (1976). 'Cyclic nucleotides in spinal cells', *Can. J. Physiol. Pharmacol.*, **54**, 416–421.

Krnjević, K., and Whittaker, V. P. (1965). 'Excitation and depression of cortical neurones by brain fractions released from micropipettes', *J. Physiol.*, **179**, 298–322.

Krnjević, K., Mitchell, J. F., and Szerb, J. C. (1963a). 'Determination of iontophoretic release of acetylcholine from micropipettes', *J. Physiol.*, **165**, 421–436.

Krnjević, K., Laverty, R., and Sharman, D. F. (1963b). 'Iontophoretic release of adrenaline, noradrenaline and 5-HT from micropipettes', *Br. J. Pharmacol.*, **20**, 491–496.

Krnjević, K., Pumain, R., and Renaud, L. (1971a). 'The mechanism of excitation by acetylcholine in the cerebral cortex', *J. Physiol.*, **215**, 247–268.

Krnjević, K., Pumain, R., and Renaud, L. (1971b). 'Effects of barium and tetraethylammonium on cortical neurones', *J. Physiol.*, **215**, 223–246.

Krnjević, K., Lamour, Y., MacDonald, J. F., and Nistri, A. (1978). 'Intracellular actions of monoamine transmitters', *Can. J. Physiol. Pharmacol.*, **56**, 896–900

Krnjević, K., Puil, E., and Werman, R. (1976). 'Is cyclic GMP the internal "second messenger" for cholinergic actions on central neurones?' *Can. J. Physiol. Pharmacol.*, **54**, 172–176.

Krnjević, K., Puil, E., and Werman, R. (1977). 'GABA and glycine actions on spinal motoneurones', *Can. J. Physiol. Pharmacol.*, **29**, 658–669.

Kruk, Z. L., Armstrong-James, M., and Millar, J. (1980). 'Measurement of the concentration of 5-HT ejected during iontophoresis using multibarrel carbon fibre microelectrodes', *Life Sci.*, **27**, 2093–2098.

Kuffler, S. W., and Yoshikami, D. (1975a). 'The number of transmitter molecules in a quantum: an estimate from iontophoretic application of acetylcholine at the neuromuscular synapse', *J. Physiol.*, **251**, 465–482.

Kuffler, S. W., and Yoshikami, D. (1975b). 'The distribution of acetylcholine sensitivity at the postsynaptic membrane of vertebrate skeletal twitch muscle: iontophoretic mapping in the micron range', *J. Physiol.*, **244**, 703–730.

Kuyihar-Csillik, E., Szucs, A., and Csillik, B. (1982). Iontophoretically applied microtubule inhibitors induce transganglionic degenerative atrophy of primary central nociceptive terminals and abolish chronic autochthonous pain', *Acta Neurol. Scand.*, **66**, 401–412.

Lake, N., and Jordan, L. M. (1974). 'Failure to confirm cyclic AMP as second messenger for norepinephrine in rat cerebellum', *Science*, **183**, 663–664.

Lambert, J. D. C., and Flatman, J. A. (1981). 'The interaction between barbiturate anaesthetics and excitatory amino acid responses on cat spinal neurones', *Neuropharmacol.*, **20**, 227–280.

Lamour, Y., Dutar, P., and Jobert, A. (1982). 'Excitatory effect of acetylcholine on different types of neurones in the first somatosensory neocortex of the rat: laminar distribution and pharmacological characteristics', *Neuroscience*, **7**, 1483–1494.

Lamour, Y., Dutar, P., and Jobert, A. (1983). 'Effects of neuropeptides on rat cortical neurones: laminar distribution and interaction with acetylcholine', *Neuroscience*, **10**, 107–117.

Large, W. A. (1983). 'Membrane potential responses to ionotphoretically applied α-adrenoceptor agonists in the mouse anococcygeus', *Br. J. Pharmacol.*, **79**, 233–244.

Lee, B. B., Mandl, G., and Stean, J. P. B. (1969). 'Microelectrode tip position marking in nervous tissue: a new dye method', *Electroenceph. Clin. Neurophysiol.*, **27**, 610–613.

Lee, H. K., Dunwiddie, T., and Hoffer, B. J. (1980). 'Electrophysiological interactions of enkephalins with neuronal circuitry in the rat hippocampus II Effects on interneurone excitability', *Brain Res.*, **184**, 331–342.

Leendertz, J., and Wright, D. M. (1983). 'A microcomputer based system for spike processing at low cost', *J. Neurosci. Meth.*, **9**, 1–7.

Leng, G. (1980). 'Rat supraoptic neurones: the effects of locally applied hypertonic saline', *J. Physiol.*, **304**, 405–414.

Levitan, H., and Tauc, L. (1972). 'Acetylcholine receptors: topographic distribution and pharmacological properties of two receptor types on a single molluscan neurone', *J. Physiol.*, **222**, 537–558.

Li, C. L., and McIlwain, H. (1957). 'Maintenance of resting membrane potentials in slices of mammalian cerebral cortex and other tissues *in vitro*', *J. Physiol.*, **139**, 178–190.

Livingston, L. G., and Duggar, B. M. (1934). 'Experimental procedures in a study of the location and concentration within the host cell of tobacco mosaic', *Biol. Bull. Mar. Biol. Lab. Woods Hole.*, **67**, 504–512.

Lodge, D., Caddy, K. W. T., Headley, P. M., and Biscoe, T. J. (1974). 'The location of neurones with Pontamine Sky Blue', *Neuropharmacol.*, **13**, 481–485.

Logan, S. D., and Cottrell, G. A. (1975). 'Responses of an identified dopamine containing neurone to iontophoretically applied drugs', *Neuropharmacol.*, **14**, 453–455.

Logan, S. D., Lovick, T. A., West, D. C., and Wolstencroft, J. H. (1982). 'Inhibitory actions of a novel endogenous tripeptide Met-Tyr-Lys on proprioceptive neurones in the lumbar spinal cord of the cat', *Neuroscience*, **7**, 2841–2847.

Lømo, T., and Slater, C. R. (1978). 'Control of acetylcholine sensitivity and synapse formation by muscle activity', *J. Physiol.*, **275**, 391–402.

Lømo, T., and Slater, C. R. (1980). 'Acetylcholine sensitivity of developing ectopic nerve muscle junctions in adult rat soleus muscle', *J. Physiol.*, **303**, 173–189.

Lorente de No, R. (1947). *Studies from the Rockefeller Institute for Medical Research* **131**, 132.

Lux, H. D., and Heyer, C. B. (1977). 'An aequorin study of a facilitating calcium current in busting pacemaker neurones of *Helix*', *Neuroscience*, **2**, 585–592.

MacDonald, J. F., and Barker, J. L. (1978). 'Benzodiazepines specifically modulate GABA mediated postsynaptic inhibition in cultured mammalian neurones', *Nature*, **271**, 563–564.

MacDonald, J. F., and Bergey, G. K. (1979). 'Valproic acid augments GABA mediated postsynaptic inhibition in cultured mammalian neurones', *Brain Res.*, **170**, 558–562.

MacDonald, J. F., and Porietis, A. B. (1982). 'DL-Quisqualic and L-aspartic acids activate separate excitatory conductances in cultured spinal cord neurones', *Brain Res.*, **245**, 175–178.

MacDonald, J. F., and Wojtowicz, J. M. (1982). 'The effects of L-glutamate and its analogues upon the membrane conductance of central murine neurones in culture', *Can. J. Physiol. Pharmacol.*, **60**, 282–296.

Madison, D. V., and Nicoll, R. A. (1982). 'Noradrenaline blocks accommodation of pyramidal cell discharges in the hippocampus', *Nature*, **299**, 636–637.

Magleby, K. L., and Weinstock, M. M. (1980). 'Nickel and calcium ions modify the characteristics of the acetylcholine receptor channel complex at the frog neuromuscular junction', *J. Physiol.*, **299**, 203–218.

Maillis, A. G. (1974). 'Interneuronal activity as a factor interfering with the interpretation of results from microiontophoretic studies', *Neuropharmacol.*, **13**, 487–494.

Mandelbrod, I., Feldman, S., and Werman, R. (1983). 'Mediobasal hypothalamic neurons are excited by the iontophoretic application of sodium', *Brain Res.*, **273**, 35–44.

Marshall, K. C., and Engberg, I. (1979). 'Reversal potential for noradrenaline induced hyperpolarisation of spinal motoneurones', *Science*, **205**, 422–444.

Martin, R. J. (1980). 'The effect of GABA on the input conductance and membrane potential of *Ascaris* muscle', *Br. J. Pharmacol.*, **71**, 99–106.

Mayer, M. L., and Straughan, D. W. (1981). 'Effects of 5HT on central neurones antagonised by bicuculline and picrotoxin', *Neuropharmacol.*, **20**, 347–350.

McBain, A. E., and Wheal, H. V. (1984). 'The piperidine analogues prevent desensitisation of glutamate receptors on crustacean muscle', *Brain Res.*, **290**, 307–310.

McCabe, B. M. (1972). 'Iontophoresis and persisting changes in neuronal firing rate in the cerebral cortex of the unrestrained rat', *J. Physiol.*, **224**, 6–7.

McCaman, R. E., and Weinreich, D. (1982). 'On the nature of histamine mediated slow hyperpolarising synaptic potentials in identified molluscan neurones', *J. Physiol.*, **328**, 485–506.

McCaman, R. E., McKenna, D. G. M., and Kono, T. J. (1977). 'A pressure system for intracellular and extracellular ejections of picolitre volumes', *Brain Res.*, **136**, 141–147.

McCulloch, R. M., Johnston, G. A. R., Game, J. C. A., and Curtis, D. R. (1974). 'The differential sensitivity of spinal interneurones and Renshaw cells to kainate and N-methyl-D-aspartate', *Exp. Brain Res.*, **21**, 515–518.

McLennan, H. (1980). 'The effect of decortication on the excitatory amino acid sensitivity of striatal neurones', *Neurosci. Lett.*, **18**, 313–316.

McLennan, H., and Hicks, T. P. (1978). 'Pharmacological characteristics of the excitatory cholinergic receptors of rat central neurones', *Neuropharmacol.*, **17**, 329–334.

McLennan, H., and Lodge, D. (1979). 'The antagonism of aminoacid induced excitation of spinal neurones in the cat', *Brain Res.*, **169**, 83–90.

Menkes, D. B., and Aghajanian, G. K. (1981). 'α_1-Adrenoceptor mediated responses in the lateral geniculate nucleus are enhanced by chronic antidepressant treatment', *Eur. J. Pharmacol.*, **74**, 27–36.

Menkes, D. B., Gallagher, D. W., Reinhard, J. F., and Aghajanian, G. K. (1983). 'α_1-Adrenoceptor supersensitivity in brain: physiological and receptor binding studies', *Brain Res.*, **272**, 1–12.

Millar, J., and Armstrong-James, M. (1982). 'The responses of neurones of the superficial dorsal horn to iontophoretically applied glutamate ion', *Brain Res.*, **231**, 267–278.

Millar, J., Armstrong-James, M., and Kruk, Z. L. (1981). 'Polarographic assay of iontophoretically applied dopamine and low noise unit recording using a multibarrel carbon microelectrode', *Brain Res.*, **205**, 419–424.

Millar, R. A., and Silver, I. A. (1971). 'Excitation of certain posterolateral hypothalamic units by cyclopropane and ether', *Br. J. Pharmacol.*, **42**, 315–327.

Miller, J. J., and McLennan, H. (1974). 'The action of bicuculline upon acetylcholine induced excitations of central neurones', *Neuropharmacol.*, **13**, 785–788.

Misell, D. L., and Richards, C. D. (1979). 'Estimates of the threshold concentration of glutamate required to excite nerve cells', *J. Physiol.*, **287**, 37–38.

Moises, H. C., Woodward, D. J., Hoffer, B. J., and Freedman, R. (1979). 'Interactions of norepinephrine with Purkinje cell responses to putative amino acid neurotransmitters applied by microiontophoresis', *Exp. Neurol.*, **64**, 493–515.

Morgan, R., Vrbova, G., and Wolstencroft, J. H. (1972). 'Correlation between the retinal input to lateral geniculate neurones and their relative response to glutamate and aspartate', *J. Physiol*, **224**, 41–42.

Morita, K., and Katayama, Y. (1984). 'Two types of acetylcholine receptors on the somata of primary afferent neurones', *Brain Res.*, **290**, 348–352.

Moss, R. L., Urban, I., and Cross, B. A. (1972). 'Microelectrophoresis of cholinergic and adrenergic drugs on paraventricular neurones', *Am. J. Physiol.*, **233**, 310–318.

Moss, R. L., Kelly, M. J., and Dudley, C. A. (1978). 'Chemosensitivity of hypophysiotropic neurones to the microelectrophoresis of biogenic amines', *Brain Res.*, **139**, 141–152.

Murakami, N. (1973). 'Effects of iontophoretic application of 5HT, noradrenaline and acetylcholine upon hypothalamic temperature sensitive neurones in rats', *Jap. J. Physiol.*, **23**, 435–446.

Myslinski, N. R., and Randić, M. (1977). 'Reponses of identified spinal neurones to acetylcholine applied by microiontophoresis', *J. Physiol.*, **269**, 195–219.

Nagler, J., Conforti, N., and Feldman, S. (1973). 'Alterations produced by cortisol in the spontaneous activity and responsiveness to sensory stimuli of single cells in the tuberal hypothalamus of the rat', *Neuroendocrinol.*, **12**, 52–66.

Napier, T. C., Pirch, J. H., and Strahlendorf, H. K. (1983). 'Naloxone antagonises striatally induced suppression of globus pallidus unit activity', *Neuroscience*, **9**, 53–59.

Nastuk, W. L. (1953). 'Membrane potential changes at a single endplate produced by transitory application of acetylcholine with an electrically controlled microjet', *Fed. Proc.*, **12**, 102.

Nelson, C. N., Hoffer, B. J., Chu, N. S., and Bloom, F. E. (1973). 'Cytochemical and pharmacological studies on polysensory neurons in the primate frontal cortex', *Brain Res.*, **62**, 115–134.

Nicholson, C., and Phillips, J. M. (1981). 'Ion diffusion modified by tortuosity and volume fraction in the extracellular microenvironment of the rat cerebellum', *J. Physiol.*, **321**, 225–257.

Nicholson, C., Phillips, C. M., and Gardner-Medwin, A. R. (1979). 'Diffusion from an iontophoretic point source in the brain: role of tortuosity and volume fraction', *Brain Res.*, **169**, 580–584.

Nicoll, R. A. (1971). 'Pharmacological evidence for GABA as the transmitter in granule cell inhibition in the olfactory bulb', *Brain Res.*, **35**, 137–150.

Nicoll, R. A., Siggins, G. R., Ling, N., Bloom, F. E., and Guillemin, R. (1977). 'Neuronal actions of endorphins and enkephalins among brain regions: a comparative microiontophoretic study', *Proc. Nat. Acad. Sci.*, **74**, 2584–2588.

Nicoll, R. A., Alger, B. E., and Jahr, C. E. (1980). 'Enkephalin blocks inhibitory pathways in the vertebrate CNS', *Nature*, **287**, 22–25.

Nistri, A., and MacDonald, J. F. (1978). 'Quantitative studies of iontophoretically applied excitatory aminoacids', In *Aminoacids as Chemical Transmitters*. Ed. F. Fonnum. Plenum Press, London, pp. 87–91.

Nistri, A., Krnjević, K., Lamour, Y., and MacDonald, J. F. (1978). 'Intracellular effects of noradrenaline, dopamine and 5HT in spinal motoneurones', In *Recent Advances in the Pharmacology of Adrenoceptors*. Eds. E. Szabadi *et al.*, Elsevier, Amsterdam, pp. 67–74.

Norcross, K., and Spehlmann, R. (1978a). 'A quantitative analysis of the excitatory and depressant effects of dopamine on the firing of caudatal neurons: electrophysiological support for the existence of two distinct dopamine sensitive receptors', *Brain Res.*, **156**, 168–174.

Norcross, K., and Spehlmann, R. (1978b). 'Decreased sensitivity of caudatal neurons to microiontophoretic dopamine in dopamine depleted caudate nucleus', *Brain Res.*, **156**, 175–180.

Norman, R. S. (1975). 'Diffusional spread of iontophoretically injected ions', *J. Theor. Biol.*, **52**, 159–162.

Normanton, J. R., and Gent, J. P. (1983). 'Comparison of the effects of two sleep peptide, DSIP and arginine vasotocin on single neurones in the rat and rabbit brain stem', *Neuroscience*, **8**, 107–114.

North, R. A. (1979). 'Opiates, opioids on single neurones', *Life. Sci.*, **24**, 1527–1546.

North, R. A. (1982). 'Electrophysiology of the enteric nervous system', *Neuroscience*, **7**, 315–326.

North, R. A., and Tokimasa, T. (1982). 'Muscarinic synaptic potentials in guinea pig myenteric plexus', *J. Physiol.*, **333**, 151–156.

North, R. A., and Tokimasa, T. (1983). 'Depression of calcium dependent potassium conductance of guinea pig myenteric neurones by muscarinic agonists', *J. Physiol.*, **342**, 253–266.

Obata, K. (1974). 'Transmitter sensitivities of some nerve and muscle cells in culture', *Brain Res.*, **73**, 71–88.

Obata, K., Takeda, K., and Shinozaki, H. (1970). 'Electrophoretic release of GABA and glutamic acid from micropipettes', *Neuropharmacol.*, **9**, 191–194.

Ogden, T. E., Citron, M. C., and Pieranton, R. (1978). 'The jet-stream microbeveler: an inexpensive way to bevel ultra fine micropipettes', *Sci.*, **201**, 409–470.

Okamoto, K., and Sakai, Y. (1980). 'Localization of sensitive sites to taurine, GABA, glycine and beta-alanine in the molecular layer of guinea pig cerebellar slices', *Br. J. Pharmacol.*, **69**, 407–413.

Okamoto, K., and Sakai, Y. (1981). 'Inhibitory actions of taurocyamine, hypotaurine, taurine and GABA on spike discharges of Purkinje cells and localisation of sensitive sites in guinea-pig cerebellar slices', *Brain Res.*, **206**, 371–386.

Oliver, A. P. (1971). 'A simple rapid method for preparing parallel micropipette electrodes', *Electroenceph. Clin. Neurophys.*, **31**, 284–286.

Ono, T., Nishiro, H., Fukuda, M., Sasaki, K., Muramoto, K., and Oomura, Y. (1982). 'Glucoresponsive neurons in rat ventromedial hypothalamic tissue slices *in vitro*', *Brain Res.*, **232**, 494–499.

Onodera, K., and Takeuchi, A. (1980). 'Distribution and pharmacological properties of synaptic and extrasynaptic glutamate receptors on crayfish muscle', *J. Physiol.*, **306**, 233–250.

Palmer, M. R. (1982). 'Micropressure-ejection: a complementary technique to microiontophoresis for neuropharmacological studies in the mammalian CNS', *J. Electrophysiol. Tech.*, **9**, 123–139.

Palmer, M. R., and Hoffer, B. J. (1980). 'Catecholamine modulation of enkephalin induced electrophysiological responses of cerebral cortex', *J. Pharmacol. Exp. Therap.*, **213**, 205–215.

Palmer, M. R., Morris, D. H., Taylor, D. A., Stewart, J. M., and Hoffer, B. J. (1978). 'Electrophysiological effects of enkephalin analogs in rat cortex', *Life Sci.*, **23**, 851–860.

Palmer, M. R., Wuerthele, S. M., and Hoffer, B. J. (1980). 'Physical and physiological characteristics of micropressure ejection of drugs from multibarrelled pipettes', *Neuropharmacol.*, **19**, 931–938.

Peet, M. J., Leah, J. D., and Curtis, D. R. (1983). 'Antagonists of synaptic and aminoacid excitation of neurones in the cat spinal cord', *Brain Res.*, **266**, 83–96.

Pellmar, T. C., and Carpenter, D. O. (1981). 'Cyclic AMP induces a voltage dependent current in neurones of *Aplysia californica*', *Neurosci. Lett.*, **22**, 151–157.

Pentreath, V. W., and Cottrell, G. A. (1974). 'Anatomy of an identified serotonin neurone studied by means of injection of tritiated "transmitter"', *Nature*, **250**, 655–658.

Peper, K., Dreyer, F., and Muller, K.-D. (1975). 'Analysis of cooperativity of drug receptor interaction by quantitative iontophoresis at frog motor end-plates', *Cold Spring Harb. Symp. Quant. Biol.*, **40**, 187–192.

Perkins, M. N., and Stone, T. W. (1980a). 'Aminophylline and theophylline derivatives as antagonists of neuronal depression by adenosine: a microiontophoretic study', *Arch. Int. Pharmacodyn.*, **246**, 205–214.

Perkins, M. N., and Stone, T. W. (1980b). 'Projections from the subthalamic nucleus and midbrain tegmentum to the globus pallidus: an electrophysiological study in the rat', *Exp. Neurol.*, **60**, 500–511.

Perkins, M. N. and Stone, T. W. (1982). 'An iontophoretic investigation of the actions of convulsant kynurenines and their interaction with the endogenous excitant quinolinic acid', *Brain Res.*, **247**, 184–187.

Perkins, M. N., and Stone, T. W. (1983a). 'Quinolinic acid: regional variations in neuronal sensitivity', *Brain Res.*, **259**, 172–176.

Perkins, M. N., and Stone, T. W. (1983b). 'The pharmacological and regional variations of quinolinic acid evoked excitations in the rat CNS', *J. Pharmacol. Exp. Ther.*, **226**, 551–557.

Perkins, M. N., and Stone, T. W. (1983c). 'Neuronal responses to 5-HT and dorsal raphe stimulation within the globus pallidus of the rat', *Exp. Neurol.*, **79**, 118–129.

Perkins, M. N., Stone, T. W., Collins, J. F., and Curry, K. (1981). 'Phosphonate analogues of carboxylic acids as aminoacid antagonists on rat cortical neurones', *Neurosci. Lett.*, **23**, 333–336.

Phillis, J. W. (1976). 'An involvement of calcium and Na-K-ATPase in the inhibitory actions of various compounds on central neurones', In *Taurine*. Eds A. Barbeau and R. Huxtable. Raven Press, New York, pp 209–223.

Phillis, J. W. (1982). 'Evidence for an A2 like adenosine receptor on cerebral cortical neurones', *J. Pharm. Pharmacol.*, **34**, 453–454.

Phillis, J. W., and Limacher, J. J. (1974). 'Effects of some metallic cations on cerebral cortical neurones and their interactions with biogenic amines', *Can. J. Physiol. Pharmacol.*, **52**, 566–574.

Phillis, J. W., and Tebecis, A. K. (1967). 'The effects of pentobarbitone sodium on acetylcholine excitation and noradrenaline inhibition of thalamic neurones', *Life Sci.*, **6**, 1621–1625.

Phillis, J. W., and York, D. H. (1968). 'Pharmacological studies on a cholinergic inhibition in the cerebral cortex', *Brain Res.*, **10**, 297–306.

Phillis, J. W., Kostopoulos, G. K., and Limacher, J. J. (1974). 'Depression of corticospinal cells by various purines and pyrimidines', *Can. J. Physiol. Pharmacol.*, **52**, 1226–1229.

Pitman, R. M., Tweedle, C. D., and Cohen, M. J. (1971). 'Branching of central neurones: intracellular cobalt injection for light and electron microscopy', *Science*, **176**, 412–414.

Poulain, P., and Carette, B. (1981). 'Pressure ejection of drugs on single neurones *in vivo*: technical considerations and application to the study of estradiol effects', *Brain Res. Bull.*, **7**, 33–40.

Purves, R. D. (1974). 'Muscarinc excitation: a microelectrophoretic study on cultured smooth muscle cells', *Br. J. Pharmacol.*, **52**, 77–86.

Purves, R. D. (1977). 'The release of drugs from iontophoretic pipettes', *J. Theor. Biol.*, **66**, 789–798.

Purves, R. D. (1979). 'The physics of iontophoretic pipettes', *J. Neurosci. Meth.*, **1**, 165–178.

Purves, R. D. (1981). *Microelectrode Methods for Intracellular Recording and Ionophoresis*. Academic Press, London.

Randić, M., and Miletić, V. (1977). 'Effect of substance P on cat dorsal horn neurones activated by noxious stimuli', *Brain Res.*, **128**, 164–198.

Reader, T. A., Ferron, A., Descarries, L., and Jasper, H. H. (1979). 'Modulatory role for biogenic amines in the cerebral cortex: microiontophoretic studies', *Brain Res.*, **160**, 217–230.

Reiffenstein, R. J., and Triggle, C. (1972). 'Sensitivity of denervated cerebral cortex to cholinomimetics', *Electroenceph. Clin. Neurophysiol.*, **33**, 215–220.

Renaud, L. P., Blume, H. W., Pittman, Q., Lamour, Y., and Tan, A. T. (1979). 'TRH selectively depresses glutamate excitation of cerebral cortical neurones', *Science*, **205**, 1275–1277.

Richards, C. D., and Smaje, J. C. (1976). 'Anaesthetics depress the sensitivity of cortical neurones to L-glutamate', *Br. J. Pharmacol.*, **58**, 347–358.

Roberts, C. J., and Walker, R. J. (1982). 'The actions of L-glutamate and putative glutamate agonists on the central neurones of *Limulus polyphemus*', *Comp. Biochem. Physiol.*, **73C**, 167–176.

Roberts, F. (1981). 'The *in vitro* iontophoretic release of radiolabelled histamine, N2-methyl-histamine and GABA from 7-barrelled glass micropipettes', *Neuropharmacol.*, **20**, 711–714.

Roberts, M. H. T., and Straughan, D. W. (1967). 'Excitation and depression of cortical neurones by 5-HT', *J. Physiol.*, **193**, 269–294.

Roberts, M. H. T., and Wright, D. M. (1981). 'The effects of chronic section of dorsal roots on the responsiveness of motoneurones to 5HT and substance P analogues', *Br. J. Pharmacol.*, **73**, 589–594.

Ropert, N. and Krnjević, K. (1982). 'Pharmacological characteristics of facilitation of hippocampal population spikes by cholinomimetics', *Neuroscience*, **7**, 1963–1978.

Rovira, C., Ben-Ari, Y., Cherubini, E., Krnjević, K., and Ropert, N. (1983). 'Pharmacology of the dendritic action of acetylcholine and further observations on the somatic disinhibition in the rat hippocampus *in situ*', *Neuroscience*, **8**, 97–106.

Rush, S., Lepeschkin, E., and Brooks, H. O. (1968). 'Electrical and thermal properties of double barrelled ultramicroelectrodes', *IEEE Trans. Biomed. Eng. Electron.*, **15**, 80–93.

Ryall, R. W., and De Groat, W. C. (1972). 'The microelectrophoretic administration of noradrenaline, 5HT, acetylcholine and glycine to sacral parasympathetic preganglionic neurones', *Brain Res.*, **37**, 345–347.

Ryall, R. W., and Kelly, J. S. (1978). *Iontophoresis and Transmitter Mechanisms in the Mammalian CNS*. Elsevier, Amsterdam.

Sakai, M., Sakai, H., and Woody, C. D. (1978). 'Intercellular staining of cortical neurones by pressure microinjection of horseradish peroxidase and recovery by core biopsy', *Exp. Neurol.*, **58**, 138–144.

Sakai, M., Swartz, B. E., and Woody, C. D. (1979). 'Controlled microrelease of pharmacological agents: measurements of volumes ejected *in vitro* through fine tipped glass microelectrodes by pressure', *Neuropharmacol.*, **18**, 209–213.

Salmoiraghi, G. C., and Weight, F. (1967). 'Micromethods in neuropharmacology: an approach to the study of anaesthetics', *Anaesthesiol.*, **28**, 54–64.

Salmoiraghi, G. C., Bloom, F. E., and Costa, E. (1964). 'Adrenergic mechanisms in rabbit olfactory bulb', *Am. J. Physiol.*, **207**, 1417–1424.

Salt, T. E., and Hill, R. G. (1980). 'The effects of microiontophoretically applied capsaicin and substance P on single neurones in the rat and cat brain', *Neurosci. Lett.*, **20**, 329–334.

Salt, T. E., and Hill, R. G. (1983). 'Excitation of single sensory neurones in the rat caudal trigeminal nucleus by iontophoretically applied ATP', *Neurosci. Lett.*, **35**, 53–58.

Salt, T. E., DeVries, G. J., Rodriguez, R. E., Cahusac, P. M. B., Morris, R., and Hill, R. G. (1982). 'Evaluation of [D-Pro^2, D-Trp^{7,9}] substance P as an antagonist of substance P responses in the rat CNS', *Neurosci. Lett.*, **30**, 291–295.

Sargent, P. B., Yau, K.-W., and Nicholls, J. G. (1977). 'Extrasynaptic receptors on cell bodies of neurones in the CNS of leech', *J. Neurophysiol.*, **40**, 446–452.

Sasa, M., Fujimoto, S., Igarashi, S., Munekiyo, K., and Takaori, S. (1979). 'Microiontophoretic studies on noradrenergic inhibition from locus coeruleus of spinal trigeminal nucleus neurones', *J. Pharmacol. Exp. Ther.*, **210**, 311–315.

Sasa, M., Igarashi, S., Fujiwara, C., and Inagaki, C. (1978). 'Comparison between fluorimetric and radiochemical assays of iontophoretically released noradrenaline from a 7-barrelled micropipette', *Jap. J. Pharmacol.*, **28**, 639–641.

Sastry, B. S. R., and Phillis, J. W. (1976). 'Antagonism of glutamate and acetylcholine excitation of rat cerebral cortical neurons by diphenylhydantoin', *Gen. Pharmacol.*, **7**, 411–414.

Sastry, B. S. R., and Phillis, J. W. (1977a). 'Metergoline as a selective 5HT antagonist in the cerebral cortex', *Can. J. Physiol. Pharmacol.*, **55**, 130–133.

Sastry, B. S. R., and Phillis, J. W. (1977b). 'Antagonism of biogenic amine induced depression of cerebral cortical neurones by Na–K-ATPase inhibitors', *Can. J. Physiol. Pharmacol.*, **55**, 170–179.

Satoh, M., Zieglgänsberger, W., and Herz, A. (1976). 'Actions of opiates upon single unit activity in the cortex of naive and tolerant rats', *Brain Res.*, **115**, 99–110.

Satoh, M., Kawajiri, S., Yamamoto, M., Akaike, A., Ukai, Y., and Takagi, H. (1980). 'Effect of tyrosyl-arginine (kyotorphin), a new opioid dipeptide, on single neurones in the spinal dorsal horn of rabbits and nucleus reticularis gigantocellularis of rats', *Neurosci. Lett.*, **16**, 319–322.

Sawada, M., Takada, S., and Yamamoto, C. (1983). 'Selective activation of synapses near the tip of drug ejecting microelectrodes, and effects of antagonists of excitatory aminoacids in the hippocampus', *Brain Res.*, **267**, 156–160.

Sawada, M., Hara, N., Ito, I., and Maeno, T. (1984). 'Ionic mechanism of a hyperpolarising glutamate effect on two identified neurons in the buccal ganglion of *Aplysia*', *J. Neurosci. Res.*, **11**, 91–104.

Sedvall, G. (1975). 'Receptor feedback and dopamine turnover in CNS. '*In Handbook of Psychopharmacology*, Vol 6. Eds L. L. Iversen, S. D. Iversen, and S. H. Snyder. Plenum Press, New York, pp. 127–177.

Segal, M. (1976). '5HT antagonists in rat hippocampus', *Brain Res.*, **103**, 161–166.

Segal, M. (1977). 'Supersensitivity of hippocampal neurones to acidic aminoacids in decommissurized rats', *Brain Res.*, **119**, 476–479.

Segal, M. (1980). 'The action of serotonin in the rat hippocampal slice preparation', *J. Physiol.*, **303**, 423–439.

Segal, M. (1982a). 'Intracellular analysis of a postsynaptic action of adenosine in the rat hippocampus', *Eur. J. Pharmacol.*, **79**, 193–200.

Segal, M. (1982b). 'Norepinephrine modulates reactivity of hippocampal cells to chemical stimulation *in vitro*', *Exp. Neurol.*, **77**, 86–93.
Segal, M., and Bloom, F. E. (1974). 'The action of norepinephrine in the rat hippocampus: Iontophoretic studies', *Brain Res.*, **72**, 79–97.
Shingyoji, C., Murakami, A., and Takahashi, K. (1977). 'Local reactivation of Triton extracted flagella by iontophoretic application of ATP', *Nature*, **265**, 269–270.
Shinozaki, H. (1980). 'The pharmacology of the excitatory neuromuscular junction in the crayfish', *Progr. Neurobiol.*, **14**, 121–155.
Shinozaki, H., Ishida, M., and Mizuta, T. (1982). 'Glutamate inhibitors in the crayfish neuromuscular junction', *Comp. Biochem. Physiol.*, **72C**, 249–255.
Shoemaker, W. J., Ballentine, L. T., Siggins, G. R., Hoffer, B. J., Henriksen, S. J., and Bloom, F. E. (1975). 'Characteristics of the release of cyclic AMP from micropipettes by microiontophoresis', *J. Cyclic Nucl. Res.*, **1**, 97–106.
Siggins, G. R., Oliver, A. P., Hoffer, B. J., and Bloom, F. E. (1971a). 'Cyclic AMP and norepinephrine: effects on transmembrane properties of cerebellar Purkinje cells', *Science*, **171**, 192–194.
Siggins, G. R., Hoffer, B. J., and Bloom, F. E. (1971b). 'Reply to Godfraind & Pumain', *Science*, **174**, 1258–1259.
Siggins, G. R., Hoffer, B. J., and Bloom, F. E. (1971c). 'Studies of norepinephrine containing afferents to Purkinje cells of rat cerebellum. III Evidence for mediation of norepinephrine effects by cyclic AMP', *Brain Res.*, **25**, 535–545.
Sillito, A. M. (1975). 'The contribution of inhibitory mechanisms to the receptive field properties of neurones in the striate cortex of the cat', *J. Physiol.*, **250**, 305–329.
Sillito, A. M. (1977). 'Inhibitory processes underlying the directional specificity of simple, complex and hypercomplex cells in the cat's visual cortex', *J. Physiol.*, **271**, 699–720.
Sillito, A. M., and Kemp, J. A. (1983). 'Cholinergic modulation of the functional organisation of the cat visual cortex', *Brain Res.*, **289**, 143–155.
Simmonds, M. A. (1974). 'Quantitative evaluation of responses to microiontophoretically applied drugs', *Neuropharmacol.*, **13**, 401–406.
Sinclair, J. G., Lo, G. F., and Harris, D. P. (1982). 'Flurazepam effects of rat cerebellar Purkine cells', *Gen. Pharmacol.*, **13**, 453–456.
Smaje, J. C. (1976). 'General anaesthetics and the acetylcholine sensitivity of cortical neurones', *Br. J. Pharmacol.*, **58**, 359–366.
Sonnhof, U. (1973). 'A multi-barrelled coaxial electrode for iontophoresis and intracellular recording with a gold shield of the central pipette for capacitance neutralization', *Pflug. Arch. (Eur. J. Physiol.)*, **341**, 351–358.
Speckmann, E.-J. (1970). 'Changes in neuronal activity on hypoxia and asphyxia', *Electroenceph. Clin. Neurophysiol.*, **29**, 206.
Spehlmann, R. (1963). 'Acetylcholine and prostigmine electrophoresis at visual cortex neurones', *J. Neurophysiol.*, **26**, 127–139.
Spehlmann, R., and Daniels, J. C. (1973). 'Acetylcholine and cortical excitation by pyramidal tract collaterals', *J. Neurol. Sci.*, **20**, 387–396.
Spencer, H. J. (1971). 'Programmable nanoampere constant current sources for iontophoresis', *Biol. Eng.*, **9**, 693–701.
Spencer, H. J., and Havlicek, V. (1974). 'Alteration by anaesthetic agents of the responses of rat striatal neurons to iontophoretically applied amphetamine, acetylcholine, noradrenaline and dopamine', *Can. J. Physiol. Pharmacol.*, **52**, 808–813.
Stanzione, P., and Zieglgänsberger, W. (1983). 'Action of neurotensin on spinal cord neurones in the rat', *Brain Res.*, **268**, 111–118.
Stephenson, R. P. (1956). 'A modification of receptor theory', *Br. J. Pharmacol.*, **11**, 379–393.
Stone, T. W. (1971). 'Are noradrenaline excitations artifacts?' *Nature*, **234**, 145–146.
Stone, T. W. (1972a). 'Cholinergic mechanisms in the rat somatosensory cerebral cortex', *J. Physiol.*, **225**, 485–499.

Stone, T. W. (1972b). 'Responses of blood vessels to various amines applied by micriontophoresis', *J. Pharm. Pharmacol.*, **24**, 318–323.
Stone, T. W. (1972c). 'Noradrenaline effects and pH', *J. Pharm. Pharmacol.*, **24**, 422–423.
Stone, T. W. (1972d). 'Noradrenaline artefacts — reply', *Nature New Biol.*, **239**, 152.
Stone, T. W. (1973a). 'Pharmacology of pyramidal tract cells in the cerebral cortex. Noradrenaline and related substances', *Arch. Pharmacol.*, **278**, 333–346.
Stone, T. W. (1973b). 'Cortical pyramidal tract interneurones and their sensitivity to L-glutamic acid', *J. Physiol.*, **233**, 211–225.
Stone, T. W. (1976). 'Responses of neurones in the cerebral cortex and caudate nucleus to amantadine, amphetamine and dopamine', *Br. J. Pharmacol.*, **56**, 101–110.
Stone, T. W. (1979a). 'Glutamate as the neurotransmitter of cerebellar granule cells in the rat: electrophysiological evidence', *Br. J. Pharmacol.*, **66**, 291–296.
Stone, T. W. (1979b). 'Aminoacids as neurotransmitters of corticofugal neurones in the rat: a comparison of glutamate and aspartate', *Br. J. Pharmacol.*, **67**, 545–551.
Stone, T. W. (1981a). 'Studies with excitatory aminoacid antagonists in rat CNS: 2APV, phenytoin and benzodiazepines.' In *Aminoacid Neurotransmitters*. Eds F. V. DeFeudis and P. Mandel. Raven Press, New York, pp. 223–230.
Stone, T. W. (1981b). 'Physiological roles for adenosine and ATP in the nervous system', *Neuroscience*, **6**, 523–555.
Stone, T. W. (1982). 'Purine receptors involved in the depression of neuronal firing in cerebral cortex', *Brain Res.*, **248**, 367–370.
Stone, T. W. (1983a). 'Actions of TRH and cyclo-(His-Pro) on spontaneous and evoked activity of cortical neurones', *Eur. J. Pharmacol.*, **92**, 113–118.
Stone, T. W. (1983b). 'A comparison of the effects of morphine, enkephalin, kyotorphin and D-phenylalanine on rat central neurones', *Br. J. Pharmacol.*, **79**, 305–312.
Stone, T. W., and Perkins, M. N. (1979). 'Is adenosine the mediator of opiate actions on neuronal firing rate?' *Nature*, **281**, 227–228.
Stone, T. W., and Perkins, M. N. (1981a). 'Quinolinic acid: a potent endogenous excitant at aminoacid receptors in CNS', *Eur. J. Pharmacol.*, **72**, 411–412.
Stone, T. W., and Perkins, M. N. (1981b). 'Adenine dinucleotide effects on cortical neurones', *Brain Res.*, **229**, 241–245.
Stone, T. W., and Perkins, M. N. (1983). 'Quisqualic acid excitation of cortical neurones is selectively antagonised by streptomycin', *Brain Res.*, **260**, 347–349.
Stone, T. W., and Perkins, M. N. (1984). 'Ethylenediamine as a GABA mimetic', *Trends Pharmacol. Sci.* **5**, 241–243.
Stone, T. W., and Taylor, D. A. (1977). 'Microiontophoretic studies of the effects of cyclic nucleotides on excitability of neurones in the rat cerebral cortex', *J. Physiol.*, **266**, 523–543.
Stone, T. W., and Taylor, D. A. (1979). 'Antidepressant drugs potentiate suppression by adenosine of neuronal firing in rat cerebral cortex', *Neurosci. Lett.*, **11**, 93–97.
Stone, T. W., Taylor, D. A., and Bloom, F. E. (1975). 'Cyclic AMP and cyclic GMP may mediate opposite neuronal responses in the rat cerebral cortex', *Science*, **187**, 845–847.
Stopp, P. E., and Whitfield, I. C. (1963). 'The influence of microelectrodes on neuronal discharge patterns in the auditory system', *J. Physiol.*, **167**, 169–180.
Straughan, D. W., Neal, M. J., Simmonds, M. A., Collins, G. G. S., and Hill, R. G. (1971). 'Evaluation of bicuculline as a GABA antagonist', *Nature*, **233**, 352–354.
Stretton, A. O. W., and Kravitz, E. A. (1968). 'Neuronal geometry: determination with a technique of intracellular dye injection', *Science*, **162**, 132–134.
Suh, T. H., Wang, C. H., and Lim, R. K. S. (1936). 'The effects of intracisternal applications of acetylcholine and the localization of the pressor centre and tract', *Chinese J. Physiol.*, **10**, 61–78.

Swartz, B. E., and Woody, C. D. (1979). 'Correlated effects of acetylcholine and cyclic GMP on membrane properties of mammalian cortical neurones', *J. Neurobiol.*, **10**, 465–488.
Szabadi, E. (1979). 'Adrenoceptors on central neurones: microelectrophoretic studies', *Neuropharmacol.*, **18**, 831–844.
Szabadi, E., and Bradshaw, C. M. (1972). 'Are noradrenaline excitations artifacts?' *Nature New Biol.*, **239**, 152–153.
Szabadi, E., and Bradshaw, C. M. (1973). 'Spread of drugs in tissue: diffusion or iontophoresis', *J. Theor. Biol.*, **42**, 185–187.
Szabadi, E., Bradshaw, C. M., and Bevan, P. (1977). 'Excitatory and depressant neuronal responses to noradrenaline, 5-HT and mescaline: the role of the baseline firing rate', *Brain Res.*, **126**, 580–583.
Talbot, R. E., Towe, A. L., and Kennedy, T. T. (1967). Physiological and histological classification of cerebellar neurones in chloralose anaesthetised cats', *Exp. Neurol.*, **19**, 46–65.
Tasaki, K., Tsukahara, Y., Ito, S., Wayner, M. J., and Yu, W. Y. (1968). 'A simple direct and rapid method for filling microelectrodes', *Physiol. Behav.*, **3**, 1009–1011.
Tauc, L., and Gerschenfeld, H. M. (1962). 'A cholinergic mechanism of inhibitory synaptic transmission in molluscan nervous system', *J. Neurophysiol.*, **25**, 236–262.
Tebecis, A. K. (1974). 'Transmitters and identified neurones in the mammalian CNS', *Scientechnica Bristol.*
Thomas, R. C., and Wilson, V. J. (1965). 'Precise localisation of Renshaw cells with a new marking technique', *Nature*, **206**, 211–213.
Thomas, R. C., and Wilson, V. J. (1966). 'Marking single neurones by staining with intracellular recording microelectrodes', *Science*, **151**, 1538–1539.
Thompson, R. F., and Patterson, M. M. (1973). *Bioelectric Recording Techniques*. Academic Press, London.
Tomita, T., and Torihama, Y. (1956). 'Further study on the intraretinal action potentials and on the site of ERG generation', *Jap. J. Physiol.*, **6**, 118–136.
Trubatch, J., and Van Harreveld, A. (1972). 'Spread of iontophoretically injected ions in a tissue', *J. Theor. Biol.*, **36**, 355–366.
Vandermaelen, C. P., and Aghajanian, G. K. (1983). 'Electrophysiological and pharmacological characterisation of serotonergic dorsal raphe neurones recorded extracellularly and intracellularly in rat brain slices', *Brain Res.*, **289**, 109–119.
Wang, R. Y., and Aghajanian, G. K. (1977). 'Recording of single unit activity during electrical stimulation and microiontophoresis: a method for minimizing stimulus artifacts', *Electroenceph. Clin. Neurophysiol.*, **43**, 434–437.
Waterhouse, B. D., and Woodward, D. J. (1980). 'Interaction of norepinephrine with cerebrocortical activity evoked by stimulation of somatosensory afferent pathways in the rat', *Exp. Neurol.*, **67**, 11–34.
Waterhouse, B. D., Moises, H. C., and Woodward, D. J. (1980). 'Noradrenergic modulation of somatosensory cortical neuronal responses to iontophoretically applied putative neurotransmitters', *Exp. Neurol.*, **69**, 30–49.
Watkins, J. C., and Evans, R. H. (1981). 'Excitatory aminoacid transmitters', *Ann. Rev. Pharmacol.*, **21**, 165–204.
Waud, D. R. (1968). 'On diffusion from a point source', *J. Pharmacol. Exp. Ther.*, **159**, 123–128.
Winokur, A. and Beckman, A. L. (1978). 'Effect of TRH, norepinephrine and acetylcholine on the activity of neurones in the hypothalamus, septum and cerebral cortex of the rat', *Brain Res.*, **150**, 205–209.
Winsbury, G. J. (1956).'Machine for the production of microelectrodes', *Rev. Sci. Instr.*, **27**, 514–516.
Wolf, P., and Haas, H. L. (1977). 'Effects of diazepines and barbiturates on hippocampal recurrent inhibition', *Arch. Pharmacol.*, **299**, 211–218.

Wong, R. K. S., and Watkins, D. J. (1982). 'Cellular factors influencing GABA responses in hippocampal pyramidal cells', *J. Neurophysiol.*, **48**, 938–951.
Woodruff, G. N., and Walker, R. J. (1969). 'The effect of dopamine and other compounds on the activity of neurones of *Helix aspersa*', *Int. J. Neuropharmacol*, **8**, 279–289.
Woolley, D. W., and Shaw, E. (1957). 'Evidence for the participation of serotonin in mental processes', *Ann. NY Acad. Sci.*, **66**, 649–667.
Yamamoto, C., and Sawada, S. (1982). 'Sensitivity of hippocampal neurones to glutamic acid and its analogues', *Brain Res.*, **235**, 358–362.
Yarbrough, G. G. (1976). 'TRH potentiates excitatory actions of acetylcholine on cerebral cortical neurones', *Nature*, **263**, 523–524.
York, D. H. (1972). 'Dopamine receptor blockade—a central action of chlorpromazine on striatal neurones', *Brain Res.*, **37**, 91–100.
Young, W. S., Bird, S. J., and Kuhar, M. J. (1977). 'Iontophoresis of methionine enkephalin in the locus coeruleus area', *Brain Res.*, **129**, 366–370.
Yurchenko, O. P., and Rozsa, K. S. (1984). 'Modulatory effect of serotonin on the acetylcholine sensitivity of identified neurones in the brain of *Helix pomatia* L.', *Comp. Biochem. Physiol.*, **77**, 127–134.
Zieglgänsberger, W., and Champagnat, J. (1979). 'Cat spinal motoneurones exhibit topographical sensitivity to glutamate and glycine', *Brain Res.*, **160**, 95–104.
Zieglgänsberger, W., French, E. D., Mercuri, N., Pelayo, F., and Williams, J. T. (1982). 'Multiple opiate receptors on neurones of the mammalian CNS: *in vivo* and *in vitro* studies', *Life Sci.*, **31**, 2343–2346.
Zieglgänsberger, W., French, E. D., Siggins, G. R., and Bloom, F. E. (1979). 'Opioid peptides may excite hippocampal pyramidal neurons by inhibiting adjacent inhibitory interneurons', *Science*, **205**, 415–417.
Zieglgänsberger, W., Herz, A., and Teschemacher, H. (1969). 'Electrophoretic release of tritium labelled glutamic acid from micropipettes *in vitro*', *Brain Res.*, **15**, 298–300.
Zieglgänsberger, W., and Puil, E. A. (1973). 'Actions of glutamic acid on spinal neurones', *Exp. Brain Res.*, **17**, 35–49.
Zieglgänsberger, W., and Reiter, Ch. (1974). 'A cholinergic mechanism in the spinal cord of cats', *Neuropharmacol.*, **13**, 519–527.
Zieglgänsberger, W., Sothmann, G., and Herz, A. (1974). 'Iontophoretic release of substance from micropipettes *in vitro*', *Neuropharmacol.*, **13**, 417–422.

Addresses of Manufacturers

Anachem Ltd, 15 Power Court, Luton (UK).
Biodata Ltd, 6 Lower Ormond St, Manchester M1 5QF (UK).
Campden Instruments Ltd, 186 Campden Hill Rd, London W8 7TH (UK).
Clark Electromedical, PO Box 8, Pangbourne, Reading RG8 7HU (UK).
Computer Institute, 17 Page St, Brunswick, Maine 04011 (USA).
Corning Glass Works, Corning Medical & Scientific, Corning, New York 14830 (USA); Corning Ltd, Stone, Staffs (UK).
Coulbourn Instruments, PO Box 2551, Lehigh Valley, Pa 18001 (USA); Sandown Scientific, 11 Copsem Drive, Esher, Surrey (UK).
Dagan Corp., 2855 Park Avenue, Minneapolis, Mn. 55407 (USA).
Digitimer, 14 Tewin Court, Welwyn, Herts. AL7 1AF (UK).
General Valve Corp., 202 Fairfield Rd, PO Box 1333, Fairfield, NJ 07006 (USA).
Haer & Co., Brunswick, Maine 04011 (USA); Campden Instruments (UK).
Harvard BioScience, Fircroft Way, Edenbridge Kent (UK).
Kopf Instruments, 7324 Elmo St, PO Box 636, Tujunga, Ca 91042 (USA).
Medical Systems Corp., 239 Great Neck Rd, Great Neck, NY 11021 (USA); or via Digitimer (UK).
Narashige, 27-9, Minami-Karasuyama 4-Chome, Setagaya-Ku, Tokyo; via Medical Systems (USA) or Optical Instruments, 166 Anerley Rd, London SE20.
Neurolog (see Digitimer).
Ortec Inc., 100 Midland Rd, Oak Ridge, Tenn. 37830 (USA).
Pierce Ltd, 44 Upper Northgate St, Chester CH1 4EF (UK). Also in USA.
R. C. Electronics Inc., 5386-D Hollister Av., Santa Barbara, Ca 93111 (USA).
Shrimpton & Fletcher, Premier Works, Redditch, Worcs. (UK).
Stoelting, 1350 S. Kostner Av., Chicago, Ill. 60623 (USA).
Sutter Instrument Co., PO Box 16385, San Francisco, Ca 94116 (USA).
Waters Associates, Milford, Mass. 01757 (USA); 324 Chester Road, Northwich, Cheshire (UK).
Wesley Coe Ltd, 32 Scotland Rd, Cambridge (UK).
WP Instruments Inc., 60 Fitch St, PO Box 3110, New Haven, Conn. 06515 (USA).

Subject index

accommodation, 89, 96
acetylcholine, 1, 2, 45, 55, 62, 94, 125, 136, 140, 145, 156 *et seq.*, 171, 174, 179
acidity, 21, 58, 59, 113, 120 *et seq.*, 166
adenosine, 86, 172
adsorption, 61
after-diffusion, 55
ageing of electrodes, 59
air bubbles, 14
amines, 45, 46, 131, 145
amino acids, excitatory, 45, 127, 128, 131, 143 *et seq.*
  mechanisms, 151
  pharmacology, 146
  receptors, 149
  sensitivity, 143
  synaptic activation, 147
amino acids, inhibitory, 153 *et seq.*
  pharmacology, 154
  receptor localization, 152, 157
  sensitivity, 157
aminoadipate, 146, 148
aminophosphonovalerate, 146, 150
anaesthetics, absence of, 129, 165
  influence of, 125 *et seq.*, 160, 165
angiotensin, 175
antagonism, 52, 99
antagonists, use of, 112, 146
  distribution, 107
antidepressants, 167
antidromic identification, 106, 166
antioxidants, 21
Aplysia, 179
artifacts, electrical, 113, 115
  osmotic, 124
  temperature, 124
ascorbate, 21
ATP, 5, 172, 173
atropine, 77, 101, 120, 158, 159
autoreceptors, 118, 169
averages, 81, 100

backing current (*see* retaining), 4

balancing current, 4, 27, 33, 114
barbiturates, 125
baseline firing, 97–100, 120
  and noradrenaline responses, 100, 165
benzodiazepines, 147, 154
bicuculline, 90, 99, 154, 156, 161
blanks, electrode, 6 *et seq.*
blood vessels, 119, 166
braking current (*see* retaining), 4
breaking tips, 12
bumping, 12

calcium, monitoring, 183
carbon fibre electrodes, 47, 48, 105
cardiac muscle, 138
cerebellum, 73, 74, 113, 147
chlorpromazine, 60
cholecystokinin, 175
cleaning pipettes, 14
cobalt, 182
cochlear nuclei, 159
computer systems, 82, 83, 100
co-operativity, 52, 138
concentration effects, 60
concentrations, threshold, 70, 107, 166
concentrations achieved, 68 *et seq.*, 84, 105, 107, 166
contamination, 13, 14, 124, 125
cortex, 126, 134, 144, 156, 159
  visual, 156, 159, 161
corticofugal neurones, 144, 148, 169
coupling, electrical, 7, 9, 16
crayfish, 134, 136, 180
critical ratio, 97
cumulative counts, 79, 80, 88
current, anionic, 3
  artifacts, 113
  balancing, 4, 27, 33, 114
  cationic, 3
  inward, 3
  outward, 3
  retaining, 4, 21, 41 *et seq.*, 52, 85, 94, 110, 115, 116, 123

testing, 4, 114, 116
current monitor, 27
current pump, 24, 25, 26
cyclic AMP, 59, 165, 171, 179
cyclic GMP, 100, 171

dendrites, 15, 16, 106, 154, 162, 168, 170
denervation supersensitivity, 167
desensitization, 89, 91, 96, 109, 111, 135
diffusion, circuit analogue, 74, 75
diffusion curves, 69
diphenylhydantoin, 147
discriminators, 78, 79
dopamine, 47, 48, 98, 101, 168, 177, 178
dose, iontophoretic, 84
  expression of, 84
dose–response curves, 87, 89, 90, 95
double layer, electrical, 3, 4, 62
dyes, 181 et seq.

efflux, diffusional, 39 et seq.
  spontaneous, 39 et seq.
ejection, by pressure, 64
  dendritic, 106, 149, 151, 153, 162, 168, 170
  iontophoretic, 39 et seq., 49
  somatic, 106, 154, 162, 168, 170
  time course, 52, 54, 55
ejection concentrations, 68 et seq.
electric field effects, 71–73
electrical double layer, 3, 4, 62
electrochemical detection, 46, 166
electrode assemblies, 15 et seq.
  blanks, 6 et seq.
electrodes, ageing, 59
  carbon fibre, 47, 48, 105
  construction, 16 et seq.
  failure, 56
  metal and glass, 18
  variation, 56
electro-osmosis, 3, 4, 44, 49, 62 et seq.
endorphins, 176
equipment, iontophoretic, 23 et seq.
error, sources of, 55
evoked response, 98, 165, 176

Fast Green, 181, 182
field potentials, 129, 162
  interpretation of, 131
filling micropipettes, 7, 12 et seq.
filtration, 20
fluctuation analysis, 135

GABA, 86, 90, 157, 180

intracellular effects, 155
  uptake, 154
ganglion cells, 141
gating, 78
geniculate nucleus, 143, 149
glass fibres, 7, 13
glia, 119, 120
glucose, 63
glutamate, 56, 70, 71, 79, 81, 85, 86, 89, 94, 102, 115, 132, 134, 138, 143 et seq.
glutamate diethylester, 146
glycine, 56, 57, 90, 157
glycosides, 165
goldfish, 177

halothane, 126, 127, 160, 165
hippocampus, 146, 147, 148, 151, 153, 162, 165, 170, 172, 175, 176
histamine, 1, 57, 101
histograms, 81, 83, 97, 100
holding current (see retaining), 4
horseradish peroxidase, 182
hydration effects, 3, 4
hydrostatic pressure, 40
5-hydroxytryptamine, 120, 127, 141, 170, 179
  antagonists, 170
hypothalamus, 113, 166
hypoxia, 119

insects, 134, 136
interphase, 41
intracellular pipettes, 9
invertebrates, 134
iontophoresis, in oil, 19
iontophoretic charge, 56
  doses, 84
  ejection, 45
  solutions, 20
isomers, use of, 122

kainate, 77, 78, 81, 89, 143, 145
ketamine, 128, 147
kynurenic acid, 147
kyotorphin, 176

lampreys, 177
latency of responses, 88, 138, 151, 159
locus coeruleus, 164
long-term potentiation, 143, 147, 148
LSD, 170

manganese, 102, 165
manipulators, 16, 18

Subject Index

Mauthner neurones, 177
medium, receiving, 57
membrane stabilization, 77
metal ions, 165
methoxamine, 46
methyl blue, 181, 182
microtap, 3, 5
morphine, 84, 141, 176
multibarrel pipettes, 2, 6 et seq., 10, 15 et seq.
multichannelled tubing, 9
myenteric plexus, 141

naloxone, 84, 141, 176
neuroleptics, 169
neuromuscular junction, 1, 109, 134
neutral red, 182
noise, 77, 135
noradrenaline, 46, 52, 56, 70, 86, 98, 102, 118, 119, 121, 127, 131, 141, 162 et seq., 168
norepinephrine (see noradrenaline)
nucleotides, 165

olfactory areas, 118, 126
opiates, 141, 175
opioids, 176
osmotic effects, 20
overdeplorization, 77

pH, 21, 58, 59, 113, 120 et seq., 166
 and pressure, 123
 effects, 113
pallidus, globus, 170
parallel electrodes, 17
parasympathetic neurones, 170
pentobarbitone, 125, 160
peptides, 141, 174
peripheral nervous systems, 134
phenothiazines, 77, 169
phenylephrine, 46
photographic records, 76
piggy-back electrodes, 17
plateau responses, 52, 75, 85, 86, 87, 91, 94
pontamine sky blue, 182
potency, 77
 comparisons of, 100, 108, 143
pressure ejection, 3, 4, 19, 36 et seq., 64 et seq., 132
 artifacts, 132
procion yellow, 182
propranolol, 77, 120
prostaglandins, 56
pullers, 10 et seq.

pump, current, 24, 25, 26
purines, 171
pyramidal cells, 101, 144, 146, 149, 154, 159, 170, 172

quinolinic acid, 77, 89, 143, 144, 151
quisqualate, 87, 95

raphe nuclei, 166, 170
receptors, 52, 146
 extrasynaptic, 110, 146
 localization, 134, 142, 149
 presynaptic, 118
 recording, 38
Renshaw cells, 2, 144, 158
resistance, 22, 24
responses, definition, 97
 excitatory and pH, 58, 166
 excitatory to noradrenaline, 58, 100, 166
 expression, 88
 measurement of, 88
 plateau, 52, 75, 85, 86, 87, 91, 94
 time course, 77
retaining current, 4, 21, 41 et seq., 52, 85, 94, 110, 115, 116, 123
retina, 148, 150, 156

sampling bias, 15
screen, electrode, 16
sensitivity, comparisons of, 100, 143
 neuronal, 76
 changes of, 174
shield, electrode, 16
signal-to-noise ratio, 15, 106
slices, 118
smooth muscle, 138
snail, 177
sodium chloride, 20
 effects, 114
sodium isotopes, 46, 57
somatostatin, 141, 175
spermatozoa, 5
spinal cord, 152, 158, 176
striatum, 98, 101, 113, 126, 144, 146, 151, 168
strychnine, 91, 154
subfornical organ, 175
substance P, 61, 67, 174, 175
 antagonists, 175
 degradation, 175
sucrose, 62, 65
sulpiride, 169
supraoptic nucleus, 158
sympathetic neurones, 170

synaptic input, 109, 147, 156
synaptic terminals, 117
synaptosomes, 5

temperature sensitive cells, 106, 158, 167
tetraethylammonium, 73
thalamus, 125
theophylline, 122
theta tubing, 9
thrombus formation, 5
thyrotropin, 174
time axes, 92, 95
tolerance, 176
tortuosity, 73
toxicity, 71
transport numbers, 13, 45 *et seq.*, 62
   and ageing, 59
   and pH, 58, 59, 122, 123
   effect of concentration, 60
   effect of filling, 59
   factors affecting, 58 *et seq.*
   measurement of, 45 *et seq.*
   values of, 48, 50, 51
trigeminal nucleus, 143, 165
tubocurarine, 154, 158

uptake, 71, 89, 91, 146
   inhibition, 143
urethane, 126–129, 160, 165

valves for pressure, 36 *et seq.*
vasoconstriction, 119, 166
vestibular nuclei, 166
volume flow, 62
volume fraction, 73

warm-up phenomenon, 55, 102, 112

zeta potentials, 62
zwitterions, 59, 63